Hairdressing

The Complete Guide

ACC NO : 048414-8
TITLE : Hairdressing : the   lete
AU OR : CU⌐⌐ING ete

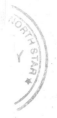

D0293811

Hairdressing
The Complete Guide

FOURTH EDITION

PETER CUTTING
RENIE ROSS

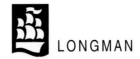

LONGMAN

Addison Wesley Longman Limited
Edinburgh Gate, Harlow
Essex CM20 2JE, England
and associated companies throughout the world

© P. Cutting, R. Ross and R. Hill 1988, 1991
© Longman Group UK Ltd 1994
© Addison Wesley Longman Limited 1996

All rights reserved; no part of this publication may be
reproduced, stored in any retrieval system, or transmitted in any
form or by any means, electronic, mechanical, photocopying,
recording or otherwise without either the prior written
permission of the Publishers or a licence permitting restricted
copying in the United Kingdom issued by the Copyright Licensing
Agency Ltd, 90 Tottenham Court Road, London W1P 9HE.

First published in Great Britain by Pitman Publishing as *Hairdressing: Theory, Science and Practice* 1988
Second edition 1991
Third edition published as *Hairdressing: The Complete Guide* 1994
Reprinted by Longman Scientific and Technical 1995
Fourth edition published by Addison Wesley Longman Limited 1996

British Library Cataloguing in Publication Data
A catalogue entry for this title is available from the British Library

ISBN 0-582-29340-5

SWINDON COLLEGE NORTH STAR
LIBRARY
O4844-8
19.10.98

Set by 30 in Palatino 10/12 and Helvetica
Produced by Longman Asia Limited, Hong Kong

Contents

*In memory of Raymond Hill –
teacher and friend*

Preface

The aim of this book is to cover all the competences of the Hairdressing Training Board/City & Guilds NVQ and SVQ at Levels 1, 2 and 3, including African Caribbean hairdressing.

We have completely revised and restructured the contents of the book to provide a single source of up-to-date and relevant material, tried and tested by our own students and taken from our own managerial experience. This has resulted in a student-oriented approach that uses accessible language, colour, charts and diagrams throughout, with an emphasis on key points, and includes a glossary for quick reference. Each unit ends with self-assessment questions and practical tasks that students can complete without specialist facilities, in their own time if necessary. Also included are safety and technical tips, and notes on the prevention of repetitive strain injury (RSI).

The structure of the book reflects the three levels of the NVQ/SVQ framework, with each section subdivided into the relevant units that cover all the competences and assessment requirements needed to successfully complete the course. This begins at the basic Level 1 and develops through Level 2 to the more specialised supervisory qualities needed for Level 3 (which also includes those elements relevant to TDLB D32 and D33 Assessor's Award).

We have also produced a completely revised *Activity Pack* to accompany the new edition of the text. This is additional material, available to tutors and free of copyright, which we have designed to support and help the trainee. It is intended to facilitate programme delivery in a variety of ways and to support workplace assessment.

We very much hope that this book will be both useful and easy to use. Whether we have succeeded in meeting these aims only our readers can tell; we would welcome any comments.

Peter Cutting & Renie Ross
September 1996

Acknowledgements

We would also like to offer personal thanks to the following:

- Adrian Greenhalgh for his photography.
- Corinne D'Souza and Pamela Goff at L'Oréal for their help and time providing photographs.
- Heather Bhebhe for her help with the African Caribbean photographs.
- Ian White for his help with the health and safety elements.
- James Newall and Brett Gilbert at Addison Wesley Longman, and Alex Whyte for copy-editing.
- John Peers at John Peers hair Studio, 1 Lord Studio, Rochdale, for supplying photographs.
- Mrs E. Middleton and Barbara Eden for proofreading.
- Nick Stephenson, Barbara Crowther and Jason Thomas for modelling.
- Sheila Jones and Pam Young for their helpful suggestions.
- The Hairdressing Training Board.
  and
- Our families, who suffered long – again, and then again.

Peter Cutting & Renie Ross

'Preventing RSI' sections written by Kathleen Dulmarge (ICE Ergonomics).

The authors and publishers are grateful to the following individuals and organisations for supplying photographic illustrations.

- Adrian Greenhalgh for Figs 2.60–2.65, 2.122, 3.52 & 3.54 and photographs on pages 244 & 350.
- Alan Edwards for the photograph on page 143.
- Daniel Gavin for the photograph on page 370.
- Dome, London (Simon Forbes) for Fig. 3.51.
- Jason Miller for the photographs on page 226.
- John Peers Hair Studio for Figs 3.50 & 3.53 and photographs on pages 165, 353 & 358.
- Shears for the photograph on page 160.
- Terry Calvert for Fig 2.23 and photographs on pages 75, 263 & 279.

All other photographs were supplied by **L'Oréal** or the authors.

CAREER ROUTES WITHIN THE HAIRDRESSING INDUSTRY

Over the last decade there has been a movement away from the traditional 'time-serving' methods of training towards training to **levels of competence**. In this way, once trainees are competent in a particular area, they progress to the next stage. Thus, particularly talented trainees will require a shorter training period than their less competent counterparts.

There are three main routes to 'qualified hairdresser' status (see Fig. I.1). The first route is via a **modern apprenticeship** (MA). The MAs are similar to previous, traditional apprenticeships in that the modern apprentice is employed by the employer who therefore decides the wage and also the terms and conditions of the employment contract. A pledge is signed by the employer, modern apprentice, the local Training Enterprise Council (TEC) and also the parent or guardian if the modern apprentice is a minor. Included within the pledge is a formal training plan, structured up to NVQ Level 3 with 'Additional skill' and 'Core skill' components incorporated within the plan to enhance the modern apprentices' effectiveness within their individual salons.

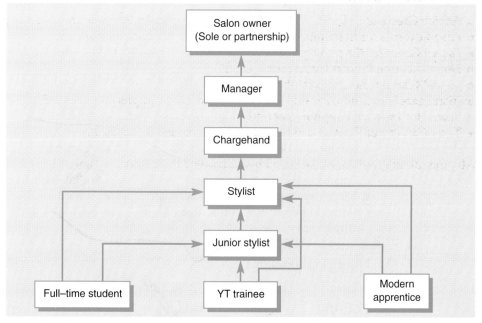

Fig. I.1 Career routes within the hairdressing industry

An alternative route is to attend a college of further education (FE) as a **full-time student** until competence in all areas of the hairdressing craft is achieved, after which time the trainee is usually employed by a salon as a junior stylist.

A third route is through **Youth Training** (YT) which may offer full-time employment in a salon and if the **trainee** (i.e. the person who is being trained through YT) is suitable and enough work is available, he or she can be retained by the salon as a junior stylist.

Most modern apprentices spend one day a week (for 36 weeks of the year) at an FE college, as do YT trainees. This allows certification and provides skills testing through various examining bodies.

After the initial training period, a stylist could progress to **chargehand**, then to **manager** and then on to **owning** a salon, either solely or jointly with one or more partners. However, not every individual dreams of becoming self-employed and there are many other options available to the aspiring stylist once the initial training period or level of competence has been achieved. If the trainee/modern apprentice is particularly talented, it is often possible to progress to 'stylist' status very quickly.

The progressive pattern of the City & Guilds of London awards can be seen in Fig. I.2.

Career options

There is a variety of options available to the competent stylist and these can be divided into seven broad areas:

- Salon-based.
- Theatrical.
- Manufacturing industry.
- Trichologist/consultant.
- Teaching/technician.
- Managerial.
- Sales.

Salon based

For obvious reasons, the majority of career opportunities within the hairdressing industry are salon based. However, salons are not always situated on the 'High Street', they can be located in a wide variety of settings and the type of service they provide will reflect the needs of a particular clientele. Hairdressing services are often required in:

- Hotels (both at home and abroad).
- Clinics.
- Health and fitness clubs.
- Health farms.
- Gymnasiums/leisure centres.
- Large department stores (as service for both the general public and the employees of the store).
- Cruise liners.
- Residential homes.
- Hospitals.
- In the client's own home with mobile hairdressing.
- Armed forces.
- Holiday camps.

Theatrical (media)

There are situations available to the stylist within the television, film and theatre industries. However, there are only a limited number of openings within the media; therefore, competition for a position in this area is great.

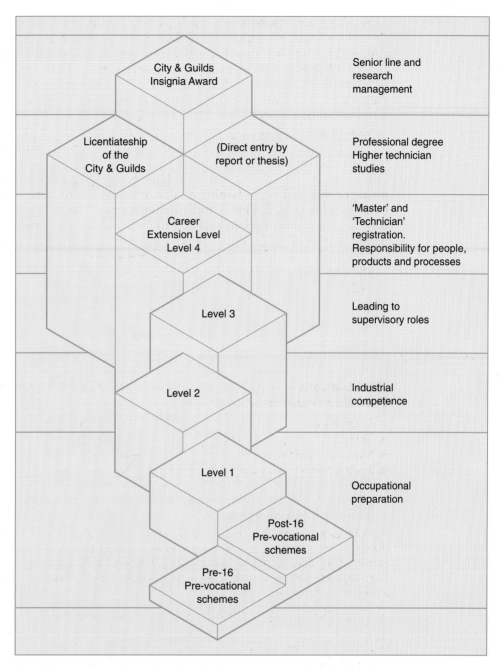

Fig. I.2 Progressive pattern of the City & Guilds awards

Entry requirements usually include competence in wigmaking, make-up, and both men's and women's hairdressing. Older candidates (over 21) with a variety of working experience are generally preferred as working hours are usually staggered and flexible – often early morning or late evening!

Opportunities are also available for specialisation in the actual making, setting and dressing of wigs and hairpieces but prospective employees must hold a relevant wigmaking certificate.

Manufacturing industry

The manufacturers of hairdressing preparations employ hairdressers to market, sell and demonstrate their products to other hairdressers. A career within the manufacturing industry usually entails a great deal of travelling throughout the country; therefore, it is easier if family commitments are minimal. Career options within this area include:

- *Technical representative*: gives technical advice and helps with the development of new products.
- *Sales representative*: sells the products by visiting salons, training centres and colleges.
- *Trade demonstrator*: demonstrates the uses of the products to hairdressers in salons, training centres and colleges.
- *Tutor in manufacturers' own hairdressing schools*: tutoring and giving advice to hairdressers who attend manufacturers' schools for specialised courses. The tutors also have to be prepared to work behind the scenes at the large national shows and seminars. Other duties often include making videos and colour slides of new techniques that they have helped to develop.

Trichologist/consultant

To practise as a registered trichologist the stylist must be an 'Associate of the Institute of Trichologists', which means that they have had a training period of three years which included a **preliminary** year, an **intermediate** year and a **final** year. This qualification can be obtained through a correspondence course with the Institute of Trichologists or by attendance at a college of further education.

The Institute of Trichologists' examination is very thorough and there is an entry requirement of four GCSE subjects (A, B or C grade or equivalent), one of which should preferably be a science subject.

The trained trichologist can practise within an existing hairdressing salon as a separate professional clinic to complement the other hairdressing services or as a separate business enterprise.

Teaching/technician

The teaching of hairdressing can be carried out in:

- Private schools.
- Manufacturers' schools.
- Training centres/colleges of further education.

The qualifications necessary to teach vary depending upon the type of establishment. Often private schools train their own instructors who are chosen because of their proven hairdressing skills. Manufacturers' schools and training centres usually require their instructors to be experienced stylists with a sound knowledge of all aspects of the hairdressing craft both theoretically and practically, while colleges of further education demand the highest hairdressing qualifications available and preferably a recognised teaching qualification as well. Provision is usually made for every college lecturer to obtain a university validated Teachers Certificate (if not already acquired) and lecturers are also encouraged to proceed to degree level, thus ensuring that they are suitably qualified to teach.

Technicians are employed in colleges of further education to give valuable assistance to the lecturers in the preparation and setting up of the teaching situation by organising stock, materials, equipment and audiovisual teaching aids. They play an important role within the college and work very closely with the teaching staff as part of a team.

Managerial

This includes **salon ownership** either solely or with one or more partner. However, there are also various other managerial options depending upon the size and type of salon and it is often advisable to gain managerial experience as an **employee** before becoming a salon owner.

Smaller salons may limit their higher management positions to either **charge-hand** (with less responsibility) or **manager** but larger hairdressing salons often require **artistic directors**, **educational directors** and **management staff** to market their salons and any courses they may run.

Sales

This area involves the selling of hairdressing and beauty products. Potential opportunities in sales include employment as:

- *Sales representative*: employed by the manufacturers to sell to the hairdressing trade.
- *Sales person*: employed by large department stores to sell the products and give advice to their customers.
- *Receptionist*: employed by the hairdressing/beauty salon and duties will include selling hairdressing/beauty products to the clients.

Level 1

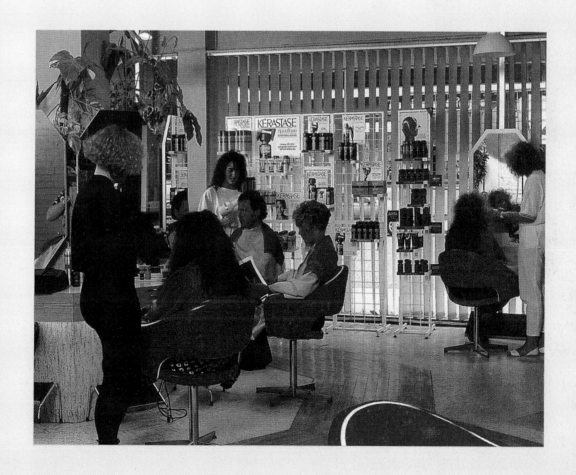

SHAMPOOING, CONDITIONING AND DRYING HAIR

Helping the stylist

The main role of the trainee is to help the stylist carry out hair services as efficiently and effectively as possible. In addition to assisting, this involves preparing the hair for further, more complex, technical services to be carried out by the stylist. Remember it is very important to listen to the stylist's instructions **carefully** to prevent any mishaps.

Shampooing hair

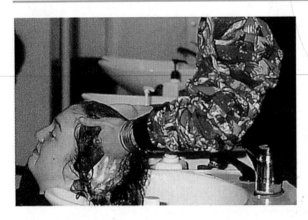

In hairdressing, to 'shampoo' hair has come to mean to clean it. Shampooing is one of the most common operations in hairdressing salons. It is typically an operation that trainees carry out very soon after starting work. (See Level 2 for more detailed information.)

What you need before you begin
- Shampoo.
- Clean gown.
- Clean towels.

Preventing RSI

When shampooing, arms and shoulders can become painful from holding the elbows out and hunching the shoulders. Be very aware of your position as you work. Keep your elbows in whenever you can and relax your shoulders. Keep your wrists as flat as you can when you massage.

How to shampoo

1 The client must be adequately protected. Clothes should be completely covered by a gown and towels tucked well down at the nape. If a front wash is to be used, a face cloth should be provided to protect the client's eyes. Check client requirements with the stylist.
2 Hair must be thoroughly disentangled prior to shampooing.
3 The temperature of the water should be checked on the wrist or the back of the hand before allowing the water to run onto the scalp.

SAFETY TIP
Make sure that shampoo does not run into the client's eyes and that water is not too hot.

4 Correct shampoo should be used for the type of hair.
5 Liquid shampoo should be allowed to run over the back of the hand then on to the scalp to minimise coldness. Do not use too much!
6 Cream shampoo should be applied to the palm of the hand before being evenly distributed over the whole head.
7 Friction hand massage should be used in circular movements from hairline to crown, across the whole scalp.
8 Hot water taps should be turned off during massage unless a mixer tap is used, in which case the whole tap is turned off. This is to conserve hot water.
9 Care must be taken to ensure that the hair is thoroughly rinsed after each massage. When it is clean it should 'squeak' under the fingers. If it does not, shampoo the hair again.
10 After shampooing, hair should be towel dried and disentangled away from the face. Never allow the client to leave the shampoo area with hair dripping on to the face. Always wrap hair in a towel to keep the head warm if the client is required to move about in the salon.
11 Tell the stylist you have finished. Complete record card.

POINTS TO REMEMBER

- Do not use too much shampoo. Use the minimum of hot water, as it is expensive to heat up.
- Long hair will need more shampoo and more rinsing.
- Avoid allowing shampoo to run into the client's eyes. Be aware that repeated use of shampoo on unprotected hands can remove the natural oil, lead to cracking and possibly dermatitis.

What to do when you have finished the shampoo
- Clean the work area.
- Place used towels and gown in correct place.
- Check shampoo left in container. Top up or replace if necessary.

Client requirements
- The client should be comfortable.
- There are a range of specialist shampoos currently on sale for various uses. Some examples are shown in Table 1.1. Read the manufacturer's instructions carefully. Any particular problem areas must be checked with the stylist or your supervisor.

Table 1.1

Type	Use
Cream	Dry, brittle, bleached, tinted, permed hair
Oil	Extremely dry, bleached, tinted, permed hair
Medicated	Mild dandruff
Egg	Sensitive scalps, children's hair
Beer	Lank, fine hair
Lemon	To adjust pH to between 4 and 6 after hair has been bleached, tinted or permed
Protein	Limp, chemically damaged hair
Herbal	To add sheen
pH balance	To adjust pH to between 4 and 6, useful on chemically damaged hair
Dry powder	Invalids, in between shampoos
Brightening	Mild bleach, e.g. to highlight dull hair
Colour	Temporary tints

Preventing RSI

Wash basins that are free-standing – set out from the wall – are a far better idea because the shampooer can stand upright behind the basin.

Potential problems

- Waste of shampoo product and hot water.
- Wrong shampoo used for hair type.
- Shampoo not thoroughly rinsed from the hair.

Conditioning hair

Hair looks at its best when it is in good condition. Exactly what 'good condition' means is hard to define, but it does involve factors such as the hair being:

- Manageable – that is, easy to brush, comb and deal with.
- Shiny (lustrous).
- Pliable and elastic.
- Soft and having body.

There are a number of factors which influence hair condition. These can be *internal* such as age, diet, drugs and illness or they can be *external* such as physical damage. Knowing which of these has caused the hair to be in poor condition is helpful in deciding which **conditioning treatment** to use. See Level 2 Unit 2 for further detail on different types of conditioners and hand massage.

Conditioning treatments

There are three basic types of conditioning lotions:

- Oil based.
- Substantive type (where ingredients 'add' to the hair).
- Acid type.

Most conditioners are applied to the hair after it has been shampooed. The stylist will assess the hair and scalp then recommend which product to use. It is very important to carry out the stylist's instructions. Directions on how to use the product will also be given by the manufacturers as it is in their interest to make sure that you use their products correctly. It is often a good idea to read the manufacturers' instructions before starting any service on the client to make sure that the correct procedure is carried out.

Carrying out a surface condition

1. Check the client's requirements with the stylist. Shampoo the hair with a suitable shampoo, one to complement the conditioning product to be used. Always follow the manufacturer's or the stylist's instructions. Some conditioners need to be left on the hair for five to ten minutes before rinsing whilst others may need to be left in the hair without any rinsing at all.
2. Pour the correct amount of conditioner into the palm of the hand. Gently place the hands together then apply the conditioner evenly onto the hair. Stroke the hands through the hair from the front through to the nape using **effleurage** massage movements to soothe and relax the client.
3. Follow the effleurage movement with a faster **rotary** (petrissage) movement to stimulate the blood vessels then end the massage with further effleurage movements.
4. Unless instructed otherwise, remove the conditioner from the hair by rinsing thoroughly with warm water when the massage is complete. Any conditioner left in the hair could make it limp, flyaway or greasy.
5. Towel dry the hair then disentangle ready for setting or blowdrying.
6. Tell the stylist you have finished. Complete a record card.

A note about 'hot oil' conditioning treatments

You may be asked to remove the oil used in this treatment from a client's hair. This is basically a shampooing operation but to make sure the oil is removed the shampoo is put straight onto the oil and rubbed gently but thoroughly into the hair.

All other points about this operation are the same as for shampooing.

POINTS TO REMEMBER

- Do not use too much conditioning product. Use the minimum of hot water.
- Be careful not to pull on long hair during the treatment. This can be very painful!
- More product needs to be used on long hair and it requires more thorough rinsing.

What to do when you have finished the conditioning treatment

- Clean the work area.
- Place the used towels and gown in the correct place.
- Clean and put away any equipment used such as dressing combs and sectioning clips.
- Check the shampoo and conditioner products left.
- Top up or replace as necessary.

> **SAFETY TIP**
> - Look out for cuts or abrasions on the scalp – ask for assistance if present.
> - Take care that the water for shampooing/rinsing and the hot towels are not too hot.

Client requirements

- The client should be comfortable throughout the conditioning treatment.
- There are a large number of different conditioning products available. The stylist will choose the most appropriate for the client following an assessment of the client's hair.

Potential problems

Potential problems which may occur include:

- Product (shampoo/conditioner) going into client's eyes.
- Cuts/abrasions on the scalp.
- Water/towels too hot.
- Waste – shampoo, conditioner or hot water and effort in massage of client's head and scalp.
- Wrong products used.
- Products not thoroughly rinsed from hair.

Things to do

1 Organise a file giving information of particular client requirements and copies of the record cards completed.

2 Look at the **potential problems**. Describe how you would avoid these problems or what action you would take.

Blowdrying hair

Carrying out a blowdry

Blowdrying is carried out on damp hair and is a method of shaping hair using brushes of various shapes and sizes. The smaller the brush that is used, the smaller the finished curl. Longer, one length hair usually needs a larger round brush otherwise there may be too much curl to cope with when dressing out the blowdry. What happens to the hair when blowdrying is covered in detail in Level 2 Unit 3.

How to blowdry the hair

1 Ask the stylist which products and equipment to use then collect all necessary equipment. Consult the client and stylist on how the client wishes the blowdry to be.
2 Protect the client with gown and towels. Check that all electrical equipment is safe to use.
3 Shampoo the hair and towel dry to remove excess water.
4 Apply any blow styling products evenly on the hair. Comb through thoroughly then comb the hair in the direction of the finished style.
5 Section the hair from forehead to nape, leaving out any fringe and using any partings, then section the hair from ear to ear across the nape area, leaving out a fine section of hair at the nape.
6 Begin blowdrying at the nape, wrapping fine sections of hair around the brush. the jet of air should be directed away from the scalp and should help to blow the hair around the brush.
7 Make sure the section of hair is dry by allowing it to cool slightly then dry the next section in the same way. Work from left to right, alternating up the sides of the head towards the front.
8 Remember that the hair will dry in the position it is placed, so always work in the direction of the finished dressing.
9 When the whole head has been completed, check that the hair is completely dry. Check the finished shape by looking in the mirror and look at the hair from all angles.
10 Tell the stylist you have finished the blowdry then complete a record card.

What to do when you have finished blowdrying

- Show the stylist the finished blowdry.
- Place used towels and gown in the correct place.
- Clean and put away the equipment used.
- Clean and sterilise the brushes and combs used.
- Clean the work area.

Potential problems

- Using too much blowstyling lotion or mousse will leave the hair 'sticky'.
- Using too high a heat may burn the client's hair.
- Blowdrying too close to the client's skin may cause burns.
- Not controlling the hair around the brush, causing it to buckle and be out of shape.
- Using the wrong type of brush.

Things to do

1 Find out about as many types of brushes for use on the hair as you can. Information can be found in trade magazines, retail and wholesale outlets.

2 Collect pictures of all the types then present them on a plain sheet of paper with a short written explanation of their use and main advantages.

3 Place your work in your portfolio as supplementary evidence of your competence.

INTRODUCTION TO PERMING, RELAXING AND COLOURING

Perming, relaxing and colouring are the main chemical processes undertaken in the salon. At level one, the trainee will mainly assist a more senior staff member by:

- Neutralising perms.
- Neutralising relaxers.
- Applying temporary rinses.
- Removing colouring and lightening products from the hair.

Neutralising hair

Neutralisation is the part of the perming process that 'fixes' the hair into the style. Without this, perming would not work. Neutralisers stop the perm lotion from working and chemically 'lock' the hair into the shape produced by the perming rods.

A major problem can arise if the hair is not rinsed thoroughly enough to remove all trace of the perm lotion before applying the neutraliser. *Always* read the manufacturer's instructions and seek guidance from the stylist *before* neutralising.

There are five main stages to neutralising the hair after perming:

1 Remove perm lotion.
2 Remove excess water.
3 Apply neutraliser.
4 Remove neutraliser.
5 Condition hair if necessary.

Stage 1: Remove perm lotion

It is important to remove all traces of perm lotion from the hair to stop it working. Because the hair is wrapped in an end paper, then possibly many times around the perm rod, a lot of rinsing with warm water is needed to make sure that the water reaches the inside hair.

Stage 2: Remove excess water

If the hair is left too wet, the water will dilute the neutraliser and stop it working properly.

Stage 3: Apply neutraliser

The neutraliser **must** be applied to each perm rod very carefully. It should be pushed well into the hair to make sure that it soaks through to the hair wrapped closest to the perm rod. It must also be left on the hair for the correct length of time otherwise it will not have time to fix the hair in its new curled shape and the hair will straighten. Always treat the hair gently throughout the process as the hair is not finally fixed until it is dry.

Stage 4: Remove neutraliser

Once the neutraliser has been left on the hair for the correct length of time, it should then be thoroughly removed from the hair. Any neutraliser left in the hair could react with the hair's colour pigment, bleaching it and making it lighter.

Stage 5: Condition hair if necessary

A special acid conditioner is usually applied to cancel out any alkali deposit left by the alkaline perm lotion. It will also close the cuticle scales on the outside of the hair which then makes the hair appear more shiny.

POINTS TO REMEMBER

- The hair is not 'fixed' in its new curled shape until it is dry so it **must** be treated carefully at all times throughout the neutralising process.
- If the neutralisation process is not carried out correctly all the hard work of the stylist will be undone. It will also be very bad publicity for the salon and will stop clients coming back for further services.

What you need before you begin

- Cotton wool, to blot hair dry and to make a protective strip around the hairline.
- Rubber gloves to protect your hands.
- Neutraliser.
- Conditioner.

How to neutralise a perm

1 To make sure that the perm has worked well enough to get the amount of curl required, the stylist will gently unwind a rod (but not remove it completely) then push the hair gently back towards the roots. If the perm is ready the hair will form an 'S' shaped movement, the size of which depends upon the amount of curl required. A large 'S' movement gives a loose curl while a small 'S' shaped movement will give a tight curl. When the perm is ready, check with the stylist which neutraliser to use.
2 Rinse the hair thoroughly for five minutes in warm water. If a front wash is used, take particular care to rinse the front rods thoroughly. If a back wash is used, particular attention should be paid to the rods at the nape.

> SAFETY TIP
> Always select the correct neutraliser for the perm used.

3 Remove excess water by blotting thoroughly with cotton wool. Take care not to disturb the wound hair. Leaving the hair too wet will dilute the neutraliser and

make it less effective. To check that enough moisture has been removed from the hair, press the palm of the hand onto the rods – if the palm is wet when it is pulled away from the head, the hair requires re-blotting.

4 Apply a strip of cotton wool around the hairline to protect the face and neck.
5 Apply the neutraliser to the wound rods, ensuring that each one is completely covered. It is important not to mix neutraliser or pour out ready-mixed neutraliser until it is required otherwise it will not work.
6 Leave for five minutes. Cotton wool around the hairline prevents the neutraliser from dripping on the face and neck.
7 Carefully remove the cotton wool and the rods. The hair should not be pulled or stretched at this stage as the curl is not yet fully 'fixed'.
8 Apply neutraliser gently to the points of the hair as each rod is removed. Do not drag the hair or massage the neutraliser into the hair as this could alter the curl. Check that all the hair has been treated with the neutraliser then leave for a further five minutes.

SAFETY TIP
Always follow the manufacturer's instructions when using chemicals on the hair.

9 Rinse the hair thoroughly and apply a conditioner.
10 Tell the stylist you have finished. Complete a record card.

How to neutralise the hair for curly perming African Caribbean hair

This has two neutralising stages:

● Neutralising the curl rearranger.
● Neutralising the curl booster (perm).

Neutralising the curl rearranger

The curl rearranger is used without any perm rods and the stylist will tell you when the hair is ready for this first neutralising stage. It is important to remember that the hair will now be fragile and you must be very careful not to rub or tangle it in any way or you could damage it.

1 Ask the stylist or technician for advice on the length of time you should rinse the hair.
2 Seat the client at a backwash basin and make sure that they are well protected with gown and towel. Some salons also use a protective face cloth for the client's eyes.
3 Rinse the hair thoroughly in warm water for the correct length of time (usually five minutes). If the hair is not rinsed thoroughly some of the curl rearranger will be left in the hair and this could damage it. Set a timer to make sure that the hair is rinsed long enough – the time always seems longer than it is!

4 When you have finished rinsing, blot the hair thoroughly to remove the excess water. If the hair is left too wet the water will dilute the perm lotion used in the next stage and the perm may not take.

5 Gently comb through the hair; it is still in a fragile state and rough handling could damage it. Place a clean towel around the client's neck.

6 Make sure that the client is seated comfortably, then tell the stylist you have finished. The hair will now be wound on perm rods by the stylist before the next neutralising stage.

Neutralising the curl booster

This is the second stage of the neutralising process. The hair will have been rewound on perm rods by the stylist or technician and left to develop until the hair has just the right amount of curl for the client. It is important to neutralise the hair immediately the stylist or technician tells you to or the hair may become over-processed and damaged.

1 Ask the stylist or technician which neutralising product to use. Always use the correct product or the perm may not take.

2 Seat the client comfortably and make sure that they are well protected as before.

3 Rinse the hair, making sure that each perm rod is well rinsed. If any rods are missed the finished curl may be uneven. Set the timer for the correct length of time (usually five to ten minutes).

4 When rinsing is completed, blot the hair thoroughly with a clean towel or cotton wool. Check that enough water has been removed by pressing the palm of the hand onto the rods, if it is wet then there is still too much moisture left in the hair.

5 Place a clean towel around the client's shoulders and tuck well down at the nape. Place strips of cotton wool around the hairline to stop the neutraliser running onto the skin and face.

6 Apply the correct neutraliser very carefully to each perm rod; if you miss any the perm will not take evenly. Push the neutraliser well into the wound hair – it has a lot of layers to soak through! Leave the neutraliser to develop, the stylist will usually tell you how long but if you are unsure then check the manufacturer's instructions.

7 When developed, carefully remove the perm rods, making sure not to pull or drag the hair as this will alter the curl movement. Apply fresh neutraliser gently to the ends of the hair that have been previously covered by the end paper. Do not pull or stretch the hair, treat it very carefully or you could spoil the curl. Leave to develop for correct length of time, usually five minutes, but check with the stylist or the manufacturer's instructions.

8 Rinse all the neutraliser from the hair very thoroughly using lots of warm water. If any neutraliser is left in the hair it could damage and lighten it.

9 Condition or moisturise the hair as directed by the stylist or technician. Towel dry the hair taking care not to rub or tangle it then comb through gently.

10 Place a clean towel around the client's shoulders, make sure they are seated comfortably then inform the stylist you have finished.

11 Clear away the products and equipment used. Clean the work station and complete a record card as directed by the stylist.

Potential problems

• Allowing the neutraliser to run onto the skin and down the face or neck. This may irritate the skin.

- Not rinsing the hair thoroughly and so preventing the neutraliser working properly.
- Not blotting the hair thoroughly to remove the excess water. This will dilute and weaken the neutraliser, again stopping it working properly. The client may return to the salon complaining that their hair has reverted back to very curly.
- Leaving neutraliser in the hair which could cause the hair to lighten or cause internal hair damage.
- Not pushing the neutraliser well down into the perm rods which will prevent all of the hair being neutralised and give an uneven finished curl.
- Pulling and stretching the hair, which will alter the finished curl

Neutralising hair after relaxing

This method of neutralising is totally different to the procedure and process of neutralising a cold perm or the curly perm described above. A cold perm alters the structure of the hair by **reduction** and the neutraliser is an **oxidation** process (this is explained in detail in Level 2 Unit 5A). A relaxer alters the structure of the hair through a process called **hydrolysis** (this is covered in detail in Level 2 Unit 5B) and the hair is neutralised by an acidic shampoo which neutralises out the alkaline cream relaxer.

The chemicals used when relaxing the hair are very strong and capable of burning the skin and dissolving the hair if not used correctly! Therefore, it is very important to follow the stylist or technician's instructions very carefully. Any mistakes can cause hair breakage and an unsatisfactory result. Remember that the relaxer can also burn your skin so always wear rubber gloves and avoid touching the relaxer cream.

Method
1 Check with the stylist which products to use and how. Collect all your equipment and the correct products. Always refer to the manufacturer's instructions if you are unsure or have forgotten what to do.
2 Take the client to a backwash station. Make sure that the client is well protected with towels tucked well down at the nape and that the client is seated comfortably.
3 Wear protective rubber gloves. Rinse the hair thoroughly with plenty of warm water. Use the force of the water to remove the relaxer and handle the hair as little as possible. Make sure that ALL the relaxer has been removed.
4 Apply the correct acidic neutralising shampoo to neutralise the alkalinity of the relaxer. Use gentle stroking massage movement; do not rub the hair or scalp as the scalp may be tender and the hair is in a fragile state.
5 Rinse the neutralising shampoo from the hair then repeat the process. The stylist or technician will tell you how many shampoos will be needed. Always follow their instructions carefully.
6 Apply a reconditioning or moisturising agent and leave for the correct time. Remove from the hair by rinsing thoroughly.
7 Blot the hair gently to remove the excess water, do not rub the hair. Place clean towels around the client. Tell the stylist you have finished.
8 Clean the workstation and clear away equipment. Fill in a record of what you have done as directed by the stylist or technician.

Potential problems

- Allowing the relaxer to go in the client's eye. This could blind the client, so be extra careful when rinsing the hair. Rinse the eye with lots of water and inform the stylist **immediately**, as the client may need medical aid.
- Not wearing protective rubber gloves. The relaxer will burn the skin – including yours!
- Not rinsing the relaxer from the hair thoroughly. Relaxers will carry on working if not removed and will break the hair.
- Rubbing the hair and scalp. This could cause skin irritation and hair breakage.
- Using the wrong product. Always use the neutralising shampoo produced for the type of relaxer used otherwise the hair may be damaged.
- Not protecting the client's clothing. If the products damage the client's clothing, then the client is legally able to claim new ones from the salon.
- Not reading the manufacturer's instructions. If you do not follow instructions correctly you could cause a great deal of damage to the client's hair and also the image of the salon.

Record cards

Always complete a client record card when the process is completed. Check with the stylist that it contains the following information:

- Date.
- Hair condition.
- Product use, including the strength of the reagent.
- Size of rod used.
- Development time.
- Any precautions necessary.
- Finished result and any comments necessary.
- Recommended after-care treatment.

POINTS TO REMEMBER

- Do not use too much neutraliser or conditioner.
- Use the correct neutraliser.
- With long hair it is important to make sure that the wound hair is well rinsed and then well blotted before applying the neutraliser. Rather than 'blotting' you may be asked to use a drier for a few minutes on the client's hair.

What to do when you have finished neutralising the perm or relaxer
- Clean the work area.
- Place used towels and gown in correct place.
- Dispose of cotton wool used.
- Clean rods/clips, combs, brushes.
- Check products used and replace if necessary.
- Carefully dispose of any partially used neutraliser.

Client requirements
The client must be **comfortable** and **protected** by gowning and cotton wool hairline strips during the process.

SAFETY TIPS
Neutralisers contain harsh chemicals. It is important to:
- wear protective gloves to avoid skin contact
- use hairline cotton wool strip on the client to prevent product running onto the client's skin
- check for cuts and abrasions on the client's scalp.

Things to do

1 Organise a file to record different client requirements and how these were met.

2 Look at the **potential problems** and explain how you would avoid these problems

What can go wrong

Problem: Curl drops out completely by the next shampoo.
Cause:
- Not rinsing hair thoroughly for the correct length of time.
- Not applying neutraliser correctly.
- Not leaving neutraliser on hair long enough.
- Neutraliser is 'off'; it may be old stock, or top not returned to neutraliser bottle correctly.

Problem: Curl looser than expected after neutralising.
Cause:
- Leaving hair too wet before applying neutraliser.
- Too much tension when pulling out the perm rods.
- Dragging the hair when applying the neutraliser.
- Massaging the neutraliser into the hair and scalp.

Problem: Uneven curl at the next shampoo.
Cause:
- Not rinsing hair evenly all over the head.
- Not applying the neutraliser evenly over the head.

Problem: Curly root hair, straight ends
Cause:
- Not rinsing thoroughly for the required time.
- Not leaving neutraliser on hair long enough.
- Not applying neutraliser to the ends of the hair.

Problem: Skin irritation around hairline.
Cause:
- Neutraliser being allowed to run onto hairline.
- No cotton wool placed around hairline.
- Cotton wool saturated in neutraliser and not removed.

Temporary rinses

Temporary rinses add colour to the hair. They coat the outside of the hair which means that they are easily removed when the hair is shampooed. If they are used on a regular basis there will be a 'build up' of colour on the hair which means that it will be more difficult to shampoo out. Temporary rinses are covered in more technical detail in Level 2 Unit 6.

Effects of temporary rinses

Temporary rinses will not lighten the hair and have a limited colour range. They will therefore also have a limited effect on the hair and will not usually show if used on a base shade that is darker than the colour of the rinse. However, they are very useful as an introduction to colour as they can be easily washed out if the client does not like the result or wants to try different colours.

Because temporary rinses are made of pure colour, their names can sometimes be misleading. For example, 'auburn' would be a red colour which is fine if used on dark hair but disastrous if used on an older client with white hair – it would go bright red/orange! **Always** check with the stylist or technician to make sure that the rinse is suitable for the client's hair colour.

Effects
- Adds a shine and brightens dull hair.
- Counteracts any lightening or fading of the hair after perming or between permanent dyes.
- Darkens the hair or adds glints and shine.
- Tones bleached or lightened hair. It will mask any unwanted golden tones.
- 'Mingles in' grey hair.
- Can give bright, vibrant, unusual colours (green, pink, orange, etc.) when used on bleached hair.

Types of temporary rinses

Types of temporary rinses that are applied to wet hair include:

- coloured setting lotion
- coloured blowdry lotion
- coloured mousse
- coloured gel

You will need
- Cotton wool to remove any stains to the client's skin.
- Rubber gloves to protect your hands.
- Suitable temporary rinse.
- Dark towel and gown to protect the client's clothing.

How to apply a temporary rinse

1 Shampoo and towel dry the hair. If a conditioner is used, it must be thorou[gh]ly rinsed from the hair otherwise it may create a barrier and prevent the[colour] sticking to the hair.
2 Ask the stylist which type of temporary rinse to use to suit the client's ha[ir] requirements.
3 Protect the client's clothing with a dark gown and towel. Do not use li[ght] towels as they will be stained by the colour rinse.
4 Apply the rinse straight from the bottle, tube or aerosol can. Apply to the roots of the hair then rub through the hair lengths. Comb through the hair with a wide-toothed comb to make sure that the rinse coats the hair evenly.

5 When using coloured mousse or gel, apply the product to the wide teeth of the comb before applying it to the hair. Again, comb through the hair thoroughly to make sure that it coats the hair evenly.
6 Remove any staining to the skin with a piece of damp cotton wool.
7 Tell the stylist you have finished the application. Complete a record card.

POINTS TO REMEMBER

- Do not use too much rinse as it could drip and stain the skin. It could also leave a sticky deposit on the hair.
- Use the correct product in the correct manner.
- Do not leave the hair too wet after shampooing – it could dilute the rinse.

What to do when you have finished applying the rinse
- Clean the work area and wipe over the surfaces.
- Place used towel and gown in the correct place.
- Dispose of the used cotton wool.
- Rinse and sterilise the comb used.
- Check products used and enter in stock book if necessary.

Client requirements
The client **must** be well protected at all times with a dark towel and gown. Any staining of the skin must be removed before the client leaves the salon.

Potential problems
- Not protecting the client's clothing properly.
- Not applying the rinse evenly.
- Allowing the rinse to run down the client's face and staining the skin.
- Not towel drying the hair enough so that the excess water dilutes the rinse.

Removing highlighting and lowlighting products from the hair

Highlighting and lowlighting are ways of changing the colour of a client's hair in a fairly subtle and natural-looking way. *Highlighting* is where hair is lightened. *Lowlighting* is where a tint darker than the natural colour is used. Both techniques are used on strands of hair which may be drawn through a cap, wrapped in foil or plastic, or streaked using other methods.

What you need before you begin
- To check with the stylist on the technique and any special client requirements.
- To gown the client, and ensure that the client is protected and comfortable.
- Shampoo and conditioner

How to remove highlighting and lowlighting products

1 Check with the stylist which products are to be used, then make the client comfortable at the wash basin.

2 Check the temperature of water on the back of your hand. If packets have been used, remove them gently, starting at the nape and working towards the front of the head.
3 Rinse thoroughly to remove all tint and/or bleach on the hair. If a cap has been used, add a small amount of conditioner to the hair and remove the cap gently.
4 Shampoo the hair with a suitable shampoo.
5 Rinse thoroughly.
6 Apply conditioner, massage and rinse thoroughly.
7 Tell the stylist you have finished.

POINTS TO REMEMBER

- Avoid using too much product, too much hot water, and too much time and effort on excessive massaging and rinsing.
- Do not use the wrong product.
- Long hair will need more product and much more rinsing than short hair.

What to do after the removal of highlighting and lowlight products
- Clean the work area and wipe surfaces.
- Wash and dry off any equipment used.
- Place tools and equipment back in proper position.
- Check products and replace or top up if necessary.

Client requirements
Check with the stylist to find out if the client has any special requirements.

SAFETY TIPS
- Make sure the client is adequately protected.
- Check the water temperature.
- Keep product out of the client's eyes.
- Wear protective gloves to avoid skin contact with colour and other products.

Potential problems
- Product running into client's eyes or water being too hot.
- Waste of product, hot water and effort.
- Long hair will contain more colour than short so it follows that more product and longer rinsing will be necessary.

Removing colouring products from the hair

Colouring (or tinting) hair involves changing the colour of the client's hair by using **colouring products** of various kinds. There is a wide variety of these available consisting of different kinds of active ingredients. One way of dividing up colouring products is on the basis of how long they last on the hair.

- **Temporary colour** – washes out at the first shampoo.
- **Semi-permanent colour** – lasts 6 to 8 shampoos.
- **Permanent colour** – will not shampoo out.

The method used to remove the colouring product depends on which type of product has been used. All the methods do, however, involve the following, although not necessarily in this order.

- **Rinsing** – warm water only is used.
- **Emulsifying** – the hair is moistened with water, hair is then rubbed and finally shampooed.
- **Shampooing** – a standard shampoo is carried out.

What you need before you begin
- To check with the stylist which techniques and products to use.
- To seat the client comfortably and protect the client with gown and towel.
- Shampoo and conditioner.

How to remove semi-permanent and permanent colour

The procedure is essentially the same for removing semi-permanent and permanent colour except that semi-permanent tints have a shampoo base so shampoo need not be applied. The steps are:

1 Check with stylist on the products to use.
2 Put a small amount of warm water onto the hair.
3 Massage well to emulsify colour.
4 Rinse thoroughly until the water runs clear.
5 Apply shampoo if needed – check with the stylist about this.
6 Rinse and condition the hair.
7 Ensure the client is seated comfortably and inform the stylist that the client is ready for the next service.

POINTS TO REMEMBER

- Do not use too much of the products involved.
- Shampoo with a suitable shampoo.
- Do not allow warm water to run to waste.
- Take care not to waste time and energy on rubbing/massaging the hair during colour removal.

What to do after the hair colour removal
- Clean the work area.
- Clean tools and equipment.
- Put items away into the correct places.
- Check tops on products, replace if necessary.

Client requirements
- The client needs to be comfortable and protected from hazards.
- The client requirement for hair colour removal will have been discussed in detail with the stylist and the client's hair condition carefully determined before the hair colour removal begins.

SAFETY TIPS
- Use dark coloured gown and towels.
- Use the correct type of shampoo.
- Follow the manufacturer's instructions.

Potential problems
- Product getting onto skin or into eyes.
- Waste – product, hot water, time and energy in rubbing and massaging scalp excessively.

Things to do

1 Make up a file of particular client requirements and copies of the record cards completed.

2 Look at the potential problems and describe how you would avoid them.

3 Carry out a survey of types of shampoo available – new ones are being marketed all the time. Are there any problems linked to their use?

5 Organise a file to record the different types of rinses you have used on clients. Describe how you have applied them.

6 Ask your supervisor if you can take a copy of the client's record card and obtain a testimony from the client and stylist stating whether the service you gave has been satisfactory and carried out competently.

7 Place your record, the client record cards and the testimonies in your portfolio of evidence for Level 1.

8 Organise a file, listing the main points when removing highlighting/lowlighting products.

What do you know?

Level 1 Unit 2

List the equipment, tools and products used in the salon. ☐

Explain the health and safety procedures for the equipment, tools and products used in the salon. ☐

How would you stop wastage? ☐

What health and safety precautions would you take when:

- *shampooing*
- *conditioning*
- *neutralising*
- *applying a temporary rinse*
- *removing highlighting and lowlighting products*
- *removing colouring products* ☐

What problems could there be when:

- *shampooing*
- *conditioning*
- *neutralising*
- *applying a temporary rinse*
- *removing highlighting and lowlighting products*
- *removing colouring products* ☐

How should the hair look and feel after a conditioning treatment? ☐

Why is it important to carry out the neutralising of a perm correctly? ☐

How should the hair look and feel after being neutralised? ☐

INTRODUCTION TO SALON RECEPTION

Hairdressing is a service industry, and as such it should be the major aim of every salon to provide a service which is:

- Professional.
- Safe – it is taken on trust that the service provided will be carried out with due regard to the client's health and safety.
- Pleasant and relaxing, so that the client's visit is enjoyable.

Each salon is a business in a highly competitive field, and everyone earning money from the salon depends on clients, regular clients being especially important.

It is sometimes difficult for younger members of staff to realise how easily a client can be offended or made angry by an offhand remark or manner. Therefore, when a new apprentice/trainee joins the staff, it is in the interest of staff and clients alike that the salon owner or manager teaches not only the practical skills but also the equally important basic skills of attitude and behaviour in the salon. A client may not actually complain at the time, but will simply not come back. They will also tell their friends about the unsatisfactory service they received, so not just one client is lost, but many. A bad reputation is extremely hard to remove.

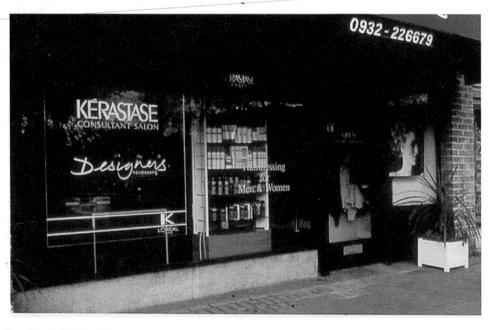

Clients and visitors at reception

The reception area usually gives the first impression of the salon so it is essential to keep it clean and tidy at all times. Many types of people visit the salon, not all of them wanting a hairdressing service. They can include sales representatives, tradesmen (e.g. window cleaner), training co-ordinators, etc., as well as new or existing clients. However, no matter who the visitor may be or the purpose of their business, they should always be attended to as soon as possible when they enter the premises.

Most people become annoyed if they are neglected or left waiting (think how **you** feel if a sales assistant ignores you or is rude and offhand) and if they are a client who has booked to have a treatment, they will not begin it in a happy, relaxed frame of mind if they have been irritated by the initial lack of service. Thus, **all** salon staff must be friendly and helpful at all times and deal with visitors promptly and efficiently.

Dealing with visitors

Greet the visitor politely and ask how you may be of assistance. Determine their name and the purpose of the visit. At this point it is usually necessary to ask questions of the visitor to make sure that their requirements are fully understood. Unless the request is of a general nature such as an enquiry regarding service prices, etc., a junior staff member will usually have to refer the visitor to a more senior person. If this is the case, make sure that the visitor is made comfortable whilst the appropriate staff member is informed of the request, then return to the visitor to explain when they can expect to be attended to. They need to know what is happening!

Dealing with expected clients

All clients must always be greeted pleasantly, preferably by name, as soon as they enter the salon. Find out the time and nature of the service required and check against the information in the appointment book. Tick off the client's name in the correct appointment column to ensure that there is a record of which clients have attended, then make the client comfortable whilst the appropriate staff member is made aware of the client's arrival. If instructed by the senior staff member, retrieve any records of the client's previous treatments and direct the client to the appropriate salon area.

If a client with an appointment does have to wait then the client should be made comfortable and told approximately how long the delay is expected to be with a simple, polite explanation. The client will then feel that they have been treated with consideration and will be less irritated by any delay.

Dealing with unexpected clients

Again, the client should be greeted pleasantly and promptly and questioned regarding their requirements. Any booking should be entered in the appointment book in pencil so that it can be easily removed if the client cancels. The name of the client and the service required must be written **clearly** so that it can be easily read by all the staff. It is embarrassing to call the client by the wrong name, so if your handwriting is poor the information should be printed instead.

See Level 2 Unit 7 for more detailed information.

Preventing RSI

Try to keep your shoulders relaxed whenever possible. Exercises will help and one of the best is shoulder shrugs. Hunch your shoulders and let them drop. In that dropped position they are relaxed. You can do six of these in ten seconds so do it every chance you get.

Gowning

It is often the duty of the receptionist or junior member of staff to gown the client after checking off their appointment. 'Gowning' is the term used when the client's clothing is protected by a gown and towels. It is carried out before any treatment and the type of towels and gown used will depend on which service is going to be carried out on the hair, e.g. dark gowns and towels are usually used when colouring the hair to minimise staining.

Before gowning the client, find out which service is required then select the correct type of gown and towels to use – always ask your supervisor if you are unsure. Position the gown over the client's clothing then place towel/s over the gown, making sure that it is tucked in snugly at the client's neckline (nape).

SAFETY TIP

Make sure that the client's clothing is *completely* covered by the gown.

Reception enquiries

During the course of the day there can be a vast variety of enquiries. Some, such as bookings, price lists or information regarding services and/or products, etc., can be attended to quite easily by junior staff members whilst other enquiries, such as official calls, people seeking employment, complaints, or business offers from manufacturers, may require the knowledge and expertise of a more experienced staff member or salon owner.

All enquiries should be dealt with promptly and professionally by finding out initially who is best suited to deal with the problem. If it requires the assistance of a more senior staff member then they should be informed immediately of the exact nature of the enquiry. However, if the appropriate staff member is unavailable it will be necessary to take a **message** which must then be passed on at the earliest opportunity.

Taking messages

Always **write down** a verbal message (Fig. 1.1) as it is often difficult to remember what has been said. An important message which has not been relayed or has been relayed inaccurately can have disastrous effects for the salon. Writing down the message acts as a **reminder** to pass on the message at a later time. The following facts should be included when writing down messages:

- Date and time.
- Name of the person giving the message.
- Name of the person to receive the message.

- Name of the person taking the message.
- Exact details of the message.

```
              TELEPHONE MESSAGE


For the attention of: Janet


Please phone Mrs Butterworth (0171 935 0121)
about her appointment tomorrow.


Message received by: Karen


Date: 24 May        Time: 11.20 am
```

Fig. 1.1 Example of a written message

When these details have been recorded, repeat the message back to the caller to make sure that it has been written down clearly and correctly. Remember that an inaccurate message can be almost as damaging as no message at all!

Preventing RSI
When you get a chance to sit, raise your feet to rest them and to help lessen the swelling caused by the accumulation of fluid.

Reception telephone calls

Always answer the telephone in a polite, clear voice. Remember to:

- Give the name of the salon.
- Give your name to the client.
- Ask how you may help the client.
- Repeat the client's request.
- Check that the client knows the correct date and time of any appointment made.

Things to do

1 Organise a file to show the systems and organisation of your salon.

2 Carry out the following task:

- Draw the layout of your salon, to scale, on a piece of graph paper.
- Label the different areas, e.g. reception, staff-room, etc., including telephone access points, cloakroom, WC and where and how refreshments are provided.
- Give a brief explanation of the function of each area.

3 Organise a file containing information to do with *reception enquiries* to show your knowledge of the services and products used in your salon.

4 Draw a format for a 'memo' pad which could be used in the salon. Create headings which will include all the relevant and necessary information for taking messages.

5 Organise a file to record the different messages that you have taken in the salon.

6 Read the following case study then answer the questions asked.

You receive an agitated telephone call from a client who wishes to speak to the salon owner regarding a previous permanent wave appointment. She refuses to speak to any other member of staff regarding her problem. Unfortunately, the salon owner will not be in the salon until the following day. What will you do?

- Explain how you feel you should act in this situation.
- Write out the procedure for recording an important telephone message. Remember to include the important points when taking telephone messages.

What do you know?	Level 1 Unit 3

What is your salon's recording system? ☐

Explain the responsibilities of the people working in the salon and where you can find them. ☐

List the services and products offered in the salon. Give their cost. ☐

Why must messages be dated, timed and addressed correctly? ☐

Who would you ask for information if you were not sure how to answer enquiries? ☐

INTRODUCTION TO WORKING RELATIONSHIPS

Communication

Effective working relationships are very important in the salon both for client satisfaction and so that you can make a worthwhile contribution to the operation of the salon team. A key factor in forming and keeping a relationship with someone is **communication**.

Communication is the passing of information from one person to another. Most people think of this as *spoken* or *verbal* communication but *body language* or *non-verbal communication* is also involved. We show our interest, attitude and how we feel by non-verbal communication and this is often more important than what is actually said!

Who are the clients?

The clients are the customers of the salon. They may belong to one of the following categories:

- Known clients who have used salon services before.
- New, unknown clients.

Any of these may have some kind of disability and may require special consideration. Clients can also be 'difficult' and it is important to notify your supervisor if you have any difficulties.

Verbal communication

The verbal communication with a client is very important. All members of staff should be pleasant, polite and helpful at all times. Remember that the client is entitled to the best possible service.

What is involved in good communication?

There is an old saying about treating others as you would like to be treated yourself. This involves putting yourself into the other's place and listening carefully to them. It also includes being reasonable and polite to them. Here are some points:

- If someone asks you to assist, respond positively and offer to help.
- If you need help ask for it politely, even if you feel pressurised.
- Try and be clear and accurate in what you say. People respond positively to this. Think about what you need to say before saying it. Clear and precise messages get you what you want.
- Make sure you show the appropriate non-verbal signals. You show your feelings in this way. Be interested, keen to find out, positive. As you listen to someone show you *are* listening.

Non-verbal communication

Non-verbal communication can be just as expressive as speaking. Postures, distances and the way in which we hold our bodies are all ways in which we express ourselves. Indeed, many psychologists believe that a person's non-verbal behaviour can have more bearing on communicating feelings and attitudes than do their words. Thus, the client must always be treated in a pleasant and polite manner not only verbally but also by the body language that is used. The main areas to consider are:

- Distance.
- Facial expression.
- Body posture.
- Eye contact.

Distance

Everyone requires their own 'space'. Touching and moving too near to the client can make them feel uncomfortable as usually only intimate relationships are allowed such close contact.

Facial expression

An expressionless face which lacks emotion will appear 'cold' and hard. However, too much emotion can make the person appear neurotic! When working in the salon, try to maintain a positive facial expression, e.g. smiling, so that the client feels that they are in a pleasant, happy environment.

Body posture

This is believed by psychologists to provide clues as to what people really think or feel. Certainly, lounging around the salon in a slovenly manner does not create a businesslike impression and will make the client question your professionalism and therefore your practical ability even if this is unfounded.

Eye contact

Eye contact with the client is extremely important as it is believed to be the basis of trust. Looking elsewhere when talking to the client will not only make him/her feel uncomfortable but will also make them doubt your sincerity.

How to manage a difficult client

This is not an easy situation to be in. Make sure you:

- Stay calm.
- Stay polite.

If these fail, refer the client to your supervisor.

When with clients, are you:

- Courteous?
- Clear and precise?
- Willing to offer help and assistance?
- Sure your non-verbal 'body language' is good?
- Able to clarify any uncertainty with the client?

If you can answer 'yes' to all of these you can be sure that you are treating your clients well!

When to seek help

A lot of communication with clients involves confidence, good training and practice. There will almost certainly be times when you need help. How will you know when this is? If this is *after* some problem with a client then it is *too late*. If in doubt ask your supervisor for help.

Many trainees are reluctant to do this and there is, of course, a balance between asking for help too often and not often enough. The best rule is to err on the side of caution. If in doubt of any kind *ask for help*!

As your experience grows this help will be needed less and less.

Confidential information

A key factor in any successful salon operation is communication which encourages trust both between client and salon staff and also between the staff. Just as a client trusts a salon to deliver a good, safe and cost-effective service they also expect information about themselves to be treated as confidential. Some of this information is deliberately gathered and entered onto record cards – either on paper or by computer. These records contain personal information yet can be accessed by other salon staff and by the clients themselves. It is therefore necessary to be careful what information is entered in these records. There have been cases of salon personnel putting insulting remarks about a client and then, at the next appointment, the client seeing it!

There is also the common situation of clients chatting to stylists and others about all sorts of things. They forget that other people may be listening, such as an apprentice tidying up or helping with the treatment. It is very important not to pass any information on. The key thing to remember here is:

See all, hear all, say nothing.

If situations arise where you feel uncomfortable about something you have overheard or you feel that others in the salon are breaking the rule of confidentiality, have a talk about this with your supervisor.

Working as part of the salon team

Liaison with the people you work with depends on forming and maintaining a good working relationship. When these exist the salon atmosphere is positive and both clients and staff benefit. There is nothing worse than a salon where problems are unresolved and there are obvious tensions and bad feeling between the staff. Some people are easier to work with than others but there are some basic things everyone can do to help develop and keep effective working relationships.

Who are the colleagues in a salon?

These may be:

- Other trainees.
- The stylists.
- Supervisor and/or manager.
- Other people who work in the salon such as a receptionist or beauty therapist.

What to do if things go wrong

There will always be problems between people working in the salon. These may be small or large, short term or long term, easy to sort out or difficult. The most important thing is that if there is a difficulty *discuss it*. Try to resolve it with the person concerned. Stay calm and polite.

If you feel you cannot discuss the problem with those concerned or have done so and the problem is still there, then take it to your supervisor. Most things can be sorted out if there is a will to do so and this is much easier if problems are resolved at an early stage.

Helping the salon team with the salon's technical services

The technical services offered by most salons will include:

- Perming (permanent waving).
- Colouring and bleaching.
- Setting.
- Cutting.
- Blowdrying.
- Dressing.

Giving skilled assistance in carrying these out is very important as they are key salon operations and generate most of the salon's earnings.

The basics of assisting the stylist are:

Before
- Getting the information needed.
- Gowning the client.
- Choosing the products, tools and equipment needed and arranging them in a suitable way.

During
- Passing the products and tools to the stylist and being 'on hand' to help when needed.

After

- When finished, ensuring that the products/tools/equipment are taken away, cleaned and stored.
- Informing the stylist.

Preventing RSI

Muscles do two kinds of work – dynamic and static. Dynamic work, when the muscles are moving, keeps the blood pumping through the muscle, carrying in oxygen and nutrients and carrying out waste products. Static work, when the muscles are holding a position, restricts the blood flow so the waste products accumulate and cause fatigue, which is felt as pain. This is why it is essential that muscles are kept as relaxed as possible and that you alternate holding tasks by using a variety of techniques. Experiment with different ways of doing each task.

Preparing for technical services

You need to know exactly what kind of operation you will be assisting the stylist to carry out. Make sure you are *very* clear about this. You cannot prepare things properly if you are not clear. If not sure – ASK. Get clarification from the stylist.

Before the operation

Gowning is carried out before starting any hairdressing procedure. It is a means of protecting the client's clothing from chemical spillage or cut hairs. Adequate care *must* be taken when gowning the client as any damage to the client's clothing will be the responsibility of the salon and the client has every right to expect a replacement of any clothing which has been damaged through negligence.

You will then need to look at **record cards** and the **appointment book**.

You will learn from experience which products, tools and equipment are needed and if particular stylists like doing things in a particular way. In addition, you will soon know how best to arrange things.

During the operation

Whatever the technical service, the stylist will operate much more effectively with efficient help. Make sure you are polite and courteous. If anything is not clear, ask for clarification.

Be careful in passing things. Scissors can be stabbed into someone! Chemical products can be spilled.

After the operation

When the service has been completed, tell the stylist that the client is ready for the next stage (if applicable), throw away disposables, clean tools and arrange in a tidy way. Clean any equipment. Wipe down the working surfaces and chair. Generally tidy up the dressing station and put things away.

Throughout the technical service

Keep in mind health and safety:

- Do not allow products to get onto skin or into eyes.
- Take care to avoid cuts when using sharp instruments like scissors.

- Be aware of the chances of *infection*.
- Look out for problems with *electrical equipment*.

Health and safety issues are covered in detail in Unit 6 (see page 40), both in terms of what to look out for and what to do.

> **Preventing RSI**
> When a dispenser has a very small hole for the solution to come out, you are forced to squeeze hard, straining the wrist and forearm, especially if your wrist is bent in any direction. Make sure that the hole is the right size for the proper flow but have it as large as possible so that you won't have to squeeze hard. Keep the bottles quite full for the same reason. Experiment with different hand grips as you apply solution and alternate them.

Care and maintenance of tools

Non-metallic tools

Brushes
Brushes should be kept as clean and sterile as possible. When not in use they should be kept in a sterilising cabinet.

Method of cleaning
1 Comb brush free from hair with a wide-toothed comb and remove any other loose particles from the bristles and base of the brush.
2 Fill a basin with lukewarm water and add a cleaning fluid (do not use too strong a cleaning fluid as this can damage the brush).
3 With the bristles pointing downwards, swish the brush about on top of the water. Do not immerse wooden brushes in the water as it will crack the protective coating of varnish and split the wood.
4 Rinse carefully in clean water to which some disinfectant has been added.
5 Towel dry the handle and base of the brush and pat the bristles on a towel to remove excess moisture.
6 Leave the brush to dry face downwards on a clean towel.
7 When dry, place in an ultraviolet disinfecting cabinet.

Combs
Combs should be thoroughly cleaned regularly to prevent loose flakes of skin and other debris lodging between the teeth of the comb at the base. When not in use and after use each client, combs should be kept completely submerged in an antiseptic solution of the correct strength or in the sterilising cabinet.

Method of cleaning
1 Brush combs with either a nail brush or a special comb brush to remove loose debris.
2 Fill a basin with lukewarm water and cleaning fluid, as for cleaning brushes.
3 Immerse combs for several minutes to loosen any grease or oil particles.
4 Scrub combs on each side individually with a nail brush.

5 Rinse in lukewarm water to which some disinfectant has been added.
6 Dry thoroughly and place in sterilising cabinet or in antiseptic solution.

POINTS TO REMEMBER

It is not always necessary to use disinfectant in the rinsing water if the brushes and combs are being placed immediately into the ultraviolet disinfecting cabinet.

Metallic tools

Scissors

These should be carefully looked after and always kept sharp. Remember the following points to ensure that they are always in good working order.

1 Always dry after use on wet hair.
2 Keep away from strong chemicals, e.g. permanent wave solution, bleach, etc.
3 They should not be dropped as this can alter the balance and could loosen the pivot or screw.
4 Each pair of scissors should be used by only one person. If the same pair of scissors is used by everybody it blunts the blades very quickly.
5 Never use them for anything except to cut hair.
6 They should only be sharpened by experts.
7 Sterilise by wiping carefully with spirit then placing them in the sterilising cabinet for the recommended time.
8 The pivots should be treated with lubricating oil from time to time to prevent stiffness.
9 Store away from dust as this is a source of possible infection.

Razors

For both safety and open razors:

- Always dry after use, otherwise the metal will rust.
- Keep away from permanent wave solution, bleach or any other strong chemicals.
- Sterilise by placing them in a sterilising cabinet for the recommended time after wiping with spirit.

Open razors must be kept sharp by **stropping** on a leather strop, or by **honing** on a special stone known as a hone.

Safety razors must have the blades changed regularly to ensure that the razor is always sharp.

Clippers

Both types of clippers are cleaned in the same manner but when using electric clippers check also for frayed wires, faulty plugs, etc., before using.

Method of cleaning
1 Remove all loose hairs with a tissue or piece of flannel.
2 Remove any grease with surgical spirit.
3 Lubricate joints with a lubricating oil.
4 Place in a sterilising cabinet for the recommended time.

Styling irons and hot brushes

Remove any grease or stains with surgical spirit. Electrical styling irons and hot brushes should be checked for frayed wires and faulty plugs.

Pressing combs

Rub the teeth of the comb with an emery board to remove any grease and stains then wipe over with surgical spirit. Check electrical pressing combs for frayed wires and faulty plugs.

Table 1.2 Summary of tools

Tools	Type	Use
Brushes	General purpose	For dressing and everyday brushing of hair
	Styling	When blowdrying the hair
	Neck	To remove cut hair from face and neck
Combs	Tail comb	Sectioning, lifting, weaving, never disentangling
	Dressing comb	Disentangling and dressing the hair
	Cutting comb	More pliable than other combs, use when cutting
	Setting comb	When setting and finger waving
	Afro comb	To style and dress curly hair, e.g. African Caribbean
Scissors	Plain straight edged	For all cutting techniques
	Very fine serrated edge	For all cutting except slither-cutting techniques
	Wide-spaced serrated edge (aesculap)	To thin hair; use on dry hair only
Razors	Open	Use mainly in men's hairdressing to cut wet hair and in shaving
	Safety razor	Same use as the open razor but has changeable guarded blade
Clippers	Hand (manual) and electric	In men's and ladies' hairdressing to cut hair close to scalp
Hot brush		To temporarily curl dry hair
Styling irons	Electrically heated	To temporarily curl, straighten or crimp dry hair
Pressing combs	Electrically heated and non-electrical	To straighten African Caribbean hair

Development within the job role

There are many things which influence 'job satisfaction'. Most of these have been mentioned in this Unit. They include relationships with and attitude towards clients and the salon team.

Another important factor is feeling that you make a valued contribution through your role in the salon. There is little satisfaction in working well below your capabilities, nor is there if far too much is being demanded of you. Both of these situations are frustrating, and feelings of being undervalued or being held in too little regard are very damaging to the operation of a team. Most people like to feel they are in an interesting, challenging (but not overwhelming) role and that a reasonable amount of trouble is taken by managers and supervisors to keep in touch with staff feelings and needs. Good management includes reviewing salon staff's current level of expertise and competence and then setting up processes to develop the salon team's skills further. One way of doing this is to have a **staff appraisal** system. Some people find the ideal of an appraisal threatening. When properly carried out a review of a person's role and development needs is a very **positive** experience. The steps in carrying out an appraisal are listed below.

Defining the job role

Is there a detailed job description including duties, responsibilities and accountability? If 'yes', is it up to day? Is it accurate? If 'no', why not?

Appraisal of job role

This should be:

- Positive.
- Identify strengths as well as weaknesses.
- Set realistic, and attainable targets within a specified time period.
- Provide support, including development opportunities to help the target to be achieved.
- A regular, supportive occurrence in the salon's operation.

Appraisal can be informal or more formal with a written record of the targets agreed and the time scale for achievement and review. The system is much better if a written record is kept.

One possible way of operating an appraisal system is:

1 The person to be appraised looks at the job description and thinks about their role in the salon. Are there areas for development? What are the strengths and weaknesses.
2 Meet with the persons who will carry out the appraisal. Discuss the appraisal, agree what should be reviewed and talked about. This is called **setting the agenda**.
3 Carry out the appraisal of those items agreed in step 2.
4 Complete a written record of agreed targets, how these are to be achieved and by when. This is called the **development action plan**. The opportunities that exist for development will vary from salon to salon but may include:

- Watching salon operations and services being carried out.
- Asking for help/guidance for other team members.
- Taking part in training activities of various kinds.

Things to do

1 Working in pairs or small groups discuss and write down:

- Reasons why client care and consideration are important.
- Some examples of good and bad practice. Explain why they were good or bad.
- What the difference is between verbal and non-verbal communication.
- Examples of non-verbal signals, both 'good' and 'bad' which a client can receive.

2 Discuss how you should fill in your personal diary/log book to cover this unit.

3 Make a list of all the tools and equipment that are used in your placement and/or training salon.

4 Collect illustrations or photographs of a selection of each type of tool and equipment including any extra or new equipment which may be available.

5 Cut out and mount the illustrations. Print a brief summary under the illustration giving the use of each.

6 Present your work neatly in the form of a portfolio.

7 Carry out review of yourself in your job role. Make a list of **strengths** and **weaknesses**, then show this to someone whose opinion you would trust. Do they agree with your assessment?

8 Are there areas of the salon's activities that you would like to take part in? List these and discuss with your supervisor.

Level 1 Unit 4

What is meant by verbal and non-verbal communication? ☐

Why is customer care important? ☐

Explain the responsibilities of the people working in the salon. ☐

List the 'line of command' in the salon. ☐

List the methods of verbal and non-verbal communication. ☐

Why is it important to have good working relationships with colleagues in the salon? ☐

Why is it important to follow instructions? ☐

What can happen if the rules of confidentiality are broken? ☐

List the opportunities by which staff in the salon can develop themselves in their jobs. ☐

INTRODUCTION TO SALON RESOURCES

Salon stock is essential to the function of a salon. Without an adequate level and range of the following it is difficult to run a hairdressing business safely, efficiently and successfully.

- Products.
- Towels.
- Personal protective equipment – such as gowns and gloves.
- Sundries – brushes and combs for sale, for example.

Hairdressing products are expensive and therefore there should be a constant 'turnover' of stock to ensure that money is not wasted by old stock remaining on the shelves. All stock should be handled carefully in accordance with manufacturers' recommendations and with due regard for the health and safety of both staff and clients.

A number of products have risks associated with their storage. A good example is not storing aerosol sprays in direct sunlight. Some health and safety practices are set up by salon policy; others are based on Health and Safety legislation, such as Control of Substances Hazardous to Health. For further details on this see Unit 6; for a more detailed account see Level 2 Unit 10 and Level 3 Unit 6.

How much stock is 'enough'?

How much stock a salon holds is determined by a number of factors, the most important of which is based on the speed at which things are used up and need replacing. Keeping a balance between having too much stock and not enough is the basis of **stock control**. If there is too much stock this represents too much money used to buy the stock. There is also the chance of not using products with a limited shelf-life before they need to be discarded. Too little stock means hairdressing operations become difficult and in extreme cases need to stop! You can imagine the reaction of a client to that! There is also the need for attractive displays of products for sale. Nothing looks worse than a display with gaps – and there are profits to be made from the sales. Because of the problem of not having enough stock most salons will, if anything, keep a small surplus rather than risk running out of key products needed for the salon's services. You supervisor will tell you what stock levels to keep.

Receipt and storage of stock

When new stock arrives at the salon it is necessary to carry out the following procedure:

- Unpack the stock carefully and check for breakages, sell-by date and discrepancies between the delivery note and the contents of the package.
- If possible, check the delivery note against the original order.
- Enter details of the new stock **accurately** in the stock book (or other salon recording system).
- Store stock carefully in the appropriate place taking into consideration manufacturers' recommendations, health and hygiene and salon procedures. When lifting or carrying heavy items, care must be taken to lift in the correct manner to avoid injury to yourself.

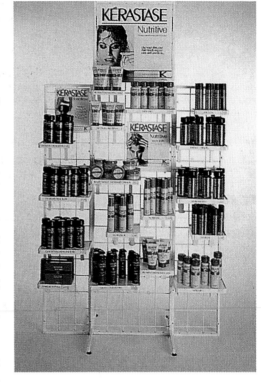

An important point to note is that stock must be used in rotation. Therefore, the new stock should be stored in such a manner that the existing older stock is used first, otherwise some products could be unfit for use because they have deteriorated and outlived their 'shelf-life'.

Lifting and carrying heavy objects

There are two main principles when lifting and carrying heavy objects. Firstly, try to use the thigh, hip and shoulder muscles as these are the most powerful muscles of the body and secondly, keep the weight as close to the body as possible.

When lifting, posture plays a particularly important part. Stand with the feet placed evenly apart to give a firm stance, keep the back straight and the head erect then bend at the knees and lift the object. Do not stoop over when lifting as this can injure the back and/or pull the weaker muscles.

Pricing stock for retail sale

Care must be taken when pricing items for sale to the public. The retail items should be clearly marked with the correct price using either tags or, more usually, a self-adhesive label. When placing the label on the merchandise remember that it should be clearly visible but should not cover any important information, e.g. what the product is or what it contains.

Always check with the supervisor/manager that the product is being correctly priced. Do not automatically assume that a new batch of stock will be the same price as before, as often it will have increased in price to the salon owner and this increase will have to be passed on to the client to maintain the profit. Alternatively, there may have been a 'special offer' and the goods could have been obtained more cheaply, in which case, the salon owner may wish to pass on these savings to the client as a promotion. Thus, before filling out any pricing labels seek the advice of the supervisor/manager to avoid costly mistakes.

There are two types of retail goods:

- Those with a sell-by date and limited shelf-life.
- Those without a limited shelf-life.

Products with a limited shelf-life such as shampoos, conditioners, gels and waxes should be sold in rotation to ensure that they do not go over their sell-by date and become ineffective. Products without a limited shelf-life such as combs, brushes and hair ornaments should also be sold in rotation, if possible, to ensure that they do not go out of fashion!

Counting and recording stock levels

Salons usually have their own individual methods of recording stock levels and these are often split into different categories including those for salon use and those for retail. It is important that all records are clear, legible and accurate and that all stock taking is checked for accuracy by the supervisor/manager.

For security reasons, stock that has been used is generally checked against both the appointment book and the till receipt, thus giving a double check as to when and where the stock has been used. However, if the stock level has been incorrectly entered in the first place it can cause many problems and misunderstandings at a later stage.

Use of resources in the salon

A salon needs certain things in order to operate. These are called 'resources' and they include:

- Stock – such as the products used on the client's hair.
- Fixtures and fittings – work stations, mirrors, heating, etc.
- Electricity – to power hair driers for example.
- Water – for shampooing, mixing products.
- Telephone and fax.
- Tools and equipment.

All of these are 'costs' to the salon. A further cost is the **time** of people who work in the salon.

All of these costs must be less than the money the salon earns in order to make a profit. This can be summarised in a single way as:

Profit = Salon income – Cost of resources (outgoings)

The bigger the difference between income and the cost of resources, the bigger the profit. It is therefore worth while to reduce costs as far as possible to make the income as large as possible. Key areas to reduce include spillages, breakages and waste.

Spillages, breakages and waste

Spillages occur even in the best-run salons! Remembering to put the caps back on containers minimises the risk of this but what if a spill does occur? The best advice is to wash it off and clean it up using lots of water. Avoid skin contact. If the spill is onto someone, wash clothes and skin under the tap. Report the spill to your supervisor.

Breakages do not happen often in the salon. Very few hairdressing products are supplied in breakable containers – most are in plastic which does not break easily. Some pieces of hairdressing equipment are more vulnerable – blowdriers for example can break if dropped. All salon lotions should be stored in well-labelled containers and not put on to high shelves where there is always a risk of dropping when taking them down. Particular care needs to be taken with stored hydrogen peroxide and pressurised aerosol sprays. Both can explode if heated so they should never be stored near heaters or in direct sunlight.

If a container has lost its label or the contents cannot be identified then dispose of it. Careful disposal of empty pressurised cans is important. These should not be punctured or burned (incinerated) as the pressure left inside could cause an explosion. Warnings about this are printed on the container.

Waste is expensive! The usual cause of waste in the salon is using too much of something, such as using too much shampoo on a client's scalp, or too much hot water which has cost money to heat up. In addition bad planning and technique can waste people's time and effort both of which cost money, cause frustration and reduce morale. Remember – always report spillages, breakages and waste to your supervisor.

Security procedures

A good salon is an open, friendly and welcoming place, but unfortunately this means that a salon is *vulnerable* to theft of stock and items belonging to staff and clients. Outside working hours a salon is also potentially under threat from break-ins, theft and vandalism.

It is therefore important that a salon has a *code of practice* on security. These are practices and procedures to protect people and property during and outside working hours.

Inside working hours

It is very important that these rules are followed. Most theft is **opportunistic**. Someone sees a chance and grabs it. To prevent this:

- Be aware at all times.
- Make sure no valuables are left about.
- Take the client's coat from them and hang it in a secure place. Ask them to describe it before you give it back.
- Take care with stock control. The stock used will be double checked against the client's receipt and the appointment book so any discrepancies will show up!
- Encourage clients to keep handbags, etc., with them at all times.
- Ensure your locker (if you have one) is securely **locked**. You should not have any valuables with you anyway.
- Report any problems with security to your supervisor.

Outside working hours

This will depend on a number of factors. There should be a *security assessment* which needs to take into account:

- Location of salon – some places are far more vulnerable than others.
- The area the salon is in.

Some routines will apply to most salons. These will include:

- Emptying the till at night and leaving the drawer open.
- Making sure no valuables are left in the salon, even if in lockers.
- Ensuring that all doors, windows and stock cupboards are locked.

In addition, items can be security marked, and the salon may belong to a local 'Crimewatch' or 'Business Watch' scheme.

Most insurance companies will give a discount if an alarm is fitted on the premises (in some areas this is essential to get insurance cover). If allowed and appropriate, in some localities salons are fitted with pull-down metal shutters to act as additional protection.

Things to do

1 Organise a file to record your salon's policy and procedures for stock control.

2 Carry out the following tasks:

- Collect packaging and manufacturers' instructions from goods for salon use and products for retail.
- Make a poster for your staff-room showing how the various products should be stored and why.

3 Carry out a *crime prevention* assessment on a salon. Consider:

- Where the 'weak spots' are. If you wanted to break in, how would you do it?
- What the salon's security arrangements are:
  – when open (working hours)
  – when closed (outside working hours)

Ask for some crime prevention information from the local police, and use this to help you carry out your assessment.

What do you know?

Level 1 Unit 5

Explain why it is important to use old stock before the new stock. ☐

To whom do you report any deficiencies and discrepancies in stock? ☐

What is the correct way to lift and carry heavy objects safely? ☐

List the stock used and sold in the salon and how it should be handled and priced. ☐

Why is it important that you check with your supervisor to make sure that stock is correctly priced? ☐

Which type of stock needs to be handled in a special way? ☐

What documents are used to show what stock has been used and what new stock needs to be ordered? ☐

Describe the characteristics of the stock you have listed above. ☐

What should you do about spillages, breakages and waste in the salon? ☐

INTRODUCTION TO SALON HEALTH AND SAFETY

The standard of the salon depends on the standards of its staff members. Taking care of your personal health and appearance will not only enable you to function more efficiently, it will also make you feel more alive and energetic!

Personal health

Eating a sensible diet which includes plenty of fresh vegetables and a balance of vitamins, minerals, fats and carbohydrates will prevent tiredness and give a glow to the skin.

Posture

Hairdressing may not seem like it, but it is a physically tiring profession and most hairdressers have to stand on their feet for a considerable length of time. Tired, irritable staff cannot give their best service to the client so it is very important that they stand and walk in such a way as to avoid too much physical strain on the body which will reduce the ability to work efficiently, and in some instances, could cause long-term problems, e.g. back strain.

Posture is the correct placing of the body in relation to the feet. If it is correct, staff will be able to work more efficiently and feel less tired. The major points for a good posture are:

- **Stand upright** – stooping causes backache, tiredness and makes it difficult to breathe correctly.
- **Balance** – the weight of the body should be evenly distributed on both feet. This reduces strain on the back and leg muscles.
- **Correct foot-wear** – shoes should be comfortable, attractive and heels should be a sensible height. Avoid open-toed shoes as hair fragments can enter under the skin and cause infection.

Preventing RSI
Keep your feet as comfortable and as cool as possible. Open shoes should be avoided because hair falls as it is being cut and may cause itching or infection. Many stylists develop calluses and corns so take precautions with your shoes – ensure that they are lightweight, have padded insoles, are a perfect fit, and have a sensible heel height for balance and comfort. Make sure you won't slip in them – there will often be water on the floor. Be sure to tend to blisters promptly and use corn plasters as needed. A pumice stone will remove hard skin and lotion will keep the skin soft.

Personal appearance

Personal cleanliness is important in any walk of life, but particularly in the salon where assistants very often work physically hard, in warm surroundings (which increases sweating), and are also in close proximity to the client.

Body odour and bad breath can be offensive to both the client and other members of staff, and steps should be taken to ensure personal freshness at all times. Listed below are a few basic guidelines which can be adapted to suit individual needs.

- Assistants should bathe regularly and always use a deodorant when necessary – at least once a day.
- Regular brushing of teeth and correct diet are essential to prevent bad breath. It is also advisable to have a dental check-up every six months.
- Avoid eating foods with an unpleasant odour, e.g. onions or garlic. They may taste delicious when eaten, but are very unpleasant second-hand!
- Assistants should always look neat and well groomed. Hair should be kept clean and well cut and if possible it should be coloured and/or permed – this encourages the client to do likewise. It is very difficult to persuade a client to be adventurous or to have perms and tints if none of the staff have had these treatments themselves. Stylists with long hair should keep it off the face but in a fashionable style.
- Nails and hands should be well cared for. Where possible, use a hand cream at night before going to bed; this will help to counteract the drying effect of degreasive shampoos and styling aids, etc., and reduces the chances of developing dermatitis. Nails must be kept clean and at a reasonable length to prevent scratching the client's scalp. If any stylists use nail polish it should be unchipped.
- Overalls or salon uniform must be spotlessly clean and fresh. Make use of tinting aprons to prevent staining when colouring or perming. Any clothes worn beneath the overall should not be allowed to show and woollen cardigans or jumpers should be avoided as these provide good conditions for skin bacteria to thrive. The best type of overall is one made of cotton or a cotton/polyester mixture. They are durable, easy to launder and do not increase perspiration. Nylon overalls do increase perspiration and can therefore be uncomfortable during busy periods.
- Avoid wearing excessive amounts of jewellery, particularly jangling bracelets – they are disconcerting to the client and hinder efficiency. A watch or a ring can be worn, but they may be damaged by the chemicals used in the salon so it is not usually worth the risk.

Salon hygiene

Hygiene is important in many industries but particularly in hairdressing when staff are dealing directly with the general public. Indeed, there is legislation on health and hygiene in the workplace, which means the salon is required by **law** to make sure that it is a safe place for both clients and staff. It is a good idea to look at leaflets published about this and these can be obtained through the local Environmental Health Department.

Each salon will have its own preferences and procedures for making sure that it is kept clean and tidy and that the tools and equipment are sterilised after use. (See Level 1 Unit 4 for details on tools and equipment.)

Everyone who works in a salon has a responsibility both to themselves and others to work in a healthy and safe manner. Much of good health and safety practice needs to be routine so that people in the salon are protected from the most likely hazards.

Routine health and safety practice and procedure

In order to work safely and help protect health the staff of the salon need to:

- Be able to recognise potential or actual hazards.
- Prevent a hazard developing and/or rectify the problem.
- Know the system for reporting hazards.

This has resulted in many salons developing a set of health and safety procedures for staff to follow, based on *government legislation* such as:

- Health and Safety at Work Act 1974.
- Control of Substances Hazardous to Health 1990.
- Workplace (Health, Safety and Welfare) Regulations 1992.
- Manual Handling Regulations 1992.
- Personal Protective Equipment at Work Regulations 1992.
- Provision and use of Work Equipment Regulations 1992.

First aid arrangements and reporting of accidents

The Health and Safety at Work Act lists recommendations for **first aid kits** and also requires that:

- a written record be kept of all accidents in an **accident record book**, which lists the sex, age and occupation of the victim and the nature of the accident and date of first absence from work (if this applies).

Control of substances hazardous to health
(COSHH – often shortened to 'cosh')

These regulations took effect from January 1990 and have been reinforced by the Health and Safety 'Framework' Regulations of January 1993. The important idea embedded in these regulations is that of *risk assessment*. This involves answering the following questions:

- What do we do in the salon? (Identify the *tasks*.)
- What are the hazards?
- How likely is a problem to arise? (Risk assessment.)
- What appropriate precautions need to be taken? (Action.)

In order to work this out, information is needed on the content of hairdressing products and what potential hazards these could be. This information has to be supplied by the manufacturer of the hairdressing product, using chemicals taken from a list of substances whose risk assessment has already been worked out.

Local by-laws

These vary in different parts of the country but often they:

- Involve registration of the salon with the local Environmental Health Department so that periodic checks by Environmental Health Officers can be made.
- Overlap with other regulations in requiring adequate ventilation in toilet and washing facilities, general cleanliness, etc.

What are the potential hazards in the salon?

Health and safety is about **recognising** the potential hazards in the salon to know which ones can be **rectified** easily and when and how to **report** their occurrence. Any account of safe practice has to be very much an outline dealing with major points only and what follows deals with some of the common problems and how to avoid them. These can be divided into four main areas:

- Physical injuries.
- Electricity.
- Chemical.
- Biological.

Physical injuries

These include:

1 **Wounds caused by scissors and razors** – by their design, scissors and razors are sharp. Scissors can cause nicks or puncture wounds if pushed in points first. Scissors should *always* be carried with points inwards and razors should *never* be carried open. Both scissors and razors should be cleaned by wiping them in a direction away from the body. Make sure scissors and razors are out of the reach of children in the salon.

2 **Tripping and falling** – there are two common causes for this:
   - Loose or broken floor coverings; these should be in good condition.
   - Trailing electric flexes; you risk not only tripping over them but the tug of the flex can cause electrical faults. There is also the danger that the pull on the flex can cause the electrical appliance supplied by it to topple over and hurt someone.

3 **Knocks** – these can be caused by a variety of reasons, often as a result of another accident, e.g. someone collapsing after an electric shock. They can also be due to:

- Equipment collapsing onto a client, e.g. infra-red octopus or steamers, when someone bumps into them or trips over the flex.
- Equipment being cleaned; there is a risk of pushing it over while cleaning it. Many salon driers have strong springs in their stands and if the drier is removed for cleaning and the spring released, the stand flies upwards with considerable force. This may strike someone cleaning the stand.

Electricity

People can be at risk for two different reasons:

- **Overheating and possibly fire** (in cables and apparatus) – the fitting of the correct fuse plugs and fuse boxes is important, as is regular and expert checking of plugs, cables and electrical equipment. It is important not to overload a circuit.
- **Electric shock** – which involves electricity flowing through a person's body.

Many of the accidents that occur when using electricity are simply due to thoughtlessness, carelessness or downright bad practice.

Do

- Make sure plugs are wired correctly and have the correct-sized fuse for the appliance.
- Have electrical equipment checked on a regular basis, repaired, or have changes made in the electrical supply by a competent electrician.
- Ensure that staff are trained to know what to do if a person receives an electric shock.

Don't

- Handle electrical appliances with wet hands or allow water to splash on to appliances.
- Overload sockets or other circuits by running too many appliances from them.
- Fit a larger fuse into a fuse box or plug if it keeps 'blowing'.
- Run flexes under floor coverings or place in a position where there is a chance of someone tripping over them.
- Pull a plug by tugging on its flex.

Chemical

Hairdressing operations very often involve the use of chemicals on the hair and some of these are sprayed onto the hair using **pressurised containers**, e.g. hair lacquers. The chemical hazards in the salon come from three main sources:

- Chemicals getting onto the skin or into the eyes.
- Storage and disposal.
- Dermatitis.

Chemicals getting onto the skin or into the eyes

The main prevention here is to be aware of the risk involved in carrying out any hairdressing operation (even shampooing) that involves chemicals and to handle chemicals with care. Chemicals can be swallowed, especially by children, so care should be taken to put these out of reach.

Storage and disposal

Accidental spills can be avoided by replacing caps and stoppers on containers immediately after use. If a spill does occur:

- Wipe up immediately.
- Avoid skin contact.
- Report the event promptly to your supervisor.

It is very important that products are stored and used in accordance with manufacturers' recommendations and that warnings are noted and followed.

Do not use *caustic soda* (sodium hydroxide) to clear blocked drains – get a plumber to do it. Caustic soda can cause severed skin burns.

Dermatitis (eczema)

Basically, this involves the body 'over-reacting' to a substance to which it has been exposed. Many of the chemicals used in hairdressing may cause dermatitis. Both the hairdresser and the client are at risk, with the hairdresser at greatest risk due to repeated and long-term exposure to hairdressing chemicals. The hairdresser can be protected by using rubber gloves for any hairdressing operation that involves chemicals, including shampooing.

Biological

These consist of infections and infestations both caused by living organisms.

They are either **infectious** or **contagious**; that is, they can be passed between people or transmitted in the salon. See Level 3 Unit 6 for detailed information.

Routine hygiene practices and procedures

The salon should always be kept clean and tidy. Well-trained staff should automatically tidy any dirty areas. A salon which has hair all over the floor and dirty towels strewn about the place is very off-putting to the client and looks inefficient. A strict code of hygiene should exist, even during busy periods – bacteria thrive in the salon's warm, moist atmosphere, and risk to the client must be minimized.

Training apprentices/trainees from the beginning to be neat and tidy, to clean up immediately and to keep equipment as sterile as possible, produces an awareness of salon hygiene. These good habits will then endure through to when they are managers or salon owners themselves and this professional attitude can only be of benefit to the hairdressing industry in general.

One point to be noted: a hairdresser works with hair and is therefore used to handling it and seeing it about. Clients feel differently – other people's hair in the wrong place can make them feel a little sick! Remember, try to see things from the client's point of view.

Good habits

- **Shop floor**. The floor should be swept and mopped each day and never left untidy. Cut hair should be swept up immediately. Check that all floor covering is sound. Any loose tiles, lino, carpet, etc., can be dangerous to staff and clients.

- **Reception area**. This should be kept clean and tidy with a cloakroom or rack for the client's coats, away from the main salon. If there is a retail sales area, the items for sale should be attractively displayed with the prices clearly marked and the display dusted regularly.
- **Work tops**. These should be kept free of litter, e.g. empty setting lotion bottles, and tidied up after each client. They should be wiped over regularly and kept free from dust.
- **Chairs**. These should be kept clean and free from hair. A vinyl covering makes cleaning easier. They should be wiped down every day, including the backs and the legs as these tend to get splashed with lotions. Any splitting or tearing of the material must be reported immediately.
- **Mirrors**. They should be cleaned every day and lacquer stains removed immediately with a lacquer solvent, such as methylated spirit or alcohol, e.g. surgical spirit. Back mirrors also need cleaning regularly to remove any lacquer stains or finger prints.
- **Towels and gowns**. Dirty towels should be placed in a linen basket after use and should not litter the salon. Clean towels only should be used on the client and any towels with holes in them are to be discarded or recycled as cleaning cloths, etc.
- **Brushes, combs and rollers**. Every client should have a clean brush and comb used on their hair. Combs should be kept in antiseptic and brushes in a sterilising cabinet. In addition, rollers and brushes should be washed and disinfected regularly to remove any stains from temporary rinses, flakes of dried skin, setting agents, etc. Any hair that has been caught in the rollers or brushes should be removed before washing.
- **Trolleys**. Trays and trolleys should be cleaned at the end of each working day and the feet of the trolleys should be checked to make sure that loose hair has not been caught in them.
- **Magazines**. Keep all magazines tidy and discard any that become 'tatty' looking.
- **Wash bowls**. Wash bowls and fittings should be kept clean and wiped over after each shampoo. Front wash bowls must be disinfected regularly to prevent unpleasant odours. Hair traps can be used to help prevent blockage – the hair should, however, be removed from these traps after each shampoo.
- **Equipment**. Steamers and infra-red lamps should be cleaned after use. Always ensure that the water bottle on the steamer has enough water in it before use (distilled water should be used) and the steamer should be cleaned out regularly. Infra-red bulbs should be checked before use and any faulty bulbs reported.
- **Vapour and ultraviolet cabinets**. Make sure that the vapour steriliser cabinet is checked each day and refilled with sterilising solution. Keep cabinets clean inside and out.

Dealing with accidents and emergencies

What to do in the event of an accident or emergency

- Stay **calm**.
- **Report** the event immediately to your supervisor or the nominated 'first aider'.
- **Assist** if you are competent to do so.

Fire and evacuation procedures

There are two main causes of **fire** in salons: smoking and electrical faults. Fires due to **smoking** can be caused by:

- Lighted cigarettes falling on to the floor, into seating, etc.
- Ashtrays with still-smouldering cigarettes being thrown into rubbish bins.

There is also a risk of fire if people smoke near a client whose hair is being sprayed with lacquer. Never allow a client to smoke when using any kind of aerosol spray on their hair.

Salon policy on fire and evacuation procedures

A well-run salon will have as a matter of policy:

- Prominent signs indicating fire exits.
- Notices stating evacuation procedure and assembly point. Active encouragement of staff to report potential hazards, both a possible cause of fire or anything which would prevent speedy evacuation of the salon. Examples could be blocked staircases, entrance halls, salon equipment in front of fire doors.
- Familiarisation of new staff with fire and evacuation procedures and the location of emergency and fire-fighting equipment in the salon as part of new staff induction.
- Regular review of the policy to take into account new developments.

In addition, it is good practice to have a 'fire drill', a simulation of a real emergency, so that all staff know clearly what to do and any weaknesses in procedures are shown up.

How to react in case of a fire in the salon

- Stay calm.
- Ensure everybody gets out of the salon and goes to the assembly point.
- Depending on the nature and extent of the fire, decide whether to tackle it or not (if in doubt **do not**). Remember that aerosol spray cans and hydrogen peroxide containers will explode if sufficiently heated.
- Try to turn off the main electrical supply. If this is not possible (or you are uncertain) do not use water to try to put out the fire. Water is a **good conductor** of electricity and electricity flowing through it could deliver an **electric shock**. The salon should have at least one suitable fire extinguisher. Use it to put the fire out if it can be used without putting anyone at risk.

Things to do   A salon fire, health and safety quiz

1   How do staff and clients get out of the salon?

2   What would you do if you noticed a fire exit, corridor or a doorway blocked by something that would hinder a rapid evacuation of the premises?

3   Where are the fire extinguishers in the salon?

4   What type are they? List which ones would or would not be suitable for use on an electrical fire.

5   In small groups describe an accident you know about or have come close to in the salon. What caused it? What action was taken?

6 Design a safety poster for display in the salon.

7 Outline a salon's health and safety policy (establishment rules).

8 Briefly list legislation (national and local) covering health and safety, and describe what to do if:
- you can see a potential hazard
- an accident happens
- there is any spillage, breakage or waste

Level 1 Unit 6

Which local by-laws affect your salon? ☐

What does 'legislation' mean? ☐

Why is it important to brush teeth and bathe regularly? ☐

Why is personal hygiene important? ☐

Explain what would happen if you stand incorrectly (wrong posture) with regard to:

- *health*
- *appearance* ☐

How does your employer expect you to dress when working in the salon? ☐

Level 2

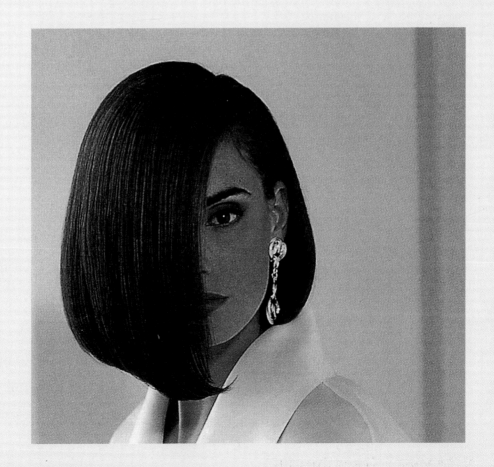

CLIENT CARE

Client care procedures start as soon as the client enters the salon, that is at **reception**.

Take the client's coat and any other belongings that will not be required whilst they are in the salon. Put these in a safe place. Be prepared to return items to the client if required either during their time in the salon or as they leave. (See Level 2 Unit 7 for details on Reception.)

Assessing the client

Assessment involves gathering information and that needs two-way **communication** with a client. To do this properly, the hairdresser needs to:

- **Look** carefully at the hair and scalp to see if any chemicals have previously been used.
- **Listen** carefully to the client's wishes and to their replies to any questions asked.
- **Feel** the hair to judge the condition, porosity and texture.
- **Assess** if these are any potential problems and whether the client's wishes match up to what is actually possible.
- **Question** the client to gather more information.

To carry the assessment further a number of factors need to be considered. These include:

- Hair growth patterns.
- Face shape.
- Age, lifestyle and hobbies.
- Conditions of the hair and scalp (such as diseases) which may influence the service that can be carried out.
- Various tests on the hair and skin.

The information gathered can then be used to judge whether the client can receive the service they are asking for and advice can be given about whether the treatment or service is appropriate for them.

These are now considered in more detail.

Communication skills

Good communication skills are required to ask a client **tactfully** for the information needed to make decisions about the appropriate service or treatment. Two important areas for good communication skills are:

- Active listening.
- Questioning.

Active listening

This is an extremely useful set of skills. Some people are naturally 'good listeners', others need to learn how to do it well. Listening skills include:

- Listening to someone without thinking about yourself or planning how you are going to reply. If you are thinking about other things you cannot listen to what the client is saying.
- Using eye contact, nods and smiles to show you are paying attention.
- Checking that you have understood. Use phrases like 'So what you are saying is...'. This gives the person the chance to clarify things to you.

Listening attentively will help the client describe their requirements with as much precision as possible and ensure that you fully understand the client's requirements.

Questioning

Questioning is used to get further information from the client. Questioning should not be carried out so as to put the client on the defensive. Good questioning, like good listening, makes the client feel valued and therefore adds to client satisfaction. Some important points about the *types* of question that can be used are:

- Negative.
- Positive.
- Closed.
- Open.

Negative

These questions should be avoided if possible as they usually elicit a negative response from the client. For example:

Trainee: 'You didn't want a conditioner on your hair did you?'
Client: 'No.'

By saying 'You *didn't...*' the trainee is inviting the client to say no.

Positive

These questions are asked in such a way as to elicit a positive response from the client. They are phrased so that it is very difficult for the client to say no. For example:

Trainee: 'I notice that you hair is very dry. Would you like me to use a conditioner to make it silky again?'
Client: 'Yes.'

In this case the client would have been unlikely not to wish to have silky hair again.

Closed

A closed question is one which usually elicits a one-word response from the client. For example:

Trainee: 'Is your hair dry?'
Client: 'Yes.'

Open

An open question is one which will elicit a much longer response and will usually encourage the client to give a lot more information or an opinion. These types of questions are useful for finding out a lot of information about the client and their hair before making any decision as to which product to recommend. For example:

Trainee: 'What other treatments have you had on your hair over the past few months?'

Client: 'Now let me think a moment...it was permed before my holidays and tinted when I got back...'

The client will then disclose more information to help the stylist to diagnose the hair condition and suggest a suitable treatment.

Client care: personal information about clients

It is good salon practice to keep information about clients stored either on a card or on computer. However, it is very important that this information is:

- Accurate.
- Up-to-date.
- Only that information needed for the salon – no personal comments about the client should be necessary.

The general rule should be:

If the client saw this record would they be completely happy with the recorded information?

Another source of information is what the client tells you or may be passed to you by other salon staff. Anything the client tells you should be treated in the strictest confidence. Only that information directly related to salon services should be passed on to other salon staff. A client overhearing or being told gossip about other clients will wonder if their confidence will be betrayed.

Keeping records on computer: the Data Protection Act

Many salons use information technology to help run the business. This includes keeping personal information, names, addressses, etc., on the salon's clients. The Data Protection Act 1984 is now fully in operation and it regulates the use of all computerised personal information relating to living individuals and places obligations on those who record and use such information (technically called 'data').

Broadly speaking, the Data Protection Act grants individuals three basic rights, which may be described as the right access to personal information held on computers; the right to compensation, through the courts if necessary, for inaccuracy, loss, destruction or unauthorised use of data; and the right to correction or erasure of inaccurate data.

Seven principles must be complied with

The Act is administered by a Data Protection Registrar in accordance with the following principles, which are embodied within the Act and are the standards by which the salon can be judged.

Personal data shall:

- Be collected and processed fairly and lawfully.
- Only be held for specified, lawful, registered purposes.
- Only be used for registered purposes or disclosed to registered recipients.
- Be adequate and relevant to the purpose for which it is held.
- Be accurate and, where necessary, kept up-to-date.
- Be held no longer than is necessary for the stated purpose.
- Have an appropriate security surrounding it.

It is now an offence to hold personal data without being registered. The register entries describe the types of data subjects to which each purpose applies, the classes of personal data held for each purpose, the sources from which any of the data may be obtained by persons or organisation to whom the data may need to be disclosed, and also the countries outside the UK to which it may be intended to transfer the data. These entries are contained in a register which the Data Protection Registrar has made widely available for public inspection through local libraries.

What is your responsibility as a salon employee?

As a salon employee you may have to handle personal data during the course of your work. You may, for example, receive a computer printed form which contains personal details or you may be involved in the collection of personal information that will eventually be processed by computer. There are very few employees who will not at some stage come into contact with sensitive personal data which has been computerised. In this situation the Act now says that you can be legally responsible for the confidentiality of the personal data, which **must only be used** to assist you to carry out your job and it must not be given to people who have no right to see it.

The importance of security measures in relation to personal data cannot be overemphasised. This extends to a number of matters, some examples of which include:

- Physical security of equipment such as computers, terminals, magnetic tapes, disks, etc.
- Data security – including the storage and disposal of output materials such as printouts, password protection, etc.

If there is a problem of any kind during the assessment of the client, their hair and the service they require, refer to your supervisor.

Face shape, age, hobbies and lifestyle

Face shape

The client's face shape is a key factor in the design of the completed style. For details of styles that are suitable and unsuitable see Level 2 Unit 3. A client suggesting an inappropriate style is a good example of where to use tact and care in subtle says to convince them that another approach would be better.

It is important to question the client closely; they may know exactly what they have in mind but have great difficulty in describing their exact wishes. If this is the case, it is often useful to keep a book of fashionable hairstyles available in the salon to show the client. Thus, the hair stylist will have a visual description of the style or 'look' that the client is aiming for.

Age, hobbies and lifestyle

The age of the client is a very important consideration. A middle-aged person does not always suit the same style as a teenager, although a current fashion trend can often be adapted to meet the needs of both, as long as it is not too extreme.

The general lifestyle and hobbies of the client also need to be considered. When assessing a client's personality, clothes, etc., it is important not to gown up until starting the procedure. Also find out if the client will have enough spare time to spend on an elaborate hairstyle or whether they will need a style that requires the minimum amount of time spent on it between salon visits. These and many other questions need to be asked to find out exactly what the client expects and requires of the salon service.

Hair growth patterns

Hair follicles

These are tiny pits in the skin (about 4 to 7 mm deep and 0.5 mm across) from which the hair grows. A diagram of a hair growing from the skin is shown in Fig. 2.1. At one time it was believed that the shape of the follicle determined the natural wave or curliness of the hair. However, more recent evidence suggests that the natural curl formation takes place in the hair bulb when the growth around the diameter of the hair is uneven, this causes the hair to bend resulting in wavy or curly hair. The angle at which the follicles lie and their distribution (or 'pattern') on the scalp produces the natural direction of the hair growth and produces natural partings and the crown on the scalp. The natural wave pattern of a person's hair is inherited from their parents (as is the colour). Typical patterns are:

- Widow's peak.
- Double crown.

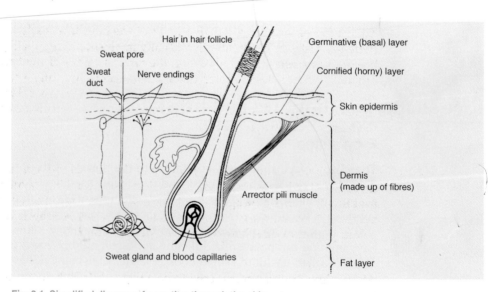

Fig. 2.1 Simplified diagram of a section through the skin

- Nape whorls.
- Cow's lick.

Useful background information

Figure 2.2 shows how hair grows from hair follicles in the skin.

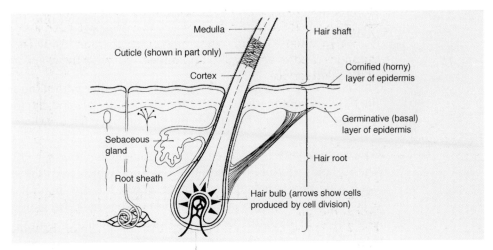

Fig. 2.2 Section through a hair folicle

Hair structure

The hair shaft is the part of the hair which protrudes above the skin and at this point it is dead. The hair is made up of three main layers:

- Cuticle.
- Cortex.
- Medulla.

The cuticle

This is the outermost protective layer of the hair. It is made up of overlapping, flattened scales of keratin and is virtually transparent. Light will pass through it as it would through frosted glass and the natural colour of the hair is seen through this layer; this is described as being **translucent**. The cuticle can be damaged by hairdressing processes, heated appliances and the weather. Where the cuticle is damaged, the hair is described as **porous** and, where much damage has occurred, the hair is likely to split and fray.

The cortex

The cortex makes up about 90 per cent of the bulk of the hair, and contains fibres made up of amino acids, twisted together. They contain **polypeptide chains** held together by **cross linkages** which are broken and reformed during setting and perming. The structure gives hair its texture, tensile strength, and elasticity. The colour pigment of the hair is also present in this layer.

The medulla

At one time this was considered to be a third, distinct layer of the hair, occupying the centre or core of the cortex. Recent findings on the detailed structure of the hair have thrown some doubt on this and the present position is not clear. If the medulla can be counted as a third layer, it is certainly not found in all hair or along the whole length of a hair. When present it appears to be a spongy area containing air spaces.

Hair root

This is the part of the hair buried in the skin. The hair follicle extends down through the upper layer of the skin (the **epidermis**) into the lower layer (the **dermis**).

Root sheath

This is the inner lining of the hair follicle. The outer part of the sheath is formed by the basal or germinative layer of the skin epidermis and the inner part interlocks with the hair cuticle which holds the hair firmly in the follicle.

Sebaceous glands

These glands produce the natural oil, **sebum**, which coats the skin and hair, keeping it waterproof and supple. In other words, it is our 'natural' conditioner. It also acts as a mild antiseptic and helps reduce the chance of skin infection by micro-organisms. Many hairdressing operations remove this natural oil from the hair, leaving it dry.

Hair bulb

This is situated at the lower end of the hair follicle. It is a swelling in the hair follicle and it encloses a knot of **blood capillaries** and **fat cells** called the **dermal papilla**. In the hair bulb (or just above it) the following processes take place:

- **Cell division** – which causes the hair to grow.
- **Hair colouring** –which is due to minute **granules** of the hair's natural pigments, i.e. melanin and pheomelanin which are almost entirely found in the hair cortex. With age or sometimes as a result of hair regrowth, after alopecia areata (form of baldness) for example, hair grows with no pigmentation, a condition called **canities** (white hair).
- **Keratinisation** – which takes place at the top of and just above the hair bulb. In this region the hair cells start to produce large amounts of the protein keratin.

The hair growth cycle

Hair grows at about 1.25 cm (½") per month due to cell hair division down at the hair root (see Fig. 2.2). There are about 100,000 hairs on a full scalp of hair, and any one of these hairs lasts for one to six years. During the time it lasts (or its 'life expectancy') the hair passes through the three stages of the hair growth cycle, i.e. *anagen, telogen* and *catagen* stages.

The details of these are summarised in Table 2.1.

About 100 scalp hairs a day are normally lost and replaced by new hairs in the anagen stage. The common forms of **baldness** are caused by the lack of new hairs being produced. For various reasons, follicles cease hair production. Baldness of various kinds is technically called **alopecia**.

Table 2.1

Name of stage	Description	Duration of stage	% scalp at stage
Anagen	Hair growing due to cell division in hair bulb.	1–5 years	80–90
Catagen	Hair stops growing as cell division stops. By end of this stage follicle has shortened by about one-third. End of hair has become separated from dermal papilla and forms a 'club' hair.	2 weeks	1
Telogen	Hair 'resting', no growth. By end of this stage new hair has started to grow from papilla. Old hair falls out.	3–4 months	13

Hair and scalp: conditions that can influence salon services

These conditions include:

- Diseases of the hair and skin.
- Infections caused by micro-organisms
- Infestations by animal parasites.
- Non-infectious hair and skin problems.

Both infections and infestations are caused by parasites. These terms are explained below:

- A **parasite** is a living organism which lives off another living thing (called the parasite's **host**) but with only the parasite benefiting.
- A body **infection** is caused by a disease-causing, or **pathogenic micro-organism**, living on the body, feeding from it and producing the 'signs' or symptoms of the disease. These parasites (commonly called **germs**) involve many different sorts of living things, but they all share the characteristic of being too small to be seen with the unaided eye.
- A body **infestation** describes an invasion by larger animal parasites which are visible to the unaided eye and mostly live at or near, the surface of the body.

A summary of the main infections and infestations is given in Table 2.2 on page 64.

Transmission

Both pathogenic micro-organisms and the larger animal parasites need to be passed or transmitted from one person to another. This transmission may take place in two main ways, which are either by contact or through the air.

Transmission by contact

'Contact' means that physical touching causes the transmission of the parasite. If a parasite can be passed in this way it is described as being **contagious**. This contact can be direct or indirect. Touching lips during kissing can transmit the micro-organism which causes **cold sores (herpes)** from one person to another. Touching heads allows the **head louse** to walk from one head to another. Both of these examples involve direct contact.

Indirect contact often involves inanimate objects which have been in contact with one person and are then touched by another; cold sores, for example, can be spread on damp towels, face cloths, etc., which have been in contact with one person and then used by another. Head lice may be transmitted from brushes and combs from one person to another.

Transmission through the air

This only involves the parasitic micro-organisms. If a parasite is passed from one person to another in this way it is described as **infectious**. The micro-organisms which cause the common cold and influenza ('flu') are spread by tiny droplets released by coughing and sneezing being breathed in by someone else. The micro-organism which causes **ringworm (tinea)** is often spread in minute **skin flakes** released by an infected person (or animal) which settle on to someone else.

Infections caused by micro-organisms

Skin and scalp conditions caused by bacteria

Many skin and scalp conditions are caused by bacteria normally found living on the skin. Two groups in particular, *staphylococci* and *streptococci*, will turn up several times as the cause of bacterial skin and scalp conditions. Both of these can also cause wound infection (or **sepsis**) which involves reddening, inflammation, swelling and pus formation.

In terms of skin conditions caused by bacteria, the following will be covered:

- Impetigo.
- Boils.
- Barber's itch.
- Folliculitis.

Impetigo (common type or impetigo vulgaris)
Cause
The skin bacteria staphylococci and streptococci.

Major symptoms
Blisters which contain a clear fluid and eventually form yellow crusts on the skin. Common on face and scalp, where the infection spreads rapidly.

- Impetigo is commonly caused by bacteria invading skin broken by scratching, e.g. as a result of head lice or itchmite infestation. This is called **secondary infection**.
- It is very contagious and spread by both direct and indirect contact. Hairdressing operations should not be started, or if they have, the stylist should stop and take care to sterilise with disinfectant any tools and equipment used.
- A different form of impetigo occurs in children (called Bockhardt's impetigo) which is caused by staphylococci bacteria invading scalp hair follicles and causing them to become inflamed, i.e. producing folliculitis. The condition appears as small red spots in the skin at the base of the hair with a 'head' of pus. The client should seek medical aid.

Boils (furunculosis)

Cause

A staphylococci bacteria invading a hair follicle or sebaceous gland and producing severe inflammation.

Major symptoms

A red raised area of the skin, very tender, with a central 'core' containing pus.

- Boils are common where clothing rubs, e.g. back or side of neck in males, where a shirt collar may rub. Staphylococcus aureus, which causes boils, is found living in the noses of between 10 and 30 per cent of the population. So it is possible to infect someone by coughing and sneezing. Sometimes a group of neighbouring follicles become involved, and this is called a **carbuncle**.
- Do not start hairdressing operations (or stop if already started) if a boil is in the area involved, e.g. scalp or beard. If the boil is not in such an area take great care not to touch it with the tools, equipment, towels, etc. This will be painful for the client and there is the possibility of picking up, and thus spreading, the bacteria.

Barber's itch (sycosis barbae)

Cause

Staphylococci bacteria invading the hair follicles in the beard area in males.

Major symptoms

Inflammation and pus formation in some of the beard hair follicles. Pain and itching in these areas.

- Barber's itch can be spread by indirect contact on shaving brushes, razors and towels.
- If scalp operations are intended, take great care not to touch beard area involved with tools, equipment or towels and gowns. Sterilise all these items after use. Do not start shaving or beard-trimming.

Folliculitis

Cause

Staphylococci bacteria.

Major symptoms

Infected hair follicles producing yellow spot with hair in centre. Itching and scratching.

Fungi

The fungi group ranges in size from mushrooms and toadstools down to microscopic varieties. Most live off dead organic material where they cause **decay**. Some microscopic types are parasites and cause skin and scalp conditions called ringworm.

Ringworm (tinea)

Ringworm can be found as:

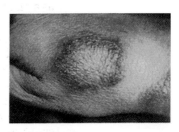

- Ringworm of the **scalp** (tinea capitis) – covered in detail below.
- Ringworm of the **body** (tinea corporis) – similar symptoms to scalp ringworm but most often caught from domestic animals.

Fig. 2.3 Ringworm

- Ringworm of the **foot** or 'athlete's foot' (tinea pedis) – a common condition, where the fungus grows through the skin between the toes causing reddening and itching (and possibly skin cracking). Commonly contracted by indirect contact through wet floors, e.g. changing rooms and swimming pools. See Fig. 2.3.

Ringworm of the scalp (tinea capitis)
Cause
The microscopic threads of the parasitic fungus growing through the cornified (horny) layer of the skin epidermis and through any hair shafts it encounters.

Major symptoms
Bald patches on the scalp with a stubble of broken off hairs (due to weakening of the hair shaft as the fungus grows through it). The bald patches are often circular and the skin inflamed.

- It is highly contagious by both indirect and direct contact and is infectious in that skin flakes breaking off from an infected person can land on another, and if they lodge for long enough they can grow from the flake into the other person's skin. It can be contracted from domestic animals.
- It is most common in children.
- Do not start (or stop, if already started) hairdressing operations. If operations have been started then disinfect tools, equipment, gowns, towels and seating.
- Sweep up (or better, vacuum) any hair clippings; place in sealed plastic bags and preferably dispose of by burning outside the salon.

Viruses

Viruses are the smallest of all the micro-organisms and unlike bacteria, moulds, yeasts and fungi, they cannot survive for long outside living cells. A common form of transmission of viral diseases is by **droplet infection**. When someone coughs or sneezes, hundreds of tiny droplets of liquid are blown into the air. These may contain living viruses which can survive as long as the droplet persists. In damp air (that is, air with a high relative humidity), the droplets evaporate slowly and this increases the chances of someone else inhaling the droplets and becoming infected. In dry air (that is, air with a low relative humidity), the droplets evaporate quickly and the viruses die. The common cold and flu (influenza) are spread in this way. Because of the large amounts of moisture entering the air in hairdressing salons (due to hot water being used, the large amount of drying, etc.) the air tends to have a relatively high humidity, unless the ventilation system can cope with its removal. This is one reason why an efficient ventilation system is important in the salon.

The various skin conditions caused by viruses are cold sores (herpes simplex) and some types of wart.

Cold sores (herpes simplex)
Cause
A virus which lives in the germinative layer of the skin epidermis (present in about 90 per cent of the population) and develops when a person's general resistance is lowered, e.g. by another disease.

Major symptoms
Often begins as a small crack in dry skin in the corner (or corners) of the mouth. It spreads rapidly with some blistering and develops into an oozing crust (like a soft scab).

- It is very common, especially in children.
- It can be passed by direct or indirect contact; therefore, care should be taken to sterilise cups, etc., used by clients or towels likely to have touched the face. If persistent, suggest the client sees a doctor. Often clears up spontaneously, but is 'carried' in the body until the next time conditions favour its growth.

Warts (verrucae)

Cause

A virus (called papova virus) which lives in the germinative layer of the skin epidermis, where it triggers a large amount of cell division in a small area. This produces the 'lumps' characteristic of common warts. On the feet the pressure causes the wart to grow inwards, which produces a plantar wart (commonly called 'verrucae').

Major symptoms

1 **Raised warts** – may be rough and rise some distance above the skin (common warts) or be smaller and smooth-topped (plane warts – common in children).
2 **Plantar warts** – grow into the skin on the feet, where the pressure caused by the weight of the body is greatest, e.g. on the 'ball' of the foot.

- Unless a client feels strongly that the size and position of the wart necessitates removal, they are best left alone. If removal is desirable, then recommend they see their doctor and do not use the proprietary 'wart removers' on the market.
- Warts often clear spontaneously as the body eventually becomes immune to the virus which causes them.
- They can be transmitted by direct or indirect contact, so take reasonable precautions.
- Plantar warts (verrucae) are spread by indirect contact in places with damp or wet floors, e.g. changing rooms and swimming pools.

Aids and Hepatitis B

AIDS is short for Acquired Immune Deficiency Syndrome which is a very dangerous disease that could, possibly, be transmitted in the salon. The chances of this happening are very small but it is worth taking reasonable precautions. The virus that causes Aids can be transmitted in body fluids and therefore could pass from one person to another in blood, such as someone being nicked with a razor, the razor not being cleaned and then someone else being nicked with the same razor. The current advice for any blood spillage is to use neat bleach on the blood and then wash away with lots of water and a detergent.

Hepatitis B is another very serious illness which can be transmitted like Aids and so the precautions are the same.

Information about both Aids and Hepatitis B can be obtained from Local Environmental Health Centres, Health Education Authority and the Department of Health.

Eye infections

These can spread rapidly by indirect contact with damp towels in the salon. The two main kinds are:

1 **Blepharitis** (or 'styes') – where staphylococci bacteria infect the eyelash follicles, causing soreness, reddening and swelling.
2 **Conjunctivitis** – which can have a variety of causes, e.g. bacteria like staphylococci and some viruses. Conjunctivitis is the inflammation of the outer,

protective layer on the front of the eyeball and can be spread by indirect contact with damp towels; some forms are very infectious. Because of the high risk of transferring the micro-organisms onto towels, hairdressing operations should be stopped and the client advised to see their doctor.

Infestations caused by animal parasites

These larger parasites are visible to the unaided eye and feed off the human body. Important examples in hairdressing are:

- Lice (especially the head louse).
- Flea.
- Itchmite (which causes scabies).

A point to remember is that anyone can become infested and it is not a reflection on personal hygiene to have picked up these parasites. In fact, head lice prefer clean scalps to dirty ones.

Lice and fleas are insects and have six legs. Both have special jaws which can pierce the person's skin and then suck blood (the mouths work rather like the hollow needle of a hypodermic syringe used to take a blood sample at the hospital). When the person's skin is pierced, the animal injects a small amount of **anticoagulant** into the tiny wound to prevent the blood from clotting. It is this action that:

- Produces the skin reddening and itching associated with lice and flea 'bites'. The scratching of these areas often breaks the skin surface and allows invasion by the skin bacteria, producing a secondary infection, e.g. **impetigo**.
- Can lead to other infections passed on by the parasite. This is unlikely in the UK, but fleas can pass on plague and lice, typhus.

Itchmites belong to a branch of the spider family and have eight legs. They are the smallest of the animal parasites with the female mite less that 0.5 mm long (the male is almost half that size). The female digs tunnels into the skin and in these lays her eggs. Chemicals released by the mites can cause intense irritation and itching and a common name for scabies is the 'itch'.

Lice

Infestation of the body by lice is called **pediculosis**. The head louse is the most important type in hairdressing:

Head lice (pediculus capitis)
About 4 per cent of the population have head lice at any one time and they are often first noticed by the hairdresser. The adults are about 3 mm long and have flattened bodies. Each leg has strong claws at the end, used to grip hair shafts. The flattened bodies and the claws make it difficult to dislodge adult lice and any lice which fall out of untreated hair are dying (due to injury or old age).

Lice pierce the skin and suck blood, causing a certain amount of irritation. Lice only have a life-span of about 30 days and events during this are outlined in Fig. 2.4.

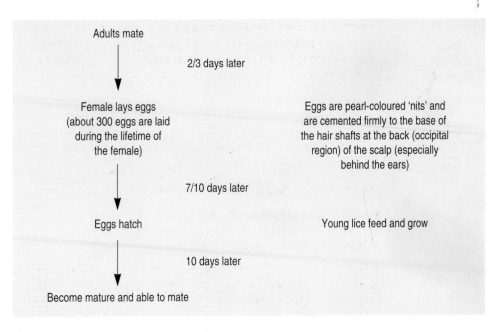

Fig. 2.4

Only a few of the eggs laid survive to maturity and a typical head infestation involves about 20 adult lice.

Head lice are contagious and can be transmitted from one person to another by direct head to head contact or indirect contact from pillows, upholstery, etc. Lice cannot jump or fly and any seen off the scalp are usually dying or dead.

Symptoms

The client will probably have noticed some itching but may be unaware of its cause. The infestation is often first noticed by the presence of the eggs or nits glued to the bases of the hair shafts and sometimes the adults are visible.

- Reassure the client that contracting head lice is nothing to do with personal hygiene (many people are horrified when they are told) and that it is easy to eradicate (the Community Health Councils hold a range of very useful pamphlets on skin disorders and body parasites, including the head louse, and these are available free from your nearest office which will be in the phone book).
- Do point out that others in the family are likely to be infected and that expert advice, e.g. doctor, health visitor or local health clinic should be sought.
- Because head lice are contagious, do not begin (or stop, if started) hairdressing operations. Take care to disinfect tools and equipment thoroughly, wipe down with disinfectant and vacuum the upholstery of chairs the client has used.
- The eggs or nits can sometimes be mistaken for flakes of dandruff. If in doubt, try to rub the flake off the hair. Dandruff flakes are easily removed, nits are not.

Non-infectious/non-contagious hair problems

In addition to the infectious and contagious conditions there are a number of non-infectious/non-contagious hair conditions.

Table 2.2 Summary of the main infections and infestations

	Name of condition	Caused by	Major symptoms	Infectious or contagious?	Stop hairdressing operations?	Medical advice needed?
INFECTIONS BY PATHOGENIC MICRO-ORGANISMS	Impetigo	Bacteria	Blisters and yellow crusts.	Yes (very)	Yes	Yes
	Boils (furuncles)	Bacteria	Red, raised area in skin. Very tender. Central pus.	Yes (if pus released)	Only if boil in scalp area	Yes, if persistent
	Barber's itch (sycosis barbae)	Bacteria	Swelling and pus formation in beard hair follicles.	Yes	Yes, on beard area (*NB* avoid contact in this area)	Yes, if persistent
	Folliculitis	Bacteria	Yellow spot with hair in centre.	Yes	Yes	Yes, if persistent
	Ringworm (tinea)	Fungus	Round bald patches. Stubble of hair, skin may be inflamed.	Yes (very)	Yes	Yes
	Cold sores (herpes simplex)	Virus	Weeping scabs around mouth.	Yes	No, but take care to prevent transmission	Not usually, but yes if persistent and extreme
	Warts (verrucae)	Virus	Lump in skin (rough or smooth).	Yes	No (but avoid nicking with scissors)	Not usually, unless removal wanted
	Conjunctivitis	Bacteria or virus	Inflamed eyes, possible weeping of fluid.	Yes	Yes	Yes
ANIMAL PARASITES	Head lice (pediculus capitis)	Head louse	Itching, eggs (nits) glued to base of hair. Sometimes adults seen.	Yes	Yes	Yes (but advice can be given by hairdresser)
	Flea (pulex irritans)	Human flea	Red spots surrounded by pink patches. Itching.	Yes	Yes	Yes
	Scabies	Itchmite (sarcopies scabiei)	Intense itching, especially in joints and at night (burrows sometimes visible).	Yes	Yes	Yes

- **Fragilitis crinium** – commonly known as split ends where the hair points are split lengthways. The only cure is to cut the ends off.
- **Trichorrhexis nodosa** – where hair is fragile due to splits along the hair shaft.
- **Monilethrix** – a very rare condition where the hair shaft has a beaded appearance due to distorted growth. Treatment for both trichorrhexis and monilethrix involves using **restructurants** and **protein treatments** (*see* below).
- **Damaged cuticle** – the most common cause of damaged cuticle is chemical treatment, but it can be caused by vigorous brushing/combing. The cuticle is important for hair condition (the cuticle in good condition makes hair shine) and porosity (in extreme cases hair is so porous that even permanent tints wash out).

A very common feature of damage to the cuticle (even relatively little damage) is hair becoming tangled. There is no treatment as such but protein based and other types of 'restructurants' in shampoo and/or conditioning treatments can help. These add to the hair in the porous areas – in other words they are **substantive**. They automatically enter the hair where needed.

Some conditions are caused by hair in areas that are normally **vellus** becoming secondary hair. Examples are **hypertrichosis**, where this happens in certain areas, and **hirsutism**, which is more general across the whole body.

A summary of non-infectious hair conditions is presented in Table 2.3 on page 69.

Non-infectious/non-contagious skin conditions

Psoriasis

This is an inherited condition and therefore is commonly found amongst members of the same family. The cause of psoriasis is not known for certain, but it may be caused by a defect in the chemical reactions taking place in the **germinative** (or basal) layer of the skin epidermis.

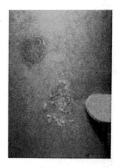

Fig. 2.5 Psoriasis

Symptoms

Patches of thickened silver-coloured scales with the underlying skin appearing red. There is no hair loss associated with the condition. (See Fig. 2.5.)

- The appearance and extent of psoriasis varies and scalp psoriasis, if extensive and severe, can be distressing to the client. They should be tactfully encouraged to seek expert advice and help.
- There is a coal tar based shampoo for this condition.

A summary of non-infectious skin conditions is presented in Table 2.3 on page 69.

Dermatitis and eczema

Both the terms 'dermatitis' and 'eczema' are used interchangeably to describe an inflammation of the skin surface.

Distinctions can be made on the basis of:

- Whether the condition is 'dry' or releases a fluid, i.e. 'weeps', where dermatitis is used for the 'dry' condition and eczema for the 'weeping' variety.
- What causes (or 'triggers') the development of the condition.
- Dermatitis is thought to be caused by both internal and external factors and eczema due to internal factors only.

Contact dermatitis

As its name suggests, 'contact' dermatitis may be produced in the skin due to contact with a chemical or chemicals. Some chemicals will produce a dermatic rash on first exposure and this over-reaction can be called an **allergy**. People may be allergic to many different substances, a common one being pollen grains in the air, causing hay fever. All allergies involve the body defence system over-reacting to a substance.

Thus, the external factor involved is the contact with the chemical and the internal factors determine the person's reaction to that chemical. Other substances can produce dermatitis after a number of exposures. This is a major problem in hairdressing as the actual number of times a person needs to be exposed to a substance until they get dermatitis varies with different individuals. Substances which may eventually produce a reaction are called **sensitisers**. The chemical in 'para' hair tints is a fairly common sensitiser and the reason for the skin test which should be carried out 24–48 hours before using such a tint is to check whether previous exposures have sensitised the client.

Symptoms

These are very variable, but include:

- Inflammation of the skin surface.
- Cracking of the skin and possibly 'weeping' of fluid.
- A certain amount of itching.

The risk to the hairdresser involves the hands in 90 per cent of cases.

The risk to the client tends to be on the face. Dermatitis triggered by the 'para' dyes, for example, tends to involve the skin of the eyelids, ears and neck.

Prevention

There is no cure once someone has developed a sensitisation to a substance, and the only action is to avoid contact with it. If a hairdresser develops a high level of sensitisation to a commonly used hairdressing chemical, often the only course of action is to leave hairdressing altogether. The best prevention is protection, particularly by using rubber gloves for all hairdressing operations involving chemicals. Barrier creams offer some protection but are not as effective as a pair of rubber gloves.

Protection of the client involves taking care to prevent hairdressing products, especially those known to be sensitisers, from touching their skin.

Seborrhoea

Seborrhoea is the general name for the over-production of sebum by the skin's **sebaceous glands**. The surplus of natural oil makes the hair greasy and the skin oily. This condition is common in people at **puberty**, where the sudden rise in the level of **sex hormones** in the blood triggers the over-production of sebum.

Seborrhoea is involved in the development of acne and in some kinds of **dandruff**. If the dandruff is linked to an inflammation of the scalp, this is called **seborrhoeic dermatitis**.

Dandruff (pityriasis)

Dandruff, or 'scurf', is a common scalp condition caused by the **flaking** of the cornified (or horny) layer of the skin epidermis. This flaking of the outermost skin layer occurs all over the body, all of the time and each person loses millions of these tiny flakes per day. The main reason for this general flaking is to remove skin bacteria, and thus keep the numbers of bacteria on the skin under control.

On the scalp, the hair tends to trap these flakes and they 'build up', or accumulate, into the large flakes which are characteristic of the condition. The damp, warm conditions under these flakes favour the multiplication of **bacteria** and **yeasts**.

At one time it was thought that dandruff was caused by bacteria. It is now known that it is not and that some people have a tendency to produce a large number of skin flakes on the scalp, while others do not. Whether bacteria are involved in the itching which often accompanies severe dandruff is not clear at the moment, but antiseptics are included in many medicated or anti-dandruff shampoos to keep the number of bacteria under control. These shampoos also contain substances like **selenium sulphide** and **zinc pyrithione**, which reduce the flaking by reducing the activities of the germinative layer of the skin epidermis.

The most common form of dandruff is where the flakes fall freely from the hair when brushed or combed (this is called dry dandruff or **pityriasis capitis**). If dandruff occurs in connection with seborrhoea (an over-production of sebum) then the oil tends to make the flakes stick to the scalp (this is sometimes called oily dandruff or **pityriasis stearoides**). This can lead to seborrhoeic dermatitis. In this case the client should be referred to their doctor.

Sebaceous cysts

These appear as raised areas on the skin and are caused by a blockage in a sebaceous gland. The sebum normally released onto the hair and skin in that area accumulates and causes the swelling. This type of cyst is sometimes called a **wen** and they are harmless.

Baldness (alopecia)

The most common type of baldness is **male pattern** baldness, which affects about 40 per cent of males by the age of 40. This condition is inherited and is not as common in females as it is in males. The necessary trigger for the hair loss is the presence of the male sex hormone and this is the reason that this type of hair loss is relatively rare in women. Older women may suffer a version of this balding as their levels of female hormones fall after the **menopause**.

How the male hormone triggers the condition is not known. For no apparent reason the hair follicles start to die when they reach the end of **telogen** in the hair growth cycle. Because of this, no new hair grows to replace the old when it falls out of the follicle. For this reason, this type of balding is a gradual process, with the hair 'thinning' and disappearing from around the crown and above the forehead. Whether high frequency treatment has a positive effect is not clear. At the moment it is not possible to prevent the hair follicles from dying, and the only effective treatment is a hair transplant.

Male pattern baldness accounts for about 90 per cent of hair loss encountered by the salon. The other 10 per cent is made up of conditions where the balding tends to be patchy or scattered; these conditions include:

- Alopecia areata.
- Diffuse alopecia (alopecia diffusa).
- Traction alopecia.
- Cicatrical (scarring) alopecia.

Alopecia areata

This is the appearance of roughly circular bald patches on the scalp. (See Fig. 2.6.) The skin of the area is soft, smooth and has no hair. These features are important in distinguishing alopecia areata from ringworm. With ringworm, the bald patches have a stubble of broken off hairs running across them and the skin is often red and inflamed. There is no itching with alopecia areata and the condition also has 'exclamation mark' hairs around the borders of the bald patches.

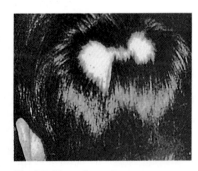

Fig. 2.6 Alopecia areata

'Exclamation mark' hairs are caused by the hair breaking and the hair root breaking down. Hairs are wider and darker near the broken end and about 0.5 cm (¼") long. They are easily pulled out and appear like an exclamation mark (!).

Alopecia areata usually disappears in two to three months, but may recur at intervals. The precise reasons for the development of the condition are not known.

Diffuse alopecia (alopecia diffusa)

This describes a general 'thinning' of the scalp hair, often most noticeable at the crown and along the parting. It can occur in young women, who find it very distressing, due to hormone changes after childbirth and sometimes as a result of oral contraception. It can also occur after serious illness and drug treatments. The hair usually regrows.

Another type of 'thinning' is **alopecia senilis** which is associated with old age.

Traction alopecia

This is a general term used to describe hair being pulled out of the scalp. This can result from the tension caused by tight rollers and due to the hair style adopted, e.g. tight plaits or hair rolled into a tight 'bun'. It can also be caused by a nervous twisting of the hair around the fingers. If the cause of the tension on the hair is removed, then the hair usually grows back.

Cicatrical (scarring) alopecia

This results from skin damage and scarred areas in which hair will not grow. There is no treatment available.

Health in the salon

Preventing the transmission of disease in the salon

The prevention of transmission of infections and infestations depends on two main factors:

- General salon hygiene.
- The ability of the salon staff to recognise which skin and scalp conditions are infectious or contagious and which are not.

Hygiene

The transmission of the parasites which cause infections and infestations can be limited by good hygiene in the salon. Good hygiene involves a number of things but these can be summarised as:

- The routine practice carried out by the hairdresser, e.g. sterilising brushes and combs, using a new neck strip, etc., for each client.
- Salon management practice, e.g. regular laundering of uniforms and gowns, regular cleaning of surfaces, training staff to carry these out.
- Salon design features which help hygiene, e.g. choice of wall and floor coverings, type of upholstery on seating, type of ventilation system.

Table 2.3 Summary of non-infectious hair and scalp conditions

Condition	Symptoms	Notes
Split ends (fragilitas crinium)	Splitting of the hair at the points.	Often occurs at the points of long hair with a tendency to be dry. Breaks can occur along the length of the hair and there is no real 'cure'. Restructurant conditioners can be used but the only real answer is to cut the split ends off.
Trichorrhexis nodosa	Swellings occur along the hair.	These are weak points and the hair tends to break. It can be caused by rollers or by strong alkaline chemicals. Can use 'restructurant' to help prevent breakage.
Damaged cuticle	Hair rough and dull and tangles easily. Difficult to untangle.	Caused by chemical treatment. Use 'restructurant' to help make hair more manageable.
Monilethrix	Bead-like swellings along the hair shaft.	A very rare condition that is inherited and appears mostly in children. Tendency for hair loss as the hair tends to break off near the scalp.
Hypertrichosis	The growth of thick secondary (terminal) hair in an area which usually shows only the fine 'down' (vellus) hair.	Can occur on a facial 'mole' for example.
Hirsutism	Where male type secondary (terminal) hair growth patterns occur in females.	Includes 'bearded ladies' of which there is a number of medically certified cases.
Psoriasis	Silver coloured scales. Reddened skin.	Inherited condition. Tends to clear up and recur.
Dermatitis and eczema	Swelling of skin. Sometimes cracking and weeping of fluid.	Terms are used interchangeably. Contact dermatitis is the major occupational risk to hairdressers.
Seborrhoea	Greasy hair and skin.	Caused by over-production of sebum. Implicated in acne.
Dandruff (pityriasis)	Flaking of scalp.	Can be dry or oily. Not caused by bacteria. Some people more prone than others.
Sebaceous cyst (wen)	Appearance of roughly circular 'lumps' on the skin.	Caused by a blockage which prevents release of sebum onto the skin. Sebum accumulates under skin.
Baldness (alopecia)	Hair loss.	Most common in 'male pattern' type. Inherited and triggered by male hormone.

What is sterilisation?

Sterilisation means the destruction of all living things including the harmful micro-organisms that cause disease ('germs'). These can be passed from one person to another and transmitted in the salon on tools and equipment particularly razors, scissors and clippers. There is some risk with *all* tools and equipment such as brushes, combs, clips, towels, etc .

Sterilisation is only really possible by using an autoclave. Autoclaves work by using steam under pressure (like a pressure cooker) at high temperatures, 125 °C for example, which is sufficient to kill *all* micro-organisms in about five minutes. Autoclaves have not been widely used in salons but their use is spreading as cheap automatic autoclaves enter the market.

What is disinfection?

Disinfection means reducing the chances of infection and techniques for this are widespread in hairdressing. They include:

- Chemicals.
- Ultraviolet rays.
- Heat – dry or moist.

Chemicals

These can either destroy or retard the growth of micro-organisms. A chemical which destroys micro-organisms is called a **disinfectant** (bacteriocide or germicide). The problems with disinfectants include:

- They rapidly go 'off' and cease to work efficiently.
- They become 'overloaded' and cease to work efficiently.
- Some are poisonous to humans.
- Some attack tools, particularly metal tools.

If they are used for washing down walls, upholstery and surfaces, the best type to use are **alcohol** based but this can cause problems as alcohol is a *fire risk* as it is *flammable*. Sterilising cabinets are still used in some salons but these suffer from all the problems listed for disinfectant.

Current thinking is that disinfectants are *not* recommended for reducing the risk of infection by tools.

Ultraviolet rays

These are used in ultraviolet 'sterilisers'. The cabinet contains a mercury vapour tube which is situated at the top of the cabinet enabling the ultraviolet rays that it gives off to fall and sterilise the equipment placed beneath them. As the rays cannot penetrate the equipment, items must be 'turned' to ensure complete destruction of the bacteria.

Ultraviolet radiation can cause burns to the skin with continual exposure; therefore most of these cabinets have some form of lid that shields the hands of the operator when tools have to be removed from the cabinet.

Heat

Very high temperatures are used in the **autoclave** which is the *only* current method of efficiently sterilising tools and equipment. Other methods which use lower temperatures to 'disinfect' rather than sterilise are:

- **Dry heat** – used in glass bead sterilisers which are useful in the salon. The higher the temperature the shorter the time tools need to be left in and the time to reach their operating temperature. Only the part of the tools covered by the beads will be treated and although good for tools such as scissors, they are less effective with clipper blades.

- **Moist heat** – used in autoclaves and boilers/steamers. Autoclaves work at very high temperatures and are very effective at killing micro-organisms. Boiling or steaming works at a lower temperature and may not kill all pathogens. Tools should be boiled or steamed for at least ten minutes.

Salon staff

The transmission of infections and infestations can also be reduced by the salon staff knowing:

- How to recognise the various scalp and skin conditions and to know which of these are contagious (spread by contact), which are infectious (spread by the air) and which are neither infectious nor contagious.
- How to deal with the client if a scalp or skin condition is thought to be of an infectious or contagious type.
- What steps to take in the salon to prevent transmission from happening.

Recognition of skin and scalp conditions

This is very much a job for an expert. Few hairdressers have the training or experience needed to be able to determine exactly what many skin or scalp conditions are. Some are relatively easy and hairdressers have an important role to play in often being the first to notice the condition and be in a position to advise the client. An infestation by head lice is a good example of this, where the client may have noticed the itching, but may be unaware of the cause. Other skin conditions involve rashes, skin scaling, crusting or weeping and these can be due to a variety of causes, some infectious or contagious and others not.

This unit covers these in outline, but the rule should be:

If in doubt do not start hairdressing operations (if they have started, then stop) and advise the client to see their doctor.

How to deal with the client

The key word here is tact. The hairdresser is in a difficult position and there are no rules for dealing with the client. Here are some general points.

- Talk quietly to the client and, if possible, speak to them alone. Find out whether they have seen a doctor about the condition. If they have not, strongly advise them to do so.
- Even if the condition has been identified, do not be too certain when discussing it with the client. It is far better that an expert confirms the nature of the condition.
- Stress that the condition is nothing to do with personal hygiene (this is particularly important with infestations) and that anyone can contract it.
- If hairdressing operations are not possible explain to the client the risk of infecting other clients (even if not sure which condition they have).
- Explain that if the condition is diagnosed by experts as non-infectious/contagious they will be welcome to return to the salon. If it is infectious or contagious, they will be welcome when it has been successfully treated.
- Stress that there are few hair or skin conditions which cannot be successfully treated.

What to do in the salon

If an infectious or contagious condition has been provisionally identified then:

- Carefully sterilise any tools or equipment used on the client.
- Take gowns, towels, etc., used on the client and soak in a strong disinfectant solution.
- Wipe down chairs they have used with a disinfectant solution (and vacuum clean if possible).
- Carefully sweep or vacuum up any hair clippings and dispose of them immediately outside the salon, by burning if possible.

Testing hair and skin

There are various tests that can be carried out on the hair and skin to make sure that there will not be any problems when carrying out further treatments or when a treatment is completed.

Always explain to the client why you are carrying out the tests – it will increase their trust in your expertise and encourage them to accept any of your recommendations. Remember to record all test results for future reference. Table 2.4 is a summary of tests.

Table 2.4

Type of test	Test used for	Further details
Curl test	To find out the amount of processing that has occurred.	Perming Unit 5A
Elasticity test	A general test of hair condition and strength, particularly of the cortex. Hair is stretched.	Perming Unit 5A Relaxing Unit 5B
Incompatibility test	To check for the presence of metallic dyes on the hair.	Perming Unit 5A Colouring/bleaching Unit 6
Porosity test	To check the hair cuticle for damage and/or being open.	Perming Unit 5A Colouring/bleaching Unit 6
Strand test	To follow the development of the colour during tinting.	Colouring/bleaching Unit 6
Skin (allergy) test	Carried out before a para dye is used. To ensure no reaction to the tint.	Colouring/bleaching Unit 6
Test curl	To check that correct rod size and lotion is used, and to find out the processing time.	Perming Units 5A and 5B
Test cutting	To check whether a chemical treatment is suitable.	Relaxing Unit 5B Colouring/bleaching Unit 6

Incorrect use of chemicals on the hair

A client may come into the salon showing the signs of a previous incorrect chemical treatment or they may ask for a service which would produce the effects of over-application or over-processing. The incorrect uses of chemical treatment are summarised in Table 2.5.

Table 2.5

Chemical treatment	Main effects of incorrect use on the hair	More details
Bleaches	Overlapping application onto previously bleached hair may weaken hair or produce uneven colouring. Uneven application will cause more bleaching in some areas than others – producing a 'patchy' look.	Colouring/bleaching Unit 6
Neutralisers	The curl will not last long-term.	Neutralising Unit 5A
Perm lotions	Uneven application will lead to uneven curl. Lotion on the scalp can cause irritation and chemical burns.	Perming Unit 5A
Relaxing chemicals	Uneven application produces uneven straightening/relaxing. Can easily cause damage.	Relaxing Unit 5B

Advising clients on after-care procedures

An important feature of client care (and the client's feelings of satisfaction with the salon) is the after-care advice they receive. This includes the salon services they may wish to use in the future and products they may wish to buy and take away with them.

After-care procedures may include:

- Advice on the use of shampoos and conditioners.
- Whether to use styling and finishing products and, if so, which ones.
- Any practical tips or precautions on using home hair-care appliances, such as curling tongs, etc.

This advice is clearly to the client's benefit but it also serves the purpose of helping to promote (or 'sell') the salon services and products. Never underestimate the power of perception (how people see things): if the client perceives you as an expert they will take your advice. However, they will not wish to attend your salon or buy goods if they do not like what they see. First impressions are important and a prospective client/buyer can be encouraged to enter the salon by its smart and clean exterior and to keep returning because of its welcoming interior and the attitude of the staff employed there. Thus, promoting the salon and selling goods can be divided into three main areas:

- Promoting the salon image.
- Promoting salon services.
- Selling retail goods.

Promoting the salon image

As stated above, it is important to first attract the client to walk through the salon doors. New clients will attend the salon either because it has been recommended by someone else or because they like the look of the salon from the outside. This being so, the exterior of the salon must always project the salon image and the type of work that takes place within. It should always be kept clean and if there is a window display this must be regularly changed to attract attention.

The type and standard of work that is produced by the salon will also present a certain image. The standard of work should be as high as possible and can be improved by regular training nights for both junior and senior staff.

In addition, the appearance of the staff will contribute to the image of the salon, so looking neat, smart and professional is very important. For example, if you were to find yourself in hospital surrounded by nurses wearing shorts and T-shirts you would not be filled with confidence. This is because they would not be projecting the image of what you 'perceive' that a nurse should look like. While their attire will make no difference to the standard of their work, it will influence how capable *you* think that person to be. The same applies to hairdressing, if the staff look the part, then clients will believe them to be competent.

Promoting the salon services

Before you can sell any salon service you must have a thorough knowledge of what these services are, how they work and what benefits they will bring to the client. Often staff are reluctant to use or recommend new products as they are unsure of these points. However, most manufacturers have trained technical staff who will come to the salon to demonstrate and instruct the staff on any of their products. They will usually run short courses at their own training centres to give any tuition needed on their products. These courses are very useful as they also give background knowledge and usually offer ways in which to promote the products. Always remember that the manufacturers are also in business and it is in their best interest to help you as much as possible as the more of their products you use then the more profit they make!

A lot of stylists feel uncomfortable about recommending further treatments to their clients. This reluctance is, however, misplaced because the client relies on the experience of the stylist to make their hair look its best. Very often the client is totally unaware of the range of services available. While they may, for example, be aware that the salon does 'tints', they could be oblivious to the very many ways that colour can be used to create effects that range from dramatic to so subtle that the hair is given only a 'sheen'. It is the responsibility of the stylist, as the expert, to guide and advise the client as to what treatments would be the most suitable and beneficial. After all, the worst that can happen is that the client will say no. The conversation below gives an indication of how a treatment can be advised to the client without giving offence:

Client: 'I like my new haircut but the top keeps going flat. I know I should have a perm but I hate curls and besides the back is now too short to curl.'

Stylist: 'Your hair is rather fine so it really needs extra bounce. A body wave or root perm would be ideal as it will only give root lift and will not make it too curly. In fact, it will not give any curl at all but it will make the blowdry hold for longer and give your style the height you like. I only need to wind the top so that the other hair will be unaffected.'

Client: 'That sounds ideal, I hadn't realised that it was possible to have a perm without curl and that I didn't need to have the whole head done. When can I book my appointment?'

Using a variety of techniques in the salon also creates interest, particularly if they are visually different from the norm. When clients see something unusual their curiosity is aroused and they will want to know all about it. For instance, when Molton Browner perm rods first came onto the market clients wanted a perm just to try the rods!

When selling salon services, keep to the golden rule of knowing your products and what they are capable of. Never promise something that is impossible to achieve. If a particular product or service is unsuitable for the client's hair, tell them so and recommend something else. In time, when clients find that your recommendations improve their hair then they will learn to trust you and it is highly unlikely that they will take their custom elsewhere.

Selling retail goods

When selling retail goods it is essential that the products are attractively displayed in a prominent place. Unless they are on show clients will not know exactly what is for sale. Large stores know the value of a good display stand where people can touch and try products. Remember; if a prospective buyer holds something they are more likely to buy it. The next time you go shopping look at how the goods are arranged and see what type of arrangement makes you stop and want to buy the products displayed.

The best place to display retail goods is in the reception area so that when the client is paying the bill they can buy the goods at the same time. Clients waiting in the reception area will also be able to look at what is displayed and people passing the salon can easily call in to purchase whatever they wish without having to go into the main body of the salon. For this reason it is a good idea to make sure that the retail display is visually attractive from the outside of the salon as well as inside.

All retail goods should be clearly marked with the price. Many people are put off buying products if they have to ask how much they are. The display should always be well stocked and *clean*; it is surprising how dusty goods can become in a very short period of time and nothing is more off-putting to a prospective buyer than to see goods which look soiled or as if they have been on the shelf a long time. Human nature being what it is we believe that if nobody else wants them then they cannot be any good!

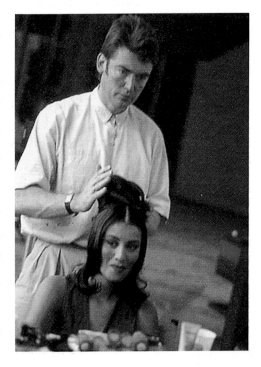

There are a multitude of products available for use on the hair and skin and it can be very confusing to be confronted by a vast range. Clients buying their hair products from other stores are often ignorant of what they should buy and this is where the stylist's expertise comes into its own. The stylist *knows* the client's hair and can therefore recommend a suitable product. They also know the effects that the various products will have on the hair and these can then be explained to the client. If making a purchase at another store, the client must make a more *uninformed* choice as the assistants will not have the same amount of professional knowledge.

Often the best way to sell retail products is to use them in the salon, explaining their use when they are being put on the hair. For example:

Stylist: 'I am just going to put some wax on to the ends of your hair to make it fall into strands and give a more tousled effect. I find that this particular wax is excellent for your type of hair as it counteracts any dryness and is very economical to use. In fact, we sell a great deal of this product and it is extremely popular with our clients. '

This stylist has covered several points here:

1 **Introducing** the client to a new product – '. . . some wax.'
2 Telling the client **where to apply** the wax for a certain effect – '. . . on to the ends of the hair.'
3 Explaining to the client the **effect** it will have on the hair – '. . . make it fall into strands and give it a more tousled effect.'
4 **Personalising** the product – ' . . . excellent for your type of hair. '
5 Giving some **benefits** of using the product – '. . . counteracts dryness and is very economical to use.'
6 **Informing** the client that the wax is for sale – '. . . we sell a great deal of this product.'
7 **Showing** that it must be effective because so many people buy it – '. . . it is extremely popular with our clients.'

Using the products in the salon has an added advantage in that the client has tried the product on their hair and therefore has an indication as to its benefits. In this way many of the products almost sell themselves.

Promotions are also an ideal way of boosting sales and there are many different ways that this can be done. For example, instead of promoting cheaper perms, why not keep the price the same but include a free specialised shampoo for home use? This will prolong the life of the perm by ensuring that the client uses the correct shampoo as well as introducing them to a new product. In addition, when the client requires more shampoo they will be more likely to purchase it from the salon than anywhere else. Other examples include selling small travel packs of the products during the summer months, or gift sets which are popular over the Christmas period. Selling two products together at a more reduced price than buying them separately or on a two for the price of one basis are also ideas for increasing sales.

Selling techniques

If you look around your salon you will probably notice that some stylists make far more sales than others. Watch carefully how they deal with the client about what they are selling and how they believe firmly in the products. This brings us back to the point made earlier, that good product knowledge is essential and the best way to find out about the products is to use them yourself.

Some people seem to be born salespeople who are able to communicate easily and persuade others as if by magic. For those who find it more difficult there are certain strategies which can be used to help overcome any initial nervousness and ask questions in the most beneficial way.

To overcome initial nervousness make sure that you have enough product knowledge; this will give you confidence. Then take a deep breath and speak calmly. Remember to sound enthusiastic and positive when you talk – you will be surprised at how well the client will respond.

Providing information to clients about the salon

If a client wishes to return to a salon they need a basic set of information to help them. Many salons provide clients with attractive pamphlets or cards giving information about the salon such as:

- Telephone/fax number.
- Contact name (or names).
- Opening times and day.
- Dates, times and prices of any repeat appointments.
- Price list of services.

With this ready to hand a client who is pleased with a salon's services will find it easy to return.

Things to do

Of the various skin and scalp complaints listed in this section there are some which you may never see and others which are far more common. The infectious conditions you will almost certainly come across are clients with head lice while common non-infectious conditions will include male baldness and dandruff. These exercises are designed to give you extra information about hair and scalp conditions and to help you tell a client that he or she has head lice. Explain your answers clearly.

1 Go to a pharmacy, chemist, hospital out-patient or local health clinic and pick up leaflets and pamphlets on hair and skin conditions. Make a summary of the information given and actions to take.

2 Contact your local area health authority and find out what activities they are involved in concerning hair and skin conditions. Do they, for example, screen school children for head lice? If so, how often, and what do they advise for the infestation? Do any other skin or scalp conditions arise?

3 Imagine you have just discovered that a client has head lice. What are the most likely signs? How can you be sure? How would you tell the client?

4 Design a poster 30 × 60 cm (12" × 24") to be used to promote a special offer in your salon. The special offer can be for either retail as goods or salon services. You may use any medium you wish to achieve your result, e.g. pastel, paint, crayon, ink, pictures and letters cut from magazines, stencils, etc. Sketch your ideas in rough before you start your final piece of work, it will help you to organise your ideas.

What do you know?

Level 2 Unit 1

Name the process which causes hair growth. ☐

What name is given to the part of the hair above the skin? ☐

What are the average width and depth of a hair follicle? ☐

What is meant by the term 'parasite'? ☐

What is the difference between an infection and an infestation? ☐

What is meant by the 'transmission' of a disease? ☐

What is the main purpose of salon hygiene? ☐

What is the key word for dealing with a client possibly suffering from an infectious or contagious scalp condition? ☐

What precautions should be taken with a client suffering from 'barber's itch' (sycosis barbae)? ☐

What are the major symptoms of scalp ringworm (tinea capitis)? ☐

What are the major symptoms of psoriasis? ☐

Why does eczema sometimes produce a secondary infection? ☐

Which **two** factors cause male pattern baldness? ☐

What is traction alopecia? ☐

With regard to hairdressing, what three areas can selling be divided into? ☐

How can the standard of work in a salon be improved and maintained? ☐

Why is it important that salon staff look neat, smart and professional? ☐

Why are staff often reluctant to use or recommend new products? ☐

How can using a variety of hairdressing techniques in the salon, which are visually different, help/promote the selling of salon services? ☐

What is the best place to display the retail goods and why? ☐

What advantage does the stylist have over the shop assistant when selling products for the hair? ☐

Name **three** ideas which could be used to promote and boost retail sales. ☐

What strategies can be used to overcome nervousness when selling? ☐

List the types of questions which are relevant to selling. ☐

SHAMPOOING AND CONDITIONING

Shampooing as a means of cleaning the hair

The cleansing process involves removing the dirt which has become stuck to the surface of the hair and skin. It requires the consideration of three factors:

1 The dirt on the hair shaft.
2 The surface of hair and skin.
3 The final condition of the hair and skin.

The dirt on hair shaft

Hair (or skin) is made dirty by a wide range of materials like skin flakes, dust particles of many types, salt from dried sweat and so on. These in themselves may rapidly dissolve in water, but they are also mixed with the oily sebum which coats the hair and skin. This combination will not dissolve easily in water and therefore water alone is not able to clean the hair or skin efficiently.

The surface of hair and skin

Skin, when viewed closely by the unaided eye, shows pits and small wrinkles. When seen through a microscope, the outer cornified layer of the skin appears as a rough, flaking surface. Similarly, the outer cuticle of the hair shaft, with its overlapping scales presents a rough surface, even when the hair is in good condition.

A rough surface, like those of skin and hair, presents a large number of places where dirt can lodge and means that the water must be able to penetrate into these microscopic hollows and cavities in order to remove the dirt.

The final condition of the hair and skin

It is important that at the end of cleaning hair and skin their outer layers are left undamaged and that some natural oil remains. Sebum has an important function in preventing skin and hair from becoming dry and brittle. A cleaning action that is too efficient will 'strip' the hair and skin of all the sebum. With hair, the hair shaft is dead and the hair can be coated with a controlled amount of oil from a conditioner. With skin, the drying and cracking of the cornified layer allows micro-organisms and chemicals to penetrate to the living cells of the germinative (basal) layer just underneath. The chemicals may cause dermatitis, and the micro-organisms, infections.

Cleaning action of shampoo

Shampoos clean by their ability to:

- Reduce surface tension of the water.
- Help the water to remove the oil and dirt from hair and skin and to prevent it being redeposited.

Surface tension

This results from the attraction of water molecules at the surfaces of the liquid, i.e. where it is in contact with other materials, towards the molecules in the rest of the liquid. This means that the water surface will tend to contract to cover the smallest possible area and form a surface 'film'. This can be seen at the air/water surface (a meniscus) on which it is possible to place an object or in the way that droplets are spherical. This surface tension film occurs when the water surface is against the hair and skin and prevents the water from penetrating into the rough surface of the skin's cornified layer or the hair cuticle.

Shampoo reduces the surface tension of water, which allows it to penetrate into all parts of the surface of hair and skin. The process of bringing the water and surface to be cleaned into more intimate contact is described as **surface activity**. Because of this, soap and shampoo are sometimes described as **surfactants** (short for *surface active agents*).

Removal of dirt

Water cannot properly dissolve oily materials, like sebum, but it can break them up into tiny droplets, i.e. emulsify them. Shampoos will attach to the oily dirt on hair and skin, remove them as tiny droplets, i.e. emulsify the oil (see Fig. 2.7) and prevent the droplets from going back on to the hair in two ways:

1 The shampoo molecules surround the oil droplets and keep them separate from one another, i.e. keep them emulsified.
2 The shampoo molecules coat the surface of the skin or hair and prevent the oil droplets from being redeposited.

To summarise, shampoos help water clean hair and skin by:

- Reducing surface tension in the water, allowing the water to wet or penetrate the surface of hair and skin more effectively.
- Acting as an emulsifying agent, causing the breaking off of the oily dirt into tiny droplets, which are then prevented from redepositing on the hair or skin.

Scalp massage

This is the name given to the rubbing action involved in cleaning hair or skin. The rubbing or the massaging of shampoo on to the scalp causes:

- A good mixing of the water and shampoo or soap.
- A good penetration by the soap or shampoo/water mixture on to the skin or hair surface.
- An emulsification of the oil and dirt as tiny droplets.

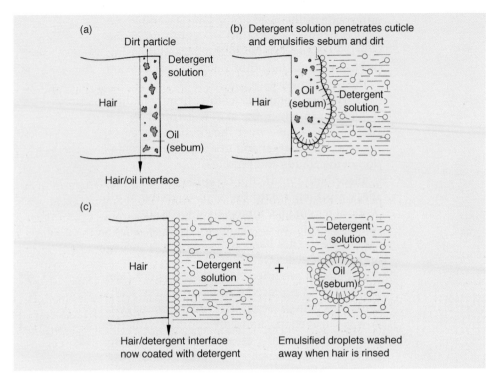

Fig. 2.7 Cleaning action of detergents on hair

There are three scalp massage techniques used in shampooing hair. They are used to work the shampoo well into the hair and to encourage emulsification of the oil and dirt.

How to carry out hand massage

Hand massage should be carried out with sure, firm movements. Nails should be kept to a reasonable length to prevent scratching the scalp and the hands and wrists should always remain flexible.

There are three main types of hand massage used in hairdressing:

- Effleurage.
- Petrissage (rotary).
- Friction.

SAFETY TIP
Jerky, uncontrolled movements can be uncomfortable or even painful to the client.

It must be stated that there are many other forms of hand massage but these are mainly used on other areas of the body and therefore do not come under the jurisdiction of the hairdresser.

Effleurage is a slow stroking movement applied to the scalp with the fingers and palms in a slow rhythmic manner. It is used at the beginning and end of each massage treatment to relax muscles and relieve tension.

Both hands are held at the centre, front of the head and then pulled firmly down the back of the head to the nape (see Fig 2.8). The hands are then placed at either side of the head at the temples and again pulled firmly back round the contours at the sides of the head down to the neck and easing out to the shoulders; thus relieving any tension in the neck muscles.

Petrissage (rotary) is a slow, firm kneading movement in which the skin is gripped by the fingers and rotated over the skull. It increases the blood circulation and gives deeper stimulation of the glands and muscles.

Place both hands in a claw-like position on the scalp then rotate the skin over the skull without moving the fingers over the scalp.

The right hand moves in a clockwise direction while the left hand moves in the opposite, anti-clockwise direction.

The hands are lifted from their position one at a time and replaced elsewhere on the scalp until the whole scalp has been massaged. Always leave one hand in contact with the scalp when removing the other to ensure continuity of the massage. If both hands are removed together the massage becomes jerky and unpleasant.

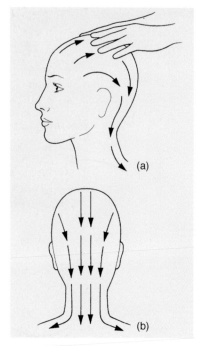

Fig 2.8

Friction is the most well known of all hand massage movements as this is the movement used when shampooing the hair. Friction is also a kneading movement and the fingers are still rotated in opposite directions for each hand. Unlike petrissage however, the movements are quite quick and vigorous with the fingers moving over the surface of the skin.

The hand is held in a claw-like position and the pads of the fingers are moved firmly over the scalp in circular movements away from the hair line up to the crown, then from the nape up to the front of the head and back down to the nape again.

Table 2.6 gives a summary of the hand massages.

Table 2.6

Movement	Description	Use
Effleurage	A gentle stroking movement.	To relax muscles and relieve tension. Used at the beginning and end of each treatment.
Petrissage	Slow, firm, kneading movement.	To increase circulation and to stimulate glands and muscles.
Friction	Quicker kneading movement with pressure applied.	To improve circulation and glandular activity, used when shampooing.

Shampoo ingredients

In addition to a soapless detergent, e.g. sodium lauryl ether sulphate, many shampoos contain the following:

1 An **auxiliary** detergent. These are weak detergents which alone are not very effective at removing oil from the hair, but they:

- thicken the shampoo
- help to maintain a rich lather
- condition the hair
- increase the solubility of the main soapless detergent

2 Common salt (sodium chloride). This is often added to thicken the shampoo.
3 Acids, e.g. **citric acid** (as lemon juice in lemon shampoo), which conditions the hair by leaving it slightly acid after shampooing. These are often called 'pH balance' or 'acid balance' shampoos.
4 Antiseptics and chemicals which inhibit the early stages of dandruff. Zinc pyrithone has both properties and is found in medicated or anti-dandruff shampoos.

Special shampoos for various types of hair

Various conditioners and additives are used in the shampoos designed for various types of hair.

Dry hair

This results from either insufficient sebum being produced by the scalp or too much sebum being removed during chemical processes like bleaching and perming.

The aim is to replace the natural oils in sebum with other oils:

- Lanolin – used in cream shampoos.
- Plant oils, e.g. olive oil used in oil shampoos (designed for very dry hair).

Note: Shampoos designed for greasy hair have a higher proportion of soapless detergent to remove the surplus oil.

Damaged hair

The aim is to coat the hair and, if possible, fill in the missing particles of cuticle. This group includes:

- **Egg shampoo** – where a raw egg is added. The egg proteins coat the hair and the scalp and act as a barrier on the scalp to other chemicals in the shampoo. For this reason, it is recommended for sensitive scalps.
- **Beer shampoo** – where beer is added. The coating slightly thickens each hair and so adds body to the whole head.
- **Protein shampoo** – these contain proteins which have been broken down into a mixture of single and short chains of amino acids. There is some evidence that these will be absorbed by the porous regions of the hair, i.e. they are substantive to the hair, but this is not entirely accepted.
- **Herbal shampoo** – may contain one or a variety of herbal extracts. Whether these substances condition the hair is far from clear, but they are usually used to add a sheen and gloss to the hair. Examples of herbal extracts include rosemary, sage, camomile, etc.

Brightening shampoo

This is a mild bleach containing a soapless detergent with 10 vol. (3 per cent) hydrogen peroxide.

Colour shampoo

This contains a temporary dye in addition to the soapless detergent. The dye belongs to the azo group and coats the hair cuticle but is easily washed off after a few shampoos.

Dry powder shampoo

This is used where it is difficult to carry out a wet shampoo; when a person is bed-bound for example. It contains a mild alkali mixed with an absorbent powder like starch. The alkali breaks down (or saponifies) a little of the sebum on the hair, so making a soap. This soap then cleans the hair during the thorough massage that follows. The powder absorbs the soap/oil mixture.

Table 2.7 gives a summary of the main types of shampoo and their uses.

Table 2.7

Type	Use
Cream	Dry, brittle hair, bleached, tinted, permed, African Caribbean hair.
Oil	Extremely dry, bleached, tinted, permed, African Caribbean hair.
Medicated	Mild dandruff.
Egg	Sensitive scalps, children's hair.
Beer	Lank, fine hair.
Lemon	To adjust pH to between 4 and 6 after hair has been bleached, tinted or permed.
Protein	Limp, chemically damaged hair.
Herbal	To add sheen.
pH balance	To adjust pH to 4–6, useful on chemically damaged hair.
Dry powder	Invalids, in between shampoos.
Brightening	Mild bleach, e.g. to highlight dull hair.
Colour	Temporary tints.

Precautions when shampooing

1 The client must be adequately protected, i.e. clothes should be completely covered by a gown and towels tucked well down at the nape. If a front wash is to be used, the client should be given a face cloth to protect their eyes (and possible make-up).

2 Hair must by thoroughly disentangled prior to shampooing.

> **TECHNICAL TIP**
> Always follow the manufacturer's instructions for shampoo type. Some conditioning-type shampoos may need to be left on the hair for a few minutes.

3 The temperature of the water should be checked on the wrist or the back of the hand before allowing the water to run on the scalp.

4 Correct shampoo should be used for the type of hair.
5 Liquid shampoo should be allowed to run over the back of the hand then on the scalp to minimise coldness.
6 Cream shampoo should be applied to the palm of the hand before being evenly distributed over the whole head.
7 Friction hand massage should be used in circular movements from hairline to crown, throughout the whole head.
8 Care must be taken to ensure that the hair is thoroughly rinsed after each massage.
9 After shampooing, hair should be towel dried and disentangled away from the face.

POINTS TO REMEMBER

- Hot water taps should be turned off during massage unless a mixer tap is used, in which case the whole tap is turned off. This is to conserve hot water.
- Never allow the client to leave the shampoo area with hair dripping on to the face. Always wrap hair in a towel to keep the head warm if the client is required to move about in the salon.

Greasy hair

Greasy hair is caused by the over-activity of the sebaceous glands which produce far more sebum than is necessary to coat the skin and hair. This excess sebum forms a sticky coating on the skin and hair enabling dirt and bacteria to adhere to it easily. Without regular attention the bacteria can cause dandruff, and if a fringe is worn, it can also be the cause of spots and blackheads on the forehead

Young teenagers, particularly during puberty, are especially prone to this condition, and unfortunately, the over-activity of the sebaceous glands is not confined to the scalp area alone. The skin on the face is often affected and this can give rise to common acne (acne vulgaris). It is possible to give help and guidance for this in three important areas.

Diet
Whether a high level of fats or sugars in the diet is linked to excessive sebum production is not clear. There is conflicting evidence for and against each view. As the majority of people take in far more fat and sugar than is necessary there is no harm in erring on the side of caution and suggesting their intake be reduced.

Drying aids
There are many products which are now manufactured especially for greasy hair. These include: shampoos, setting lotions and special conditioners without the addition of oils or waxes. Common salt also has a drying effect on the hair. However, it is well worth remembering that bleaching, tinting and perming are all processes that dry the hair and can be used to combat oiliness. They also have the added advantages of making the hair look better and also increase trade in the salon.

Shampooing
There is no evidence that frequent shampooing results in the excess production of sebum. Most oily hair requires washing every two or three days. A dry shampoo used between shampoos is often useful to absorb some of the unwanted sebum

but vigorous brushing of the hair should be avoided at all times as this stimulates the sebaceous glands and distributes the excess sebum along the entire length of the hair shaft.

Shampoos containing oils or creams should be avoided. A soapless shampoo with no additives is the most effective, but it should not be used at too high a concentration, particularly if the hair has to be shampooed frequently.

Shampooing African Caribbean hair

The basic operation is the same as for European hair but African Caribbean tends to be dry and therefore specially formulated products often contain lanolin as a substitute for natural oils. Particular care must be taken in combing through. Always use an 'Afro' type comb which slides through the hair more easily.

Conditioning the hair and scalp

Hair condition

The hair shaft is dead and cannot repair itself in the way that living parts of the body can. Yet the condition of each individual hair shaft determines the overall condition of the whole head of hair.

In the average life of a typical scalp hair, it may have been:

- Brushed and combed nearly 10,000 times.
- Washed (using a shampoo) about 600 times.
- Blowdried (after the shampoo) about 600 times.
- Permanently waved about 16 times.
- Tinted (perhaps with a bleach included) 40 times.

It says much for the toughness of the hair structure that it can stand up to all this punishment without disintegrating. Hair does 'age', however, and the oldest hair is that at the hair points, which has usually suffered more damage than that near the scalp. This needs to be considered in terms of the processing time in bleaching, tinting and perming hair.

A key factor in hair condition is the degree of **cuticle damage**. This can result from a number of factors which will be classed here as 'internal' and 'external'.

Internal factors influencing hair condition

Age
General slowing down of hair growth and production of the natural sebum results in dry hair and scalp. Unpigmented hair may have a coarser texture than pigmented hair which can also create difficulties when styling hair.

Diet
A well-balanced diet is essential for healthy hair. It has been suggested that there is a link between high sugar and oil intake and greasy hair and skin. However, expert opinion tends to be divided on this.

Drugs and illness

Both can have a profound effect on the hair, and even an illness as simple as the common cold can alter hair condition. With more serious illnesses, the drugs and treatment used can cause rapid thinning and even baldness, e.g. chemotherapy. A hormone imbalance or fever illnesses, e.g. glandular fever, can also cause thinning of the hair.

Internal reasons for hair in poor condition are largely beyond the control of the hairdresser. However, even if the hairdresser is only able to improve the hair superficially, there are still psychological benefits to the client by improving the hair visually.

External factors influencing hair condition

These can either be physical (or mechanical) damage – caused by brushing, combing and heat or chemical damage – caused by the chemical treatments and the ultraviolet rays in sunlight.

In reality both types will almost certainly be involved in determining the condition of a client's hair.

Physical (or mechanical) damage

When the hair is in good condition the cuticle scales of the hair shaft are tight into the hair. This makes the hair smooth and shiny. When combing or brushing (and especially backcombing or backbrushing) hair, the mechanical scraping of the brush bristles or comb teeth across the cuticle roughens it. This leaves the hair dull and liable to further mechanical or chemical damage. The increased friction caused by roughened hair can lead to the production of static electricity in the hair and this can cause 'hair fly', thus making the hair less manageable.

Tight rollers, pins or clips on the hair can cause physical damage, especially on chemically treated hair. The hair normally contains some water, chemically bound to the cortex fibrils and some of this water can be lost from the hair by blow-drying or by the drying effect of the atmosphere. Reduction in the water content of hair reduces its elasticity and this influences the movement of the hair.

Chemical damage

This includes both the 'natural' damage caused by the ultraviolet rays in sunlight and that caused by the chemical treatments used in hairdressing.

The pH scale and hair condition

The pH scale is a 14-point scale which measures acidity or alkalinity.

- pH 7 is neutral, neither acid nor alkaline
- below pH 7 is acid
- above pH 7 is alkaline

Hair is in its best condition if slightly acid (pH 5.5) but many hairdressing processes upset this pH 'balance' as can be seen in Fig 2.9.

Details on how conditioners are used to restore or balance hair pH are given in the section on acid-type conditioners on page 89.

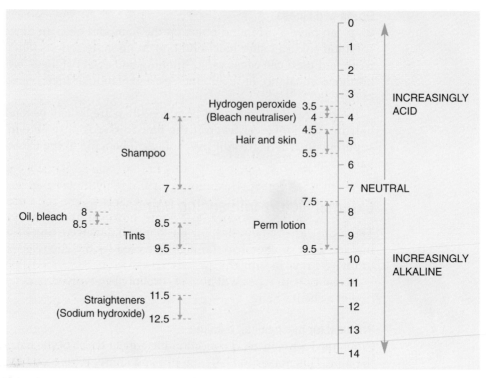

Fig. 2.9 Effects of chemicals on the pH balance

Types of conditioners

There are three general types of conditioners, based on their main ingredients and actions. These are:

- Oil based – which are the traditional conditioners.
- Substantive type – where material 'adds' to the hair.
- Acid type.

Oil-based conditioners: external or surface conditioners

Sometimes called **emollients** or **conditioning creams**, these are the simplest method of conditioning. The oil added to the hair, in a measured dose, is to replace the natural oils removed by shampooing, perming, tinting or bleaching. The oils used are often in the form of an **emulsion** in water, which makes spreading on to the hair easier, and are left coating the hair when the water evaporates. **Lanolin** (from sheep's wool) or slightly altered forms of lanolin are a good substitute for human sebum and are often used.

To ensure that the conditioning effect lasts beyond the next shampoo, moist heat, e.g. hot towels or a steamer, can be used to swell the cuticle allowing the conditioner to penetrate deeper into the hair shaft. As the hair cools, the cuticle scales close, trapping some of the conditioner between them, thus preventing complete removal at the next shampoo.

Substantive-type conditioners: internal conditioners

These become fixed to, or absorbed into, the hair shaft, mainly due to the **electric charge** on the conditioner molecule and the hair shaft. This category includes some soapless detergents and **polyvinylpyrrolidone** (PVP) which acts as both a setting agent and a conditioner.

Other materials which appear to be absorbed by the hair include the protein conditioners (sometimes called **restructurants**). Because the hair is dead it cannot be 'fed', but does have the ability to absorb small polypeptide chains and single amino acids. These are produced by breaking down animal or plant proteins and the evidence is that some is deposited on the cuticle and some passes through the cuticle into the cortex. The amount absorbed by the hair seems to increase in the more damaged areas of the hair shaft, which is a very good property for a conditioner to have. The evidence does show, however, that this type of conditioner is most effective at protecting the hair from damage; so it is best applied before a perm, tint or bleach is carried out. Whether protein conditioners used after the treatment in any way increase the tensile strength or elasticity of the hair is not clear, although some evidence seems to indicate that they do.

Acid-type conditioners

These are based on the natural skin and hair secretions (e.g. sebum and sweat) having a pH of between 4 and 6. They produce an **acid mantle** over the hair and since pH does influence hair condition in that at acid pH the cuticle scales are flat, the hair is then smooth and shines. In alkaline pH the cuticle swells and the scales open slightly so the hair is rough and dull and more liable to both physical and chemical damage. Acids also help to hold the water soluble products produced by perm lotion and peroxide attacking the hair. Without an acid pH these can be washed from the hair during shampooing and weaken it.

There are two types of acid conditioners:

- **pH restorers** – contain organic acids, e.g. **citric acid**, and have a pH of about 3. They are used to chemically neutralise the alkaline deposits left on the hair after perming, bleaching and tinting and are formulated to leave the hair with a pH of about 4.
- **pH balancers** – are mildly acidic, e.g. pH 6. They are used, for example, in pH balance shampoos to ensure the final pH of the hair is acidic. Organic acids are used, e.g. **citric**, **tartaric** and **lactic acids**.

Conditioning treatments

This involves practical methods used to improve the hair's condition and a first step is to find the cause of a client's hair being in poor condition.

How to find the cause of poor hair condition

Before starting any treatment, first make a visual and tactile analysis of the hair and scalp. This assessment will give a good indication as to the extent of the damage and will also indicate the depth of treatment that will be needed to restore the hair to a natural, healthy state.

Question the client as to the possible reason for the damage. Very often the client will have a good idea as to the cause of the hair's present condition, particularly if prompted with suggestions from the hairdresser. However, always remember to question the client tactfully and sympathetically – they obviously know that their hair is not at its best otherwise they would not want the treatment!

Consider the following areas when assessing the hair and scalp:

Hair assessment
- *Hair types*: Is the hair dry, brittle, greasy or wiry?
- *Hair texture*: Is the hair fine, medium or thick?
- *Hair porosity*: Is there a high degree of porosity? If so, has this been caused by chemical or physical factors such as bleach, tint, straighteners, permanent wave solution, sunlight or heat? Or is it because the client's hair has above average porosity?

> **TECHNICAL TIP**
> Know the products and treatments available, their uses *and* their limitations.

- *Hair abnormalities/diseases*: Are there any of the following present: fragilitis crinium (split ends), monilethrix (beading), alopecia (baldness)? If so, what has caused this?

Scalp assessment
- *Skin type*: Is the skin dry, greasy or normal?
- *Skin abnormalities/diseases*: Are any of the following present: psoriasis, pityriasis capitis (dry dandruff), seborrhoea (greasy dandruff)?

Choosing the treatment

Before choosing any treatment the hairdresser must have a sound knowledge of the products available and must be aware of their limitations. Never promise the client instant, lustrous locks if the hair is badly damaged – instead, explain what the treatment will do, how many treatments will be needed and why. Hair can be so badly damaged as to be almost beyond repair and the only real remedy would be to remove it from the head by cutting until new, undamaged hair takes its place! However, even this type of hair can be made more supple and therefore easier to handle by careful and thorough use of restructurants, conditioners, oils, etc. Knowing which product to use and how to make it more effective is essential if the client is to have confidence in the hairdresser's judgement.

The intended effect of any hair/scalp treatment is to make the hair more supple and to improve the circulation of the blood. An improved blood supply brings more food and oxygen to the hair and scalp which encourages hair growth and makes the sebaceous glands more active.

Heat and massage increase the blood supply to the scalp by causing the blood capillaries in the skin to dilate so that more blood flows into the skin; this can be clearly seen when the scalp turns pink in colour.

Heat treatments

A heat treatment can be carried out in various ways depending on the source of heat.

Sources of heat
1 **Steamer** – produces warm, moist heat.
2 **Hot towels** – produce warm, moist heat. Their temperature should be 60 °C.
3 **Accelerator or infra-red** – produces heat only, therefore has a more drying effect.

TECHNICAL TIP
Use distilled water in the steamer kettle to prevent any limescale deposit reducing the efficiency of the equipment.

4 **Rollerball machine** – this produces infra-red and has a fan to speed up the processing. The advantages of these machines are that the:
   - source of heat moves around the machine so hair is heated evenly
   - hairdressing operations can still be carried out while the client is sitting under the rollerball
5 **Climazone** – produces even, warm heat.

Massage treatments

Massage is a form of manipulation which can be achieved either with the hands or mechanically with either the vibro or high frequency machine. The psychological value of massage has been very underrated in the past and this is one area in hairdressing that salons have not exploited to the full. Very few salons provide treatments which include the use of all the forms of massage, particularly when carrying out oil or conditioning treatments.

POINTS TO REMEMBER

A good massage, expertly carried out, not only benefits the hair and scalp but also gives the client a feeling of well-being.

Uses of massage
- To soothe and relax the client.
- To stimulate the sebaceous glands of the scalp to produce the natural oil, sebum.
- To increase blood circulation in the skin capillaries and therefore to aid nourishment of the hair and scalp.
- To soften and improve skin texture by making it more pliable.
- To ease contracted tissue, e.g. in the neck muscles.

Types of massage available
There are two types of massage:

- Hand massage.
- Vibro massage.

Hand massage
The types of hand massage are:

- Effleurage.
- Petrissage.
- Friction.

These are covered earlier in this Unit – see page 81.

Vibro massage

Vibro massage is a mechanical massage that uses electricity as its source of power. The vibration produced by the machine causes friction between the applicators and the scalp which stimulates the scalp. Do not be tempted to use added pressure when massaging with the vibro machine as this could be uncomfortable for the client.

There are three main rubber applicators for use with the vibro machine (see Fig. 2.10):

- Spiked applicator.
- Sponge applicator.
- Rubber-domed bell or flat vulcanite applicator.

The spiked applicator (rubber pronged) is the attachment most commonly used in hairdressing as the rubber prongs will move through the hair quite easily. It is used on the scalp in either circular or straight movements (see Fig. 2.11).

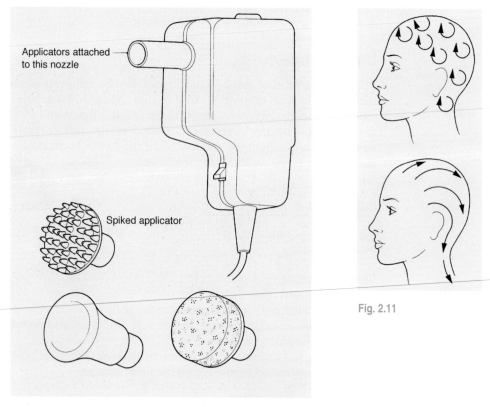

Applicators attached to this nozzle

Spiked applicator

Fig. 2.11

Fig. 2.10

Types of conditioning products

The hairdresser should not only know which conditioning products are available but also how they work before the client can be advised as to which is the most suitable for their particular hair type.

Hairdressing manufacturers spend a lot of money and research to produce whole ranges of hair care products for particular hair types and common hair or scalp disorders, the choice of which depends largely upon personal preference.

However, before buying a whole new range of products, try them first to assess the results. Most manufacturers are only too willing to provide a sample of the product to prove its worth. It is very important that the hairdresser has every confidence in the product used and knows exactly the limitation of that product. Remember that the client will be disappointed if the results are not as good as they were led to expect. Do not be afraid to explain to the client how a course of treatments may be necessary to achieve a good result – if the hair or scalp has been mistreated or neglected it is unfair to expect it to be miraculously transformed overnight!

It would be virtually impossible to list every kind of hair/scalp disorder and give a full account of each treatment. However, the two most popular types of treatment will be dealt with in more detail as these can be adapted to meet a variety of needs.

A basic conditioning treatment

A conditioning treatment will have a more lasting effect on the hair than a conditioning rinse which is merely rinsed through the hair after shampooing. Any types of conditioning agent may be used for the treatment, either a pH balance or the more traditional type depending upon the requirements of the hair.

Uses of a conditioning treatment

- To replace the natural oil of the hair and scalp.
- To ensure that the hair has the correct pH.
- To lubricate and moisten dry hair, thus making it more supple and easier to handle.
- To soften and improve the texture of the skin by making it more pliable.
- To relax the muscles and relieve tension.
- To increase sebaceous activity if this is necessary.
- To increase the blood circulation and stimulate the glands and muscles of the scalp allowing them to be more effective.

Hot oil treatment

Oil treatments are of maximum benefit to the client who suffers from a dry, tight scalp and dry brittle hair due to the inactivity of the sebaceous glands.

Vegetable oil is used in preference to mineral oil as it is more easily absorbed into the skin and hair than mineral oil. Deep massage movements with a combination of hand and vibro massage is recommended with this type of treatment to loosen the scalp and stimulate the sebaceous glands helping them to produce more sebum. The massage also helps to remove any flakes of dry skin that may adhere to the scalp.

Purposes of hot oil treatment

- To lubricate the scalp thus making it more supple and elastic.
- To soften brittle hair caused by lack of sebum, giving it a healthier shine.

- To loosen the scalp by relaxing the muscles and relieving any tension.
- To increase sebaceous activity.
- To increase the blood circulation and stimulate the glands and muscles of the scalp allowing them to be more effective.

Method of application

1 Adequately protect the client with a gown and towel, making sure that the towel is tucked firmly down at the nape.
2 Assemble the equipment and heat the oil by pouring it into a small bowl then placing this in a larger bowl filled with hot water. This is known as a water bath. The oil should be heated to a temperature of 55 °C.
3 Disentangle the hair and check the scalp for cuts and abrasions.
4 Divide the hair into six sections as for a conditioning treatment. (See Level 1 Unit 1.)
5 Wrap a hot moist towel around the head or steam the hair for five minutes under a steamer. This swells the hair and opens the cuticle scales thus aiding absorption of the oil.
6 Check the temperature of the oil and, while the hair and scalp are still warm, apply the warm oil to the scalp using a cotton wool swab or brush.
7 Application should commence at the nape and continue up towards the front, working from side to side as quickly as possible.
8 When application is complete, draw the oil through the lengths of the hair by massaging the scalp. First with the effleurage movements, to soothe and relax then with a petrissage hand massage to stimulate the sebaceous glands and loosen the scalp.
9 Apply the steamer for 10–15 minutes or use several hot moist towels.
10 Massage the scalp again while the hair and scalp are still warm. The vibro machine may be used at this point but the massage should be concluded with an effleurage hand massage.
11 To remove the oil, add soapless shampoo directly onto the hair before applying water. Massage the shampoo into the hair using friction movements until it emulsifies with the oil. This can be seen to happen when the oil becomes white and creamy and the hair no longer lathers.
12 Rinse the hair thoroughly in warm water and shampoo again with soapless shampoo. It is often necessary to shampoo the hair several times to completely remove all traces of the oil from the hair. Should any be left on the hair, the hair will become lank and greasy when it has been dried.
13 After the final rinsing, towel dry the hair then distangle ready for setting or blowdrying.
14 Complete a detailed record of the work carried out.
15 Advise the client on the after-care of the treatment.

Record keeping

A detailed record should be kept of all hairdressing treatments, particularly those that will be carried out over a period of weeks. This builds up a very clear picture as to how the hair is reacting and progressing with the treatment and any modifications to the treatment, e.g. increasing or decreasing the massage time or even changing the product can be done without getting in a muddle. (See Fig. 2.12 for an example.)

RECORD CARD
HAIR/SCALP TREATMENT

Name: .... Tel No: ....

Address: ....

....

Hair assessment	Type	Porosity	Diseases/abnormalities
Scalp assessment	Skin type		Diseases/abnormalities
Cause of damage			

Date	Conditioner/ lotion	Type of massage	Time	Source of heat	Time	Result

Fig. 2.12

Things to do

1 The following table has been devised to help you to recognise various hair types, to choose the correct shampoo and to be aware of necessary safety procedures when shampooing.

Collect hair cuttings of the following types of hair then attach them to a piece of paper. Select a suitable shampoo for each type giving reasons for your choice. Set out your work in the format shown below.

Hair type	Hair cutting	Suitable shampoo	Reasons for choice
Permed Fine textured Coarse textured Tinted Bleached			

Next take samples of five (or more) different shampoos. Try to make these a range of types and prices. You may also find it interesting to include your own favourite type.

On small sections of your own or someone else's hair, try out shampooing with equal amounts of each shampoo. Compare them in terms of:

- thickness
- colour
- scent
- lathering
- cleaning action
- hair condition after shampooing

Put your findings into table form.

You can set the shampoos a more difficult task by moisturising the fingers with a little mineral or vegetable oil and putting this on to the hair first. This will produce hair which is very greasy. Wash the small sections as before.

2 The condition of the hair has an important effect on all of our hairdressing services. This assignment aims to help you to identify the characteristics, both visual and tactile, which show whether the hair is in good or poor condition. You will need:

- two sheets of A4 card
- scissors, pencils, ruler
- chosen materials for the collage
- glue or cow gum

Now read the following two statements before beginning the task:

Hair in poor condition feels rough, dry and brittle. It looks dull, lifeless and without shine.
Hair in good condition feels supple, bouncy and pliable. It looks shiny, healthy and gleaming.

Using the above descriptions of the hair, create two collages: one to illustrate hair in poor condition and one to illustrate hair in good condition.

Each collage must be on an A4 size card with a 2.5 cm (1″) border. You may work with any medium to create the effect that you want, e.g. silver paper, foil, egg boxes, fabrics, dried pulses or pasta, empty cartons, tacks or nails and/or any other materials which you feel will give the visual and tactile (touch) illusion of the two hair conditions.

Assemble all your equipment and materials then work out your designs in rough before placing the materials on the card. Do not glue or stick your materials to the card until you are completely satisfied with the result. When the design is finished and firmly glued in place, either draw a 2.5 cm (1″) border around it or mount it on another larger piece of card which will give the same size border.

3 Design a record card similar to Fig. 2.12 and fill in the details of a real or an imaginary client.

What do you know?

Level 2 Unit 2

What is meant by the term 'surface tension'? ☐

Shampoos reduce surface tension. Explain why this is important in cleaning hair. ☐

What is meant by the term 'emulsify'? ☐

Why should the water used for a shampoo be run over the hairdresser's hand before spraying onto the client's head? ☐

After shampooing, why should hair be dried and disentangled away from the client's face? ☐

*List **three** common additives in shampoo and explain what each does.* ☐

What is a 'pH balance' shampoo? How do such shampoos work? ☐

What types of shampoo should be avoided with a client with greasy hair? ☐

List **four** factors involved in hair condition. ☐

What effect does heat have on hair condition? ☐

Explain why backcombing or backbrushing hair may cause more damage than brushing or combing. ☐

Why is hair that has been made alkaline by chemical treatments, rough and dull? ☐

In what form are most oil-based conditioners applied to the hair? ☐

Distinguish between 'pH restorers' and 'pH balancers'. ☐

Why is a well-balanced diet important to maintain healthy hair? ☐

Why does age play an important part in the condition of the hair? ☐

Which layer of the hair directly affects its porosity? ☐

What is the purpose of a pH conditioner? ☐

Name the layer of the hair which is most affected by restructurant conditioners. ☐

What is the natural oil of the hair and scalp called? ☐

Which type of vibratory application is most suitable for use on the head? ☐

What effect does massage have on the blood capillaries? ☐

DRYING HAIR

How it works

Hair is **hygroscopic**, which means that it is capable of absorbing moisture. When the hair is shampooed, a small amount of water penetrates the outside cuticle of the hair and enters into the cortex. Once inside the cortex, the water breaks some of the weak, water breakable 'H' (hydrogen) bonds that help to hold the polypeptide chains in position. Breaking these bonds enables the polypeptide chains to move slightly past each other allowing the hair to be moulded into a new position. The action of drying the hair then removes the water from the cortex, refixing the 'H' bonds in a new position and holding the hair in whatever shape it has been moulded into.

When hair is in its normal, unstretched state it is known as **alpha (A) keratin** and when it is moulded or stretched and then dried into a new shape it is referred to as **beta (B) keratin**. Thus, a physical change takes place in the hair when it goes from A (unstretched) to B (stretched).

However, as stated previously, hair is hygroscopic and will, over a period of time, absorb any moisture from the atmosphere around it. This moisture again breaks the 'H' bonds causing the hair to revert back to its natural, unstretched state which is why a blowdry or set appears to 'drop out'.

Drying and dressing aids contain water-repellent substances which coat the hair and help to prevent the absorption of atmospheric moisture allowing the hairstyle to 'last' longer.

Before drying the hair

Each head of hair is different and before deciding on how it should be dried other factors such as type of equipment and the most suitable products to use must also be decided upon. Factors which will influence the decisions the stylist makes will include:

- Head and face shape.
- Problem features.
- Texture of hair and hair cut/shape.
- Hair growth patterns.
- Personality and lifestyle of client.

Head and face shape

The shape of the hair can alter the shape of the face by emphasising good features and minimising others.

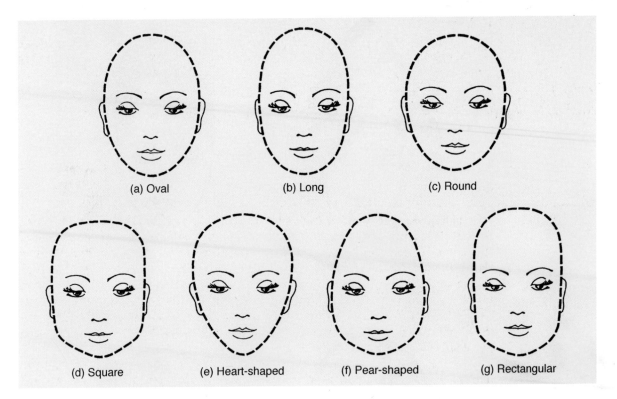

Fig. 2.13 Basic face shapes

Facial structure

It is important that the professional stylist is able to recognise the various facial shapes. An oval face shape (see Fig 2.13(a)) is believed to be the perfect shape and the stylist must aim to achieve the illusion of an oval shape on their client. Other face shapes are shown in Fig. 2.13.

Long face

To avoid a long face effect, create width at the sides using loose soft waves or curls. Medium length hair is best with the fullness around the ears. Fringes can shorten the effect of an over-long face. This is shown in Fig. 2.14.

Round face

Short hair is most suitable for a round face, with height on top of the head and the side hair flat, preferably covering the cheeks. An asymmetrical hairstyle or a parting will minimise the roundness but a full fringe across the forehead will emphasis the roundness of the lower face. This is shown in Fig. 2.15.

Square face

A soft design is needed to reduce the angular jawline. Fullness at the temples and cheekbones gives an illusion of roundness and the face shape can be softened by covering the jawline if possible. This is shown in Fig. 2.16.

Heart-shaped face

Play down width at the temples and create fullness round the chin. An asymmetrical style or a side parting also looks effective on this face shape, as shown in Fig. 2.17.

Drying Hair 99

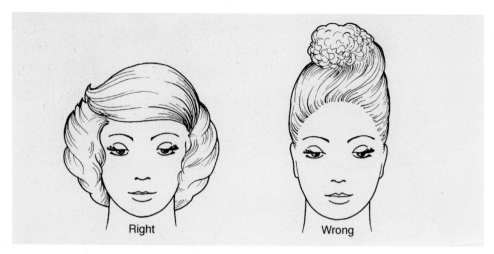

Fig. 2.14 Possible styles for a long face

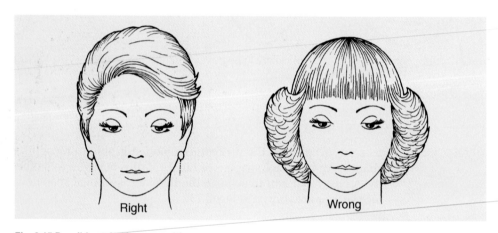

Fig. 2.15 Possible styles for a round face

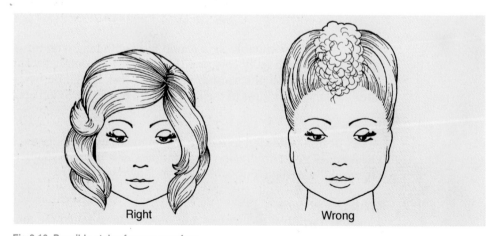

Fig 2.16. Possible styles for a square face

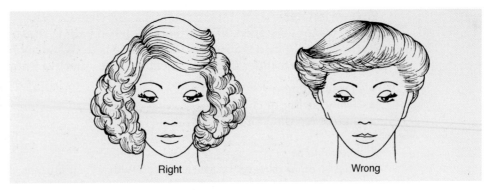

Fig. 2.17 Possible styles for a heart-shaped face

Pear-shaped face

Hair should be given width above the chin and left soft at the nape to soften the lower part of the face This is shown in Fig. 2.18.

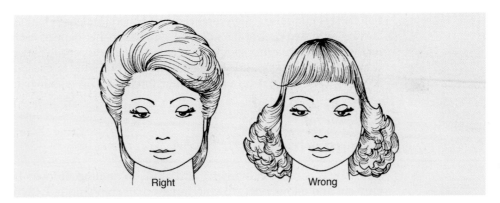

Fig. 2.18 Possible styles for a pear-shaped face

Rectangular face

Longer than a square-shaped face but with the same strong jawline that should be disguised with softness around this area. A fringe will help reduce the length of the face and a side parting offsets the angular features of this face shape. This is shown in Fig. 2.19.

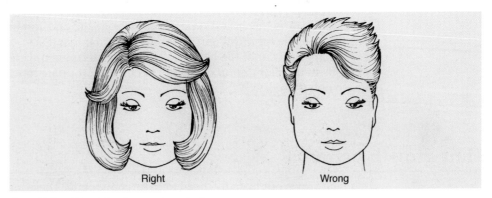

Fig. 2.19 Possible styles for a rectangular face

Problem features

Where features are good, the hair may be pulled back to reveal them but problem features should be disguised so that the eye is drawn away from them and the more attractive features then gain attention. Less attractive features include:

- Prominent nose.
- Heavy jawline or chin.
- High or receding forehead.

Prominent nose

Emphasise other parts of the face and head with soft curls at the chin line or hair that hugs the face. If a fringe is worn it should be full and loose. Avoid centre partings as this emphasises the length of the nose and draws attention to it. (See Fig. 2.20.)

Heavy jawline or chin

A smooth definite style that clings to the jawline should be used. Fringes help to balance the face. Hair that is drawn back from the face will accentuate the jawline. (See Fig. 2.21.)

High or receding forehead

Full fringes minimise a high forehead and a medium length hairstyle, either smoothly curving or flicked back at the sides will emphasise the shape of the head rather than the forehead. Centre parting should be avoided but a side parting may be used if the hair is draped across the forehead. A side parting will make the forehead appear broader and so will only be effective on a narrow high forehead. This is shown in Fig. 2.22.

Texture of hair and hair cut/shape

Fine hair is narrow in diameter and tends to be limp. It looks its fullest when it is club cut and allowed to grow no longer than chin length. Extremely fine, lank hair may also require a soft perm to give it extra body without a great deal of curl. Finger drying this type of hair can be problematic as it is difficult to obtain enough root lift or volume by this method. Blowdrying on smaller brushes is often more effective.

Coarse hair has a larger diameter and is usually strong and wiry. It can be allowed to grow longer unless it is also very curly in which case it will go very bushy. Coarse hair may have to be layered or thinned to make it more controllable. When drying coarse, bushy hair is may be necessary to use a larger brush. Avoid giving the style too much root lift as this can increase its 'bushiness' unless, of course, the style requires a lot of volume.

Medium hair is the easiest type of hair to manage and combined with medium body it is suitable for most hairstyles and most hair lengths.

The shape and cut of the hairstyle will also determine the most effective drying technique to use. For example, it is not usually appropriate to scrunch, finger dry a smooth bob style.

Hair growth patterns

Each hair grows out from the head at a different angle. These angles determine the way the hair 'falls' and gives it a hair growth pattern. Whenever the hair is

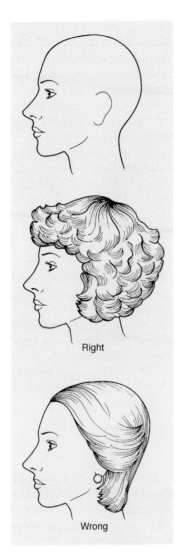

Fig. 2.20 Styling for a prominent nose

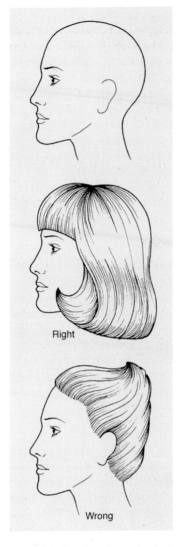

Fig. 2.21 Styling for a heavy jawline

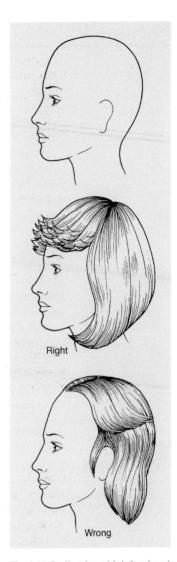

Fig. 2.22 Styling for a high forehead

moulded into a shape either by finger, blow or natural drying, the direction of the hair's growth pattern **must** be taken into account before starting the treatment.

Always try to incorporate the natural fall or any movement of the hair into the finished style, this will make it last much longer. Any imperfections such as double crown, awkward hairline, etc., should be carefully camouflaged by the way it is styled.

Preventing RSI

Create mini-breaks (30 seconds or so) to move around and rest your hands and arms. You might use this time to explain to your client how to maintain the style, which conditioners or shampoos to use, etc. Be resourceful – your client will appreciate the special attention, so the time is not wasted. Making the client's next appointment gives you a rest and encourages your client to return.

Personality and lifestyle of the client

The client's finished hairstyle should meet their needs, and therefore their lifestyle and personality will have a definite effect on the type of style they require. Sporting hobbies create the need for a sleek, well-cut, easy-to-manage hairstyle, whereas a client who entertains a great deal will probably require a more elaborate hairstyle. Likewise, a quiet, subdued person will not thank the stylist for an outrageous style whilst a person with an extrovert personality probably would!

When the client arrives, look at the style of clothes and the image they currently project, find out if they wish to change their image and what they expect of the style. In other words, look and listen very carefully to the client *before* beginning the treatment. Client consultation is extremely important to enable the stylist to use the correct products, equipment and techniques to give the best results.

Choice of product

There are many products available to make the hair more manageable, in better condition or to prolong the life of the style. It is often easier for a salon to carry the full range of one particular manufacturer, as this ensures that the needs of any type of hair can be met and also enables the staff to have a more in-depth knowledge of a full range of products. The types of products which aid the drying process include mousses, gels, hair thickeners, blowdry lotions, restructurants, moisturisers or activators. The types of finishing products which help to dress the hair and maintain the hairstyle include hair sprays, waxes, gels, dressing creams, moisturisers or activators. A description of these products and how they work can be found in Unit 11 on setting.

Tools and equipment used when drying hair

Hair is usually dried with a drier. Hand-held driers are used when blowdrying, blow waving or finger drying the hair whilst a stand drier is used when the hair has been set. Alternatively, infra-red heat produced by the 'octopus', climazone or roller ball machines is usually used when the hair requires natural drying.

Tools used when drying the hair include:

- Brushes.
- Styling irons.
- Hot brushes.
- Pressing combs.
- Combs.
- Diffuser.

Brushes

Natural bristle brushes are kindest to the hair. Both hair and bristle are composed of keratin and so neither wears against the other. Nylon brushes have a harsher effect on the hair and tend to increase static electricity and cause 'hair fly' but they are useful in hairdressing because they are easily cleaned and sterilised, thus cutting down on the risk of infection between clients. The bristles of any brush should have even tufts or rows to allow loose, shed hair to collect in the grooves without interfering with the action of the bristles. Styling brushes are used when blowdrying the hair. These can be obtained in various sizes and shapes depending upon the result required. Nylon, bristle or a combination of both is the material used.

TECHNICAL TIP
If the bristle tufts of brushes are spaced too close together, they will not penetrate the hair.

Styling irons

Electrically heated styling irons include:

- **Hair tongs** – round and usually obtained in small, medium and large sizes and used to create curl or movement, e.g. after blowdrying, between sets, etc.
- **Crimping irons** – specifically designed to produce a crimped effect on the hair.
- **Straightening irons** – originally designed to temporarily straighten African Caribbean hair but now also used on Caucasian (European) hair to produce straight or flattened results.

POINTS TO REMEMBER

Metal tools should not be left in a vapour-type sterilising cabinet for too long, as the chemicals used in these cabinets can cause corrosion.

Hot brushes

These work on the same principle and have the same use as round styling irons except that instead of just a smooth electrically heated barrel, the hot brush also has vulcanite prongs attached that act as a brush. Thus, the hair can be combed and curled into position more easily.

Preventing RSI
Take care when blowdrying as the wrist motion with the brush can result in painful inflammation of tendons at the elbows. Learn to alternate hands for the drier and the brush.

Pressing combs

There are two types of pressing combs: electrical and non-electrical. The comb has metal prongs (steel or brass) and a wooden or vulcanite handle. These are used to temporarily straighten African Caribbean and extremely curly hair. The comb is heated then combed through the hair.

Combs

These are useful when drying short hair when a brush would give too much lift. A comb is often used when blow waving men's hair as it allows more control particularly in conjunction with the flattened nozzle attachment of the hand drier.

Diffuser

This is an attachment which fixes onto the end of the hand drier in place of the nozzle. The diffuser disperses the air over a larger area instead of concentrating it in a stream onto the hair. It also lessens the force of the air, making it easier for the stylist to manipulate the hair with the fingers when either finger drying or scrunch drying.

Drying techniques

There are a variety of drying techniques available to the stylist. They may be used individually or combined to produce various effects on specific hair types. The most common drying techniques in current use include:

- Blowdrying.
- Finger drying.
- Blow waving.
- Natural drying.

Blowdrying

Blowdrying is used to create a natural, soft effect and the finished result should be smooth and 'bouncy' (see Fig. 2.23).

There are many methods of blowdrying the hair and each operator may use slight variations to achieve the same result. However, there are certain precautions to take, regardless of the method used, to ensure a successful finish.

Before commencing a blowdry

1 *Always* talk to the client to find out their requirements before beginning the treatment.
2 Client must be well protected with gown and towel.
3 Hair must be scrupulously clean and in good condition. The use of a conditioner after shampooing is often beneficial (use an oil-free conditioner if the hair tends to be greasy) and will give a healthier, shinier finish to the style.
4 Note the texture of the hair. Fine hair will require more body than thick hair, therefore the finer the hair the smaller the diameter of the brush to be used.
5 Note the amount of curl present in the hair. Curly hair requires more control (especially at the roots) than straighter hair. Taking smaller sections of hair when drying helps to overcome this problem.
6 Note the direction of the hair growth. Do not work against hair growth as hair could stick up, become unmanageable and the style will not last.

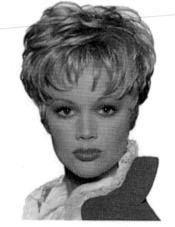

Fig. 2.23 Style created by blowdrying

7 A conditioning blowstyling lotion ensures a more durable style and helps reduce static electricity.
8 The sectioning of longer hair helps the operator to work more quickly, methodically and efficiently.
9 Combing hair in the direction of the desired style, particularly short hair, helps the operator to dry the hair in the correct direction.

While blowdrying

1 The jet of air should follow the direction of the brush and hair. Never blow against the cuticle of the hair as this can be damaging and give a rough finish to the style.

2 Never allow the jet of air to flow onto the client's scalp as it can cause burns to the skin.

3 Maintain plenty of lift at the roots, particularly at the crown area unless the style dictates otherwise.

4 Ensure that each section of hair is completely dry before proceeding to the next. If the hair is not sufficiently dried then a capillary action takes place between this damp hair and any dry hair and the shape of the style will not last.

5 The size of the sections depends on the size of the brush. The smaller the brush, the smaller the section. Taking too large a section and dragging the hair can make the style flat.

6 Greater curl and body can be achieved by winding the hair around the brush, drying with a hot jet of air and then allowing the hair to cool still wrapped around the brush. For speed, the brush is left in the hair while cooling takes place and another brush of the same size is used on the next section of hair.

7 Ensure that the points of the hair are dried evenly around the brush. Rotating the brush while drying helps to prevent 'kinking' of the hair. Remember that hair will dry where it is placed and if the points or roots of the hair are buckled while drying, the finished result will be buckled.

8 In the case of very short hair, finger drying (i.e. drying the hair with the fingers instead of a brush) is sometimes more effective. Short hair at the nape, on the sides or on the fringe is often better dried by this method as a brush gives too much lift to this length of hair.

9 Blowdrying long hair can be tedious and time consuming. To save time it is often easier to dry off the roots of the hair by brushing it in the opposite direction than the finished style and allowing the jet of air to dry the root section only in this position. When the hair is combed back into its original position there is then a good degree of lift at the roots. The points of the hair are then dried in the direction of the style.

After blowdrying

1 When blowdrying is completed, allow the hair to cool thoroughly then check that the hair is completely dry. Warm hair often gives the illusion of dryness while it is still damp.

2 Comb or brush the hair into the finished style. Check that the sides are blended into the back and that all partings are straight and clean. Pay particular attention to the nape area to ensure that the shape is pleasing and check the balance of the finished dressing from the front, sides and back of the head, making full use of the mirror.

3 Apply a fine spray of lacquer or shine and smooth down any flyaway hairs with the back of the comb or palm of the hand.

Blowdrying African Caribbean hair

The technique of blowdrying is essentially the same for all types of hair. However, African Caribbean hair does not usually blowdry successfully unless it has been temporarily straightened by 'soft pressing' first (see Level 3 Unit 8). The hair can then be moulded into shape using round brushes and heat from the drier in place of curling tongs.

Finger drying

This is drying the hair with the fingers to create a tousled, natural effect. The hair is combed in the direction of the finished style and the fingers are then used to create lift and movement when needed. A hand drier with a diffuser attachment is often used and the air is directed to the roots of the hair as it is moulded by the fingers (see Fig. 2.24). The hair may also be squeezed between the fingers whilst it is dried to give more movement. This is known as 'scrunch' drying the hair. This is particularly useful for clients who prefer a more 'natural' look to their hair.

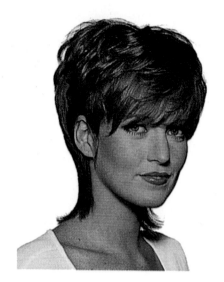

Fig. 2.24 Style created by finger drying

Blow waving

Blow waving the hair is a method of waving the hair, producing soft natural movements with the aid of a comb or brush and heated air from a hand hair drier. The hair is held in a wave position and a flattened nozzle drier attachment directs and concentrates the flow of heated air. The control required to form wave shapes is determined by movements of the comb or brush and drier, in relation to the hair position. It is mainly used in men's hairdressing.

> **SAFETY TIP**
> Take care not to burn the fingers with the jet of air when finger drying the hair.

Method

1 Commence at front hairline and follow any natural movement.
2 Insert the comb in the hair, using the coarse end of the comb, and with a backward combing movement, grip and hold the hair in a wave crest.
3 Direct the hot air on to the centre of the wave in the opposite direction to which the comb is held.
4 The comb movement is similar to a finger waving movement and half strength air flow should be used or the force will blow the hair out of the comb.
5 Continually move the drier along the hair; in this way the heat is evenly directed and does not burn the head.

Natural drying

As its name suggests, this is leaving the hair to dry naturally. Comb the hair into the position of the finished dressing. It is sometimes easier to use a very wide toothed comb to do this, particularly if the hair is curly. It is often useful to lift the hair out from the head at the root to give some lift to the style. Putting the head upside down then letting it fall back is also a way of achieving root lift. When the hair is in position the client is placed under an infra-red heat machine to speed up the drying time.

Do not be tempted to recomb or brush the hair whilst it is drying; curly hair will frizz and the effect will be spoilt.

Health and safety

- Check that electrical wires on equipment are safe before use.
- *Always* dry hands before using any electrical equipment.
- Take care not to have trailing electrical wires; either you or the client may trip and be injured.
- Take all necessary precautions when using electrical equipment (see Level 2 Unit 10 for greater detail).
- Be aware of any adverse effects of the products being used.
- Do not splash or spill any product onto the client, especially into the eyes, or on the floor. Either will create a safety hazard.
- *Always* follow the manufacturers' instructions for the products being used.

Things to do

Talking to clients can be a very daunting prospect for some trainees. To help you to overcome any initial shyness, fill in the following checklist for each client over a period of one week. At the end of this time you should then feel more comfortable when talking to the clients.

Checklist for client consultation

1   Is the client: New ☐

    Been once before ☐

    Regular ☐

2   What is the client's name?

3   Where does the client live?

4   What is the client's occupation?

5   Does the client have any hobbies? If yes, what?

6   Does the client have a family (including pets)? If yes, what?

7   Is the client going somewhere special? If yes, where?

8   Is the client going on holiday? If yes, where and when?

9   What product/s does the client usually use on their hair? (e.g. mousse, gel, lacquer, etc.)

10 Does the client's hairstyle usually 'stay in' well? If no, what could be the cause?

11 Does the client's hair need a perm/conditioning treatment/colour?

12 If yes, what have you recommended?

13 What after-care advice have you given to the client?

14 Are there any retail sales suitable for the client's hair? If yes, what?

15 Has the client made another appointment?

What do you know?

Level 1 Unit 4

List five influencing factors which need to be considered before drying the hair ☐

What type of style favours a long face? ☐

How can a style be designed to minimise a heavy jawline or chin? ☐

What type of drying makes hair appear fullest? ☐

What contrast could there be for a hair design for a person who regularly:

- *plays sports?*
- *entertains guests?* ☐

List the different hair textures. ☐

What are the reasons for considering the hair growth direction when drying hair? ☐

Explain what happens inside the hair when it is wet, moulded then dried. ☐

Explain what is meant by 'hygroscopic'. ☐

List the drying techniques currently available to the stylist. ☐

CUTTING HAIR

The cutting of hair is one of the most important of all the hairdressing skills. A good haircut, skilfully executed, can transform the most mediocre head of hair into something special. To cut hair proficiently the hairdresser must be aware of where and how the length and bulk (thickness) need to be removed from the hair in order to create a desirable shape with good line and balance. Each head of hair differs in some way and each haircut should be carefully cut to emphasise any good points and minimise any defects.

Remember that a good haircut is the basis for all good hairdressing. When a blowdry or set has 'dropped' from the hair, all that remains is the shape of the haircut!

The various methods and techniques of cutting hair can be seen in Table 2.8 on page 126.

Haircutting tools

These include:

- Scissors.
- Razors.
- Clippers.
- Combs.
- Neck brush.

Scissors

These may be obtained in a variety of lengths and weights. The choice of length and weight is entirely up to the individual but it is important that the scissors feel comfortable. When purchasing a new pair of scissors, test them first by holding between the thumb and the third finger, as this is how they should be held when cutting the hair – they should feel as if they are an extension of the fingers.

Hairdressing scissors should only be used for cutting hair. Using them for cutting string, paper, etc., will blunt the blades very quickly and blunt blades will tear the hair.

> **Preventing RSI**
> Choose your scissors carefully, making sure that they fit your hand; operate smoothly with the minimum of effort; are a proper size for the job; are as light as they can be while being sturdy enough for the amount of use they will get; are balanced for easy control; and can be sharpened easily. Get the best you can afford and replace them when you find a better pair.

Types of scissors

- **Plain straight edged** – used for normal cutting including both club and taper cutting techniques. The longer blade lengths are used in men's haircutting. (See Fig. 2.25.)
- **Very fine serrated edge** – these scissors are intended to be self-sharpening. They can be used for all cutting techniques except when 'slither cutting' the hair, e.g. taper cutting or slide cutting. In this case the finely serrated edge of the scissors tends to drag on the hair and does not cut it as cleanly as the straight-edged scissors.
- **Wide-spaced serrated edge** – these are known as aesculap scissors. Either one blade or both blades are serrated to allow a limited amount of hair only to be cut. This type of scissor is usually used to remove bulk or weight from the hair, i.e. thinning. However, there are many different types of aesculap scissors, some designed to remove far more hair than others. The choice of aesculap depends upon the required result and also the stylist's own personal preference. They must only be used on dry hair – if used on wet hair they can remove too much bulk as the wet hairs tend to stick together. (See Fig 2.26.)

TECHNICAL TIP

Scissors should always be used by the same person and should not be dropped on the floor as this can alter the balance.

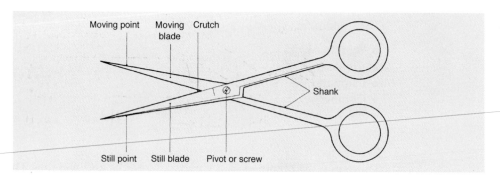

Fig. 2.25

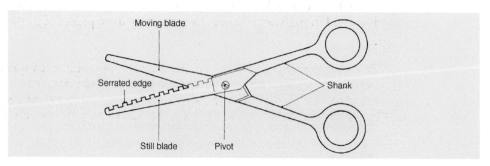

Fig. 2.26

Razors

Razors are used to cut wet hair. There are two types:

- Open.
- Guarded or safety razor.

Open razor

An open, or cut-throat, razor requires far more attention than a safety razor and is more commonly used in men's hairdressing. The blade of the razor must be kept very sharp, by what is known as **razor setting**. This involves sharpening the blade on a special stone, known as a **hone**, and then stropping on a leather **strop**. An open razor is shown in Fig. 2.27.

The solid bladed French razor is the most suitable open razor for cutting hair as it is more rigid than the hollow-ground razor and is, therefore, more stable on the hair.

> **SAFETY TIP**
> The blade of the safety razor must be changed frequently and the old blade discarded, as a blunt blade will tear the hair and is painful to the client.

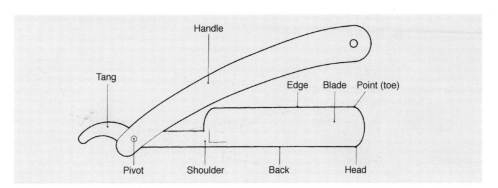

Fig. 2.27

Guarded or safety razor

The guarded razor differs from the open razor in that it has a replaceable blade which is protected by a metal guard and is attached to a fixed or movable handle. It is either what is known as a 'shaper' razor or it is shaped like an open razor, and it is used in preference to the open razor by most present-day salons.

Clippers

There are two types of clippers: hand clippers and electric clippers. Both types consist of two blades with sharp edged teeth. One blade remains fixed while the other moves across it. The distance between the blade teeth determines the closeness of the haircut. Used in men's and ladies' haircutting to produce very short haircuts.

> **SAFETY TIP**
> Combs with broken or irregular teeth should not be used as they may scratch the scalp or tear the hair.

Combs

Cutting combs are smaller and thinner than other combs. They are also more pliable and allow the hair to be cut nearer to the scalp; for example, men's graduation, short back and sides, shingle.

> **SAFETY TIP**
> When not in use and after use on each client, combs should be kept completely submerged in an antiseptic solution of correct strength or in the sterilising cabinet

Neck brush

These are used to remove the loose hairs from the face and the neck after cutting the hair. Made from bristle, nylon or a combination of both.

Basic haircutting techniques

There are three main haircutting methods that can be employed to produce particular effects on the various types of hair. Blowdrying and the movement towards natural looking hair has helped to encourage a greater responsibility on the part of the hairdresser to produce better haircutting. To this end, it is necessary to become proficient in the various methods of cutting to enable the hairdresser to adapt these methods to any fashion changes.

The basic techniques are:

- Tapering.
- Thinning.
- Clubbing.

Tapering

This method removes bulk and length from the hair, in other words, it will thin the hair at the same time as removing the length. By thinning the hair, a lot of the hair bulk (or weight) is also removed, thus it will allow the hair to curl more easily. Obviously, this type of cutting will not make straight hair curly, but it can encourage any natural curl or wave movement already present in the hair.

Hair can be tapered either wet or dry. The scissors are used in a slithering movement to taper dry hair. Taper cutting wet hair with the scissors can tear the hair and may also cause 'steps' because of the hair's tendency to stick together when wet.

When taper cutting wet hair the razor is used. Using a razor to cut dry hair is undesirable because the blade of the razor tends to pull the hair, making it a painful experience for the client!

Taper cutting dry hair

Hold the section of hair to be cut firmly between the first and second fingers. Then, using a backcombing or slithering action with the open blades of the scissors near to the crutch, direct the scissors from the points of the hair to the middle lengths. The blades should be closed very slightly during the stroke towards the scalp, then opened again drawing the scissors away from the scalp. Never completely close the scissors during the stroke towards the scalp as this could remove too much hair and create 'steps' in the haircut.

Alternatively, the section of hair may be backcombed slightly before cutting. This will produce less taper than without using backcombing. The more the hair is backcombed, the less taper is produced .

Taper cutting wet hair

Take the mesh of hair to be cut and with the razor blade held at a slight angle to the mesh, make a light slicing movement from the mid-lengths to the points of the hair, either on top or underneath the section of hair. The pressure on the blade will determine how much of the hair is cut away and the length of the stroke will determine the amount of taper. (See Fig 2.28).

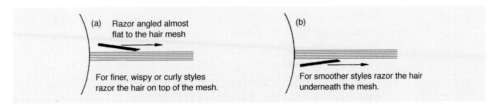

(a) Razor angled almost flat to the hair mesh

For finer, wispy or curly styles razor the hair on top of the mesh.

(b)

For smoother styles razor the hair underneath the mesh.

Fig. 2.28

Uses of tapering

- To remove excess length and bulk (thickness) from thick hair.
- To encourage natural curl and wave movement by removing the weight from the points of the hair.
- To re-introduce natural taper into over-clubbed hair.
- Before a basic permanent wave, to aid winding – hair which has finer, tapered points will bend much more easily around a perm rod than thicker, clubbed hair.
- To produce a lighter, feathered effect to the hairstyle.

Thinning (or bulk reducing)

This method removes unwanted bulk, but not length from the hair. It may be done with the scissors, razor or aesculap scissors but it must be remembered that the scissors and aesculap scissors should only be used to thin out dry hair and the razor used to thin out wet hair.

Check the hair carefully to decide where on the head the bulk needs to be reduced, as it is not always necessary to thin out the whole head. "

The following areas on the scalp should never be thinned because of their growth direction patterns and the possibility of unwanted spiky effects or odd hairs sticking out from the scalp if the hair is cut too short:

- The hairline, particularly at the front.
- Along a parting.
- The crown area.

Preventing RSI

Take note of your hand and wrist positions and motions. Try to keep in neutral position and to alternate motions.

Thinning dry hair using scissors

Divide off the areas that should not be thinned, then taking approximately 10 mm (½") width sections, hold the hair out from the scalp at right angles. Using the points of the scissors, remove a few hairs from the root area and along the hairshaft. Continue in this manner until the whole head, or the parts that require thinning, have been completed. Take care not to remove too much hair at the root area as these hairs will tend to 'spike out' when they grow if too many have been removed.

Thinning dry hair using aesculap scissors

Divide off the areas that should not be thinned, then taking larger width meshes than thinning with the scissors, approximately 2 cm (1") in depth, hold the hair out from the scalp at right angles. The aesculap scissors are then inserted into the sections at an angle. The hair is cut in a zig-zag pattern along the length (see Fig. 2.29). Continue in this manner until the whole head, or the parts that require thinning, have been completed.

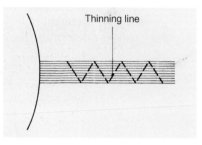

Fig. 2.29

Thinning wet hair using a razor

Divide off the areas which should not be thinned, then taking approximately 1 cm (½") sections hold the hair out from the scalp at right angles. With the tip of the razor, remove a few hairs at the root and along the hair shaft. Alternatively, the hair may be thinned out by using shorter and extra slicing movements on each hair mesh while actually razor cutting the hair (removing length at the same time); in this case, the slicing movements are commenced closer to the scalp.

Uses of thinning

- To remove excess bulk from the hair.
- To give a finer, feathered effect to certain areas of a hairstyle.
- To remove the weight from over-clubbed hair.

Club cutting

Club cutting is a method of cutting the hair bluntly straight across, thereby removing the length from the hair but retaining the bulk. Because the weight is left on the points of the hair it tends to discourage any natural tendency of the hair to curl. Hair can be club cut wet or dry, either using the scissors or a razor. However, club cutting with a razor requires a lot of practice and should only be attempted when the operator is fully proficient in razor cutting.

Club cutting allows the hair to be cut very precisely, but it must always be remembered that the head is a curved object, and although the hair may be cut in a straight line, the angle at which the hair is held away from the scalp is very important to produce the correct shape for the finished haircut.

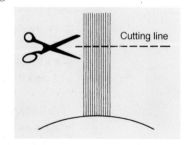

Fig. 2.30

Club cutting wet or dry hair

Vertical or horizontal sections of hair are held from the scalp at an angle and the points of the hair are cut straight across either between fingers or, if the hair is to be cut very close to the scalp, over the comb, with the scissors (see Fig. 2.30).

Uses of club cutting

- On fine hair, to retain as much bulk and weight in the hair as possible.
- To discourage curl on over-curly hair.
- For fashion cutting, where weight needs to be retained.

Haircutting shapes

There are various shapes that can be cut into the hair using either taper or club cutting:

- Solid form.
- Uniform layering.
- Low layering.
- Reverse graduation.
- Increased layering.

Solid form

Most commonly known as a 'bob' where all the hair is cut to the same base line. This gives a 'chunky' effect to the ends of the hair and produces a square shape. There is no graduation in this hair shape and it is very useful for finer hair to make it appear as thick and dense as possible (see Fig. 2.31).

Uniform layering

This is when the inner hair length is the same as the outer hair length. This is achieved by lifting the hair out from the head at a 90° angle and cutting to the same length all over, i.e. the same length at the front, sides, nape, crown, etc. This results in a rounded effect which is to the shape of the head. (see Fig. 2.32).

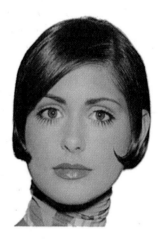

Fig. 2.31 A 'bob' haircut

Low layering

A haircut with the inner hair length longer than the outline hair length. Pulling the hair down at a 45° angle, as opposed to lifting it up, creates less graduation. It is interesting to note that the less graduation there is in the hair, the more of the hair bulk remains see (Fig. 2.33). Thus, finer hair can have as much thickness as possible retained by club cutting the hair into a style with very little graduation, while thicker hair can have some of the weight or thickness removed by thinning and cutting the hair into a style which requires layering.

A 'wedge' is an example of this hair shape and the low graduation of this cut creates a triangular shape (see Fig. 2.34).

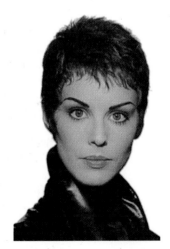

Fig. 2.32 Uniform layering

Reverse graduation

This technique is used when the top layers or inner length of the hair are longer than the underneath layers of the hair, e.g. a bob or pageboy style (see Fig 2.35). But in this case the inner hair length is also longer than the base line.

Increased layering

This is when the inner hair length is shorter than the outer hair length. Increased layering on long hair is a good example of extreme angles, where the hair is cut from short on the top or front, to long at the nape (see Fig. 2.36). The difference in lengths at these two points is very great and therefore the angle of the haircut is very steep. By cutting a guideline at the shortest point, then combing all the hair up to this guideline and cutting straight across at this point, very steep graduation is achieved. To cut the hair vertically and to hold the fingers at this steep angle would be very difficult and it is unlikely that each section of hair could be cut at exactly the same angle all round the head.

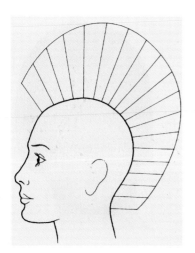

Fig. 2.33

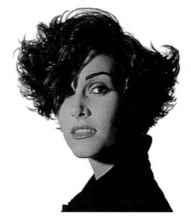

Fig. 2.34 Wedge cut

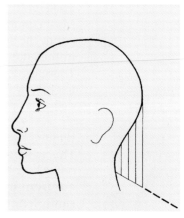

Fig. 2.35 Reverse graduation

What is graduation?

Graduation is sometimes referred to as **layering**. Increased layering is when the hair is steeply graduated and low layering is when there is little graduation. Graduation can be achieved by either club cutting or taper cutting, whichever is the most suitable for the hair type and the finished dressing. It is attained when the top layers of the hair lie above the lower layers. The top layers may lie well above the lower layers, in which case there would be a high degree of graduation, but if all the top layers lie just above the lower layers then there is less graduation.

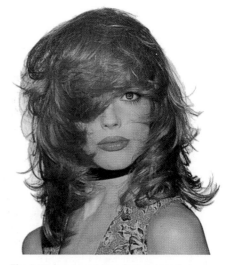

Fig. 2.36 Increased layering on long hair

Increasing graduation

By increasing the graduation the amount of layering in the hair is also increased. The more the hair sections are lifted, the greater the graduation. When the hair is held down close to the head, at a 0° angle, a bob effect is the result, which contains no graduation. At each degree of lift of hair away from the head the more graduation is achieved. To help with the understanding of the degrees of lift, it is useful to remember that a 90° lift means that the hair is held straight out from the head at right angles. Thus, a 45° lift is half this amount and a 180° lift is twice the lift of 90°.

- **45° lift** (see Fig. 2.37(a)) – this will create slight graduation, usually used for wedges, etc.
- **90° lift** (see Fig. 2.37(b)) – this will create twice as much graduation, usually used for short, uniform layered shapes.
- **90°–180° lift** (see Fig. 2.37(c)) – this will create a great deal of graduation, usually used for long, high layered styles.

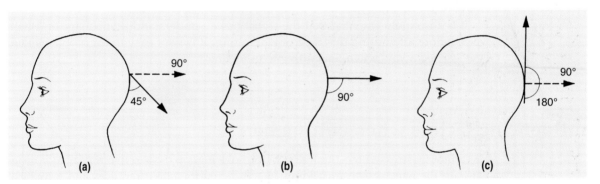

Fig. 2.37

Scissor over comb

This technique can cut the hair extremely short and was originally used in men's haircutting and the ladies' shingle of the 1920s.

A fine, pliable comb is used to allow the hair to be cut as close to the scalp as possible. The hair is combed upwards from the nape and the hair which protrudes through the teeth of the comb is cut off. If scissors are being used, they should rest along the length of the comb and should open and close quickly whilst the comb is moving up the head. If the scissor movement is too slow then steps will occur in the haircut.

Alternatively, the clippers may be used with the comb in place of the scissors. If this is the case, make sure that the clipper head is in the correct position to enable it to remove all of the hair protruding through the comb.

The angle at which the comb is held will determine the length of the hair, if it is held next to the scalp then the hair will be very short, the further away from the scalp that it is held then the longer the hair.

Electric or hand clippers can be used on their own in place of the scissors and comb. The clipper heads have attachments which are numbered according to their depth, thus the lower the number the shorter it will cut the hair.

A special comb known as a *Brian Drummer Flat Topper* can also be used with the clippers in place of the attachments. It has a spirit level incorporated into it so that the stylist can make sure that the hair is completely level when cutting.

POINTS TO REMEMBER

No matter what type of haircut is being carried out it is very important to keep the client's head in the correct position. If it is inadvertently held to one side during cutting then the finished haircut will be lopsided!

Cutting hair freehand

Cutting hair freehand requires skill and confidence as it involves cutting the hair without holding it in place. Many of the more advanced cutting techniques such as slither cutting or chipping into the hair are done by this method as is the majority of clipper cutting and the cutting of African Caribbean hair.

It is absolutely essential that the stylist has an understanding of shape and balance before attempting this type of haircutting. It is very easy to hit problems and get 'carried away' when not cutting to guidelines!

Influencing factors when cutting hair

It cannot be stressed too often that before placing a pair of scissors near to a head of hair, the hairdresser must know exactly what the client requires and how best to achieve that result. It is too late when the hair has been cut to realise that the client's requirements have been misunderstood, or even ignored!

Clients are often nervous when they visit a salon for the first time, particularly when they require a haircut. Talking to the client and discussing the requirements enables the hairdresser to find out exactly what the client needs and expects from the haircut. It also helps to build up a relationship of trust and confidence between the client and the hairdresser. Remember that the client is a very important person and if displeased with the finished result the client will not return to the salon, nor will they recommend the salon to their friends.

To prevent unnecessary mishaps, and to gain enough information to allow the hairdresser to proceed with confidence, two main areas must be explored:

- Assessment of the client.
- Assessment of the hair.

Assessment of the client

This is meant to determine the client's requirements and enables the hairdresser to advise the client on any modifications of the chosen haircut that may be necessary.

It is important to question the client closely; they may know exactly what they have in mind but have great difficulty in describing the exact haircut. If this is the case, it is often useful to keep a book of fashionable hairstyles available in the salon to show the client. Thus, the hairdresser will have a visual description of the style or 'look' that the client is aiming for.

The following factors must also be taken into consideration as they will influence the suitability of the chosen haircut:

- Face shape and prominent features.
- Neck length.
- Body size.
- Age, hobbies and lifestyle.

Face shape and prominent features

The finished shape of the haircut should suit and flatter the client. This seems a very obvious statement, but it is surprising how many hairdressers disregard the shape of the client's face when restyling the hair. Take a good look at the client's face by drawing the hair away from the face to determine whether it is round, square, long, oval, etc.; this can affect the amount of hair that needs to be removed and will also help to determine the shape of the finished haircut. Next, check whether there are any prominent features or blemishes that need to be camouflaged, e.g. a receding chin. Some prominent features can be attractive and therefore need to be emphasised, e.g. the eyes can be emphasised by a fringe.

Neck length

If the client has a very long neck the hair needs to be left longer in the nape. Alternatively, a very short neck looks less obvious if the hair is kept shorter in the nape or is swept up towards the top of the head to make the neck appear longer.

Body size

The finished haircut should be part of a total look, not just a separate item that happens to be attached to the client's head! For example, a very tall, slim client with a small head would look ridiculous with a short, scalp-hugging haircut.

Age, hobbies and lifestyle

The age of the client is a very important consideration. A middle-aged person does not always suit the same style as a teenager, although a current fashion trend can often be adapted to meet the needs of both, as long as it is not too extreme.

The general lifestyle and hobbies of the client also need to be considered. When assessing a client's personality, clothes, etc., it is important not to gown up until starting the procedure. Also find out if the client will have enough spare time to spend on an elaborate hairstyle or whether they will need a style that requires the minimum amount of time spent on it between salon visits. These and many other questions need to be asked to find out exactly what the client expects and requires of the haircut.

Assessment of the hair

This is to determine the type and method of cutting to use. Remember that it is sometimes necessary to combine a variety of haircutting techniques on one head to achieve the required shape.

Whenever possible, use the type of hair to its best advantage – it is very difficult, if not impossible, to create a long, smooth bob style on very thick, wiry, naturally curly hair. It is far better to utilise the curl and thickness of the hair to create a style that requires these features. Consider the following:

- Hair texture.
- Hair volume.
- Hair length.
- Amount of natural curl or movement present in the hair.
- Growth direction of the hair.

Hair texture

The texture of the hair refers to the diameter of the hair and can either be fine, thick or medium. Fine hair will need all the bulk retained, heavy clubbing helps to do this. Thick or coarse hair may need to have some of the bulk removed, in which case it may be necessary to thin, taper or high layer the hair, depending upon the finished style. Medium-textured hair is usually no problem and adapts to most cutting techniques, again depending upon the finished style.

Hair volume

This is the amount of hair on the scalp, or how densely the hair grows. A client may have fine-textured hair, but with plenty of hairs on the scalp making it quite abundant or they may have thick, coarse hair which is very sparse. The density of hair can vary throughout the head, e.g. hair may be denser at the nape than the crown. Therefore, there are many combinations making each head slightly different.

Hair length

Clients do not always realise that some haircuts require a lot of length in certain areas and often do not appreciate how long it takes for the hair to grow to the length they require. Often it is necessary to compromise with a hairstyle, and it may take a few months and quite a few haircuts to achieve the final effect. A good example of this is when a client has had a layered or steeply graduated haircut and wishes to 'grow out' the top layers until the hair is all one length. This can take up to twelve months, depending upon how short the hair was originally. Advice should be given to the client on the type of styles and haircuts they can have during this period, in order to keep the hair well shaped without loss of length from the areas which need to grow longer.

Amount of natural curl or movement present in the hair

Always try to use any natural curl or movement in the hair. Ignoring or fighting against the curl can often ruin a haircut. By using and incorporating any natural curl or movement the haircut will stay in shape longer and will be easier for the client to manage.

Growth direction of the hair

Strong growth direction patterns can cause some difficulties when cutting the hair, e.g. a double crown, strong napeline, etc. Cutting the hair when wet without tension allows extra length in these areas and prevents an uneven line when the haircut is finished.

Sections for cutting

Sections are necessary when cutting hair to allow the hairdresser to proceed with the haircut in a neat and methodical manner. When cutting hair it is often more efficient to commence cutting at the nape. Sectioning is necessary therefore to hold the remaining hair firmly out of the way for greater ease when working.

Cutting angles around the hairline

The hair may be cut at many angles around the hairline to create different shapes and styles. But always remember to take into consideration any strong hair growth direction patterns, e.g. strong napeline, cow's lick, etc.

The areas to consider when cutting angles around the hairline are:

- The forehead or fringe (see Fig. 2.38).
- The sides of the head (see Fig. 2.39).
- The nape of the neck (see Fig. 2.40).

TECHNICAL TIP
When using the features of the face or ears, etc., as a guide to form the cutting angles, always check that they are even on either side.

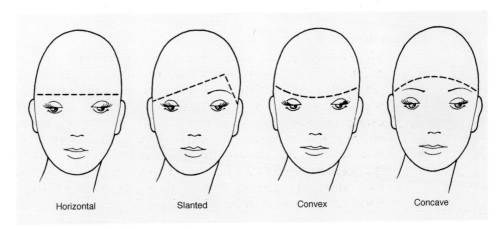

| Horizontal | Slanted | Convex | Concave |

Fig. 2.38 Fringe outline shapes

Cross checking the hair

After cutting any head of hair the haircut should be checked very thoroughly across the sections to ensure that the haircut is level and even from all angles. This is known as **cross-checking**. However, remember when cross-checking a fashion cut not to get too enthusiastic and alter the line or shape of the style, particularly if the angles already cut are very steep.

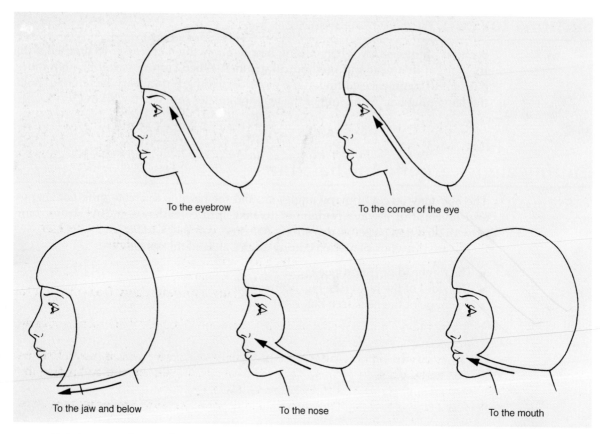

To the eyebrow

To the corner of the eye

To the jaw and below

To the nose

To the mouth

Fig. 2.39 Cutting shapes around the face

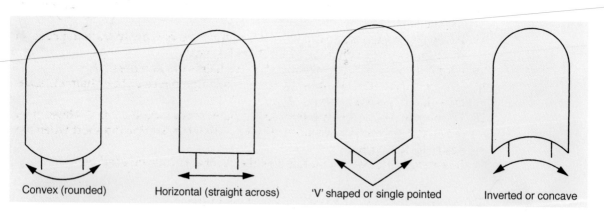

Convex (rounded)

Horizontal (straight across)

'V' shaped or single pointed

Inverted or concave

Fig. 2.40 Nape shapes

Check carefully around the hairline at the sides, front and nape. If the hair has been held and cut away from the head, the underneath hair will be slightly longer, leaving wisps of hair which can make the finished line untidy. Unless this was intended to be part of the finished style they should be removed.

Preventing RSI

Try not to bend or twist your neck. Adjust and turn the chair so you can be exactly centred at the section you are doing. This also gives you the best results. Try to face straight ahead and look down slightly. If you bend your neck forward, you can easily put a 60 degree slant on it and this leads to headaches and backaches. After 20 degrees of slant, the weight of your head (8–12 pounds) is transferred from your skeleton to your muscles and that is a great strain. Imagine carrying 8 pounds of sugar around and you will get the idea. Let your bones carry the weight – they don't strain.

Basic guidelines when cutting hair

1 Decide the exact shape of the finished haircut before starting to cut the hair.
2 Choose the correct type of cutting necessary for the type of hair.
3 Always cut a guideline from which to work.
4 Cut the guideline at the shortest point of the haircut.
5 Comb each section of hair to be cut cleanly and thoroughly from the root to the point.
6 Do not take cutting sections that are too large. The guideline must be clearly visible through the mesh.
7 Try to cut the hair on a straight line as this gives a more precise result. Use the fact that the head is a round object to create the angles, rather than holding the hair, scissors or fingers at an awkward angle.
8 Cut with the hair growth direction and utilise any natural curl or movement to enhance the style.
9 Never cut the hair too short. It is easy to remove more hair but impossible to put it back on again.
10 When cutting wet hair, allow for the fact that hair will lift 5 mm ($\frac{1}{4}$″) when dry.
11 When precision cutting, do not allow the hair to dry out – always keep it wet.
12 When cutting around the ear, allow for ear protrusion and do not cut the hair too short.
13 Always cross-check a basic haircut by lifting the hair away from the head in the opposite direction from which it has been cut.
14 Give a final check to the haircut when the hair is dry and dressed.
15 Always advise the client on the care and maintenance of their haircut, especially if they have had a new style.
16 For beginners – if the guideline at the nape is cut with the client's head bent forward it will help to avoid the risk of cutting the hairline too short when the head is lifted upright.
17 Be aware of the health and safety of the client and yourself at all times.

Example – Cutting a short graduated haircut

Commence the haircut at the shortest point which in this particular case is at the side of the head. Section off a small section of hair and if the hair is to be cut very short at the sides, comb the section smoothly from root to point then rest the fingers against the scalp. The hair is then cut to the width of the fingers. This will be the guideline.

Work up the side of the head to the temple, bringing the hair down in fine meshes and cut to the guideline. The more the hair is lifted away from the head the greater will be the graduation.

Create a guideline from the sides through to the nape by taking a section of hair parallel to the hairline, above and just behind the ear and combing it towards the sides. Use a small section of the previously cut hair to give the required length then cut the hair down towards the nape with the scissors parallel to the hairline. Continue down the side back to the nape in the same manner. All the hair is then brought to this perimeter guideline until the centre of the head is reached.

Cut the other side of the head in the same manner, working up the sides to the centre of the head.

Create graduation in the hairstyle by lifting the hair out from the head at right angles and cutting straight across to the desired length.

A guideline is then cut to the length required down the centre back and through to the front but omitting the fringe.

To cut a slanted fringe, take a diagonal section across the front of the head and comb the hair in the opposite direction to the longest point of the fringe. Cut the hair parallel to the section parting. When the hair is combed back the opposite way it will graduate from short to longer. To check where to commence cutting, comb the fringe area down on to the face. Decide which is the longest point of the fringe and cut a small piece of hair at this point, then take the cut piece of hair across the forehead to the opposite side. This will show where the hair has to be cut.

Cut in the shape at the nape, taking off any stray neck hairs.

Check all of the hairline, removing any stray hairs that may spoil the line of the haircut. Cross-check the entire haircut.

SAFETY TIP

Take particular care if the hair is cut short around the ears to protect the ears with the fingers.

Table 2.8

Method/technique	Description	Effect
Tapering	Slithering movement with scissors on dry hair. Slicing movement with razor on wet hair.	Removes length and bulk. Encourages curl.
Thinning	Aesculap scissors or scissors on dry hair. Razor on wet hair.	Removes bulk only.
Clubbing	Cutting straight across the hair section.	Removes length only. Retains bulk and discourages curl.
Solid form	All the hair is cut to one length at a single base line.	Gives a square 'chunky' effect.
Graduation	Cutting the hair so that the top layers lie above the underneath layers. Increased layering – steep graduation. Low layering – very little graduation.	Can give a layered effect or a full effect depending upon the degree of graduation.
Reverse graduation	Cutting the hair so that the top layers are longer or lie below the underneath hair.	Gives hair maximum volume where the ends turn under, e.g. pageboy, bob.
Scissor over comb	Cutting the hair through the teeth of the comb or with the clippers	Can create very short haircuts on both men and women.

Hair growth patterns

This assignment should help you to get used to diagnosing the hair growth patterns of your clients and give you practice in selecting suitable haircuts.

1 Look carefully at the hairgrowth of *two* of your friends or family members then draw the position of the hair growth pattern at the front, nape, sides and crown area.

2 Compare the different growth patterns for each person and write a brief summary of each.

3 Describe a suitable haircut for each and give reasons for your choice.

4 Draw or cut out from magazines haircuts which would be suitable for someone with a:

- double crown
- strong upward-growing napeline
- cow's lick at the front of the head

Give reasons for your choice of haircuts.

Level 2 Unit 4

Which method of cutting reduces length and bulk? ☐

Which method of cutting reduces bulk only? ☐

Which method of cutting retains the bulk? ☐

Which method of cutting encourages any natural wave movement or curl present in the hair? ☐

What is the correct name for thinning scissors? ☐

What is meant by graduation? ☐

What is meant by reverse graduation? ☐

What safety precautions would you take to protect both the client and yourself whilst cutting hair? ☐

How does sectioning the hair prior to cutting aid the hairdresser? ☐

How is the basic haircut cross-checked? ☐

PERMING

Perming and setting both involve the breaking of some of the cross-linkages between the polypeptide chains of hair keratin.

The type of cross-linkage broken in setting is different from that broken in perming, in that:

- In setting, some of the weak water-breakable cross-linkages between the polypeptide chains are broken and re-formed.
- In perming, some of the stronger linkages are broken and re-formed.

Perming is most often used to wave or curl the hair. The style is permanent in that it can only be removed by 'growing out' or by straightening the hair with perm lotion. There are several methods of perming hair, the most common being **cold permanent waving (cold perm)** as it is cold in comparison to other methods that use heat to permanently curl the hair.

Cold perming

Much practical expertise is needed in perming but the basic operation can be thought of as three stages:

1 **Softening** – by using the **perm lotion**.
2 **Moulding** – in practice this consists of rolling or combing the hair to give the required amount of curling or straightening.
3 **Fixing** – this permanently 'fixes' the hair in the styled position. This last stage is often called **neutralisation** and the chemical used, a **neutraliser**, but technically it is not really a chemical neutralisation at all. These three stages will now be considered in more detail.

Stage 1 – Softening

Traditional cold perm lotion has a pH value of 9 to 9.5 (it is alkaline on the pH scale). This dissolves some of the cement-like keratin which usually holds down the hair cuticle scales. The alkaline factor in turn allows the lotion to get into the hair cortex and to then work on the cross-linkages between the polypeptide chains in the cortex. First, the water in the perm lotion breaks some of the water-breakable cross-linkages (in the same way as wet setting) and second, and more importantly in perming, a chemical called **ammonium thioglycollate** attacks and breaks the water-unbreakable cross-linkages made up of sulphur bonds (about 60–70 per cent of them).

In 'acid' perms, another chemical is used, called **glycerol thioglycollate**, which has a pH value of about 4, but the hair is made alkaline first to cause the outside scales to open and the lotion to penetrate the hair cortex. Another point about 'acid' perms is that only about 10 per cent of the sulphur bonds are broken, because these bonds are stronger in acid conditions.

In both cases, the sulphur bonds are broken by the perm lotion forcing some of the sulphur atoms making up the cross-linkages to take hydrogen atoms instead of linking together between the polypeptide chains.

Sulphur atoms can only form two links or bonds with other chemicals, i.e. one is used up holding the sulphur atom on to the polypeptide chain and the other is used to link to a sulphur atom of a neighbouring chain (i.e. from a cross-linkage). Accepting the hydrogen from the perm lotion means the bond that is used to form the cross-linkage is taken up by the hydrogen atom and the cross-linkage is broken. This is shown in Figs 2.41(a) and (b).

In chemistry, the adding of hydrogen atoms like this is called a **reduction**, with the chemical giving the hydrogen called a **reducing agent** (in this case the perm lotion) and the substance accepting the hydrogen being said to be reduced (in this case the hair keratin).

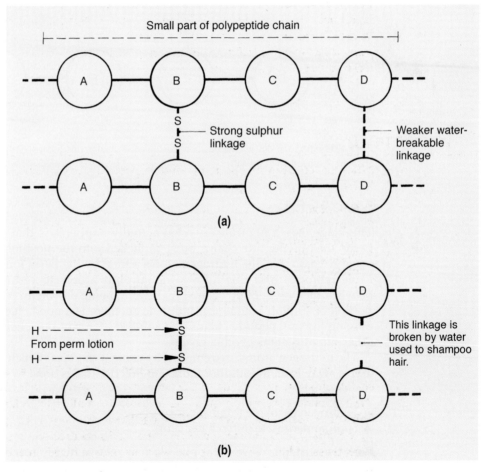

Fig. 2.41 Hair structure: (a) before shampooing and applying perm lotion; (b) after application of perm lotion – hydrogen (H) released from lotion attacks sulphur atoms (S) of sulphur linkage

Stage 2 – Moulding

Most often, this involves winding hair around rollers. The hair is stretched slightly and **tension** is applied. Since some of the water-breakable and non-water-breakable sulphur cross-linkages are broken in Stage 1, the stretching causes the polypeptide chains to slip past each other very slightly. This very tiny movement on the minute scale of polypeptide chains adds up, by slightly moving millions of chains, and allows the individual hairs, and therefore the hair in general, to be styled. How much the chains are caused to slide determines just how much curl will be in the hair when the perm is finished. This sliding of the polypeptide chains is shown in Fig. 2.42.

The hair is then rinsed thoroughly to remove the perm lotion.

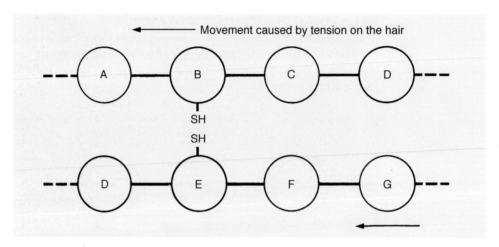

Fig. 2.42 Winding hair causes the polypeptide chains to change positions slightly (A, B and C of lower chain have moved off to the left)

Stage 3 – Fixing

This stage uses a neutraliser. What actually happens, is that in order to fix the perm, the polypeptide chains must be locked into the positions they are in after Stage 2. To do this, the hydrogen atoms added by the perm lotion in Stage 1 have to be removed and this allows the sulphur atoms to re-form cross-linkages between the polypeptide chains. As keratin, being a protein, contains a high proportion of sulphur-containing amino acids, there is a good chance that even after moving the polypeptide chains, the sulphur atoms of one chain will still be near other sulphur atoms of other chains.

The hydrogen atoms are removed by using a chemical which can pull hydrogen atoms away from the sulphur atoms. In practice this is done by one or other of two reagents, which are:

- Hydrogen peroxide (often 6 per cent).
- Sodium perborate (often 5 per cent).

Both these chemicals when applied to hair release highly reactive single atoms of oxygen (called nascent oxygen) which pull the hydrogen off the sulphur, allowing the cross-linkages to re-form. In fact, each atom of nascent oxygen pulls two hydrogen atoms off and combines with them to form water. All this is shown in Fig. 2.43.

In chemistry, the removal of hydrogen atoms in this way is called **oxidation**, with the chemical doing the removal called an **oxidising agent**, and the substance the hydrogen is removed from being described as **oxidised**.

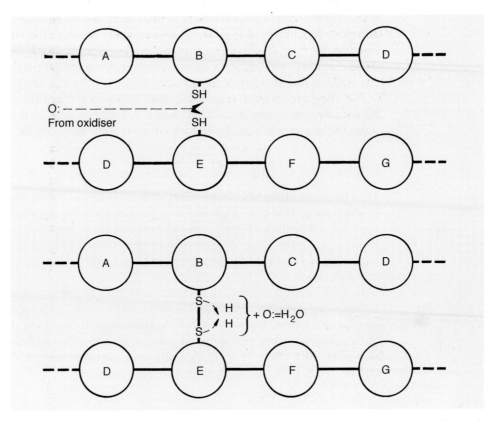

Fig. 2.43 Nascent oxygen removes hydrogen from the sulphur atoms and joins with them to form H_2O (water)

The cold perming process

Hair and scalp analysis

Consultation with the client *before* starting the perming process is essential to allow the client's requirements to be thoroughly discussed and understood.

Examine the hair carefully to make sure that it is really suitable for perming and question the client on any previous treatments, referring to record cards if the client has attended the salon previously. If in any doubt as to the suitability of the hair for permanent waving always carry out a pre-perm test to support the analysis.

The client's scalp must also be checked for the presence of any inflammation, excessive dryness, cuts or abrasions (this can be done when disentangling the hair prior to shampooing). If these conditions are minor they can be protected with barrier cream but if they are major then the treatment must be postponed. Remember, if in doubt postpone the treatment.

Preparation of the operator

Rubber gloves should be worn by the operator while applying the permanent wave lotion to prevent contact dermatitis of the hands. However, if the rods are wound with water and the lotion applied after the rods have been wound (post-damping technique) it is not always necessary to wear the rubber gloves when winding the hair. In this case it is often a good idea to apply barrier cream to the hands as it will protect them if they should come into contact with the lotion at any stage of the perming process.

A tinting apron worn over the overall helps to prevent the lotion from splashing and drying on the overall. Although it does not stain in the same way as tint, perm lotion can leave an unpleasant odour if allowed to dry on any clothing.

Preparation of the client

The client's clothing should be protected at all times during the perming process. A gown should be placed around the client in such a way as to cover all the clothing and a towel should be securely tucked in at the nape to prevent it from slipping on to the floor. A neck strip or strip of cotton wool may be placed at the nape as a precautionary measure to prevent any lotion or water from seeping down the neck.

Barrier cream applied to the skin around the hairline protects it from any lotion that may accidentally run on to this area and prevents burning or sensitising of the skin by the lotion. This is particularly important if the client already happens to have a sensitive skin. But remember that the barrier cream must be applied to the skin only. Any cream that accidentally coats the hair will prevent lotion penetration of that hair and will therefore affect the curl.

Preparation of the hair

The client usually, but not always, requires the hair to be cut when having a perm. It is the decision of the operator whether the hair is cut before or after the permanent wave. However, for a basic perm it is usual to shape the hair before winding the perm. Taper cut hair is easier to wind than hair that has been club cut because the points of the hair are finer and have had some of the weight removed, thus allowing them to be curled more easily around the rod.

Most cold permanent waves are wound on wet hair but the hair should not be over-saturated with water as this could dilute the perm lotion and makes it less effective. Towel drying the hair after shampooing removes the excess water but leaves the hair damp enough to give better absorption of the lotion.

The hair should be shampooed with a soapless shampoo as this not only cleans the hair and scalp but also removes any natural sebum that may be coating the hair. If the sebum remained, it could create a barrier between the lotion and the hair which would prevent the lotion from entering the cortex and the perm would not produce a satisfactory curl.

If the hair is structurally damaged or porous it may be necessary to apply a restructurant or special pre-perm treatment after shampooing to even out the porosity of the hair and to strengthen the cortex. Always take a test curl if the hair is very porous or damaged to make sure that it can withstand the perming process. If in any doubt at all, do not perm until the hair is strong enough.

Preparation of the tools and equipment

All the equipment and tools that you will need should be assembled before beginning the permanent wave. A lot of time and energy can be saved if everything is to hand when it is needed.

> **Preventing RSI**
> Winding perm rods or rollers uses small muscles of the hands that tire quickly, as well as putting a strain on the tendon at your elbow, so try to avoid several winding tasks one after the other.

Contra-indications for permanent waving

The hairdresser should not go ahead with permanent waving if:

- Incompatible chemicals are present on the hair shaft.
- Hair is excessively porous or weakened, e.g. over-bleached.
- The tensile strength or elasticity of the hair has been impaired.
- If previous permanent wave is present – remember that a permanent wave will remain in the hair until it is cut off. However, specialised techniques like 'blocking-out' with conditioner or specially designed restructurants may be used over the old curl in some cases.
- Hair or scalp suffers from contagious or infectious disease, e.g. tinea, pediculosis capitis, etc.
- After childbirth. The nutrients in the blood which are usually given to the hair to feed it are required to return the body to normal, leaving the hair in poor condition. It is usually more successful to perm the client's hair before the birth of the baby, during pregnancy.
- After/during illness or when the client is taking drugs. Perming hair during this time is often unsuccessful. If in doubt, always take a test curl.

Sectioning for a basic cold perm

Reasons for sectioning
- Ease of working.
- Minimum of wasted time.
- Cuts down the risk of over-processing.
- Divides the hair into neat, controllable divisions.
- Helps rod selection.
- Keeps the size of the rods balanced by dividing the head into smaller areas.

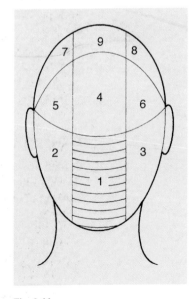

Method of sectioning
1 After shampooing with soapless shampoo, towel dry and disentangle the hair.
2 Divide the hair into nine sections as shown in Fig. 2.44. The numbers refer to the order in which the sections are wound, Section 1 being divided into sub-sections. Note how the sections curve to the shape of the head. Start at the centre front.

Fig. 2.44

Each section should be the same width and slightly longer than the perm rod.

3 Next, move on to the front, side section, checking for width with the perm rod at the top and the bottom of the section to ensure that the width is even along the length of the section. Allowance should be made for any problem hairlines.

4 When the side section has been completed, the other side can be sectioned in the same way, remembering to check the width at the top and bottom of the section.

5 When the front sections have been completed, commence sectioning the crown area by extending the top front section down the back of the head. The length of this section is determined by an imaginary line from the top of both ears which curves round the back of the head. Secure the section. Next check that the side sections are the correct width for the rods.

6 Join both side sections to the centre back section, from the top of both ears. Make sure that all partings are straight and neat and that the hair is securely held with the sectioning clips.

7 Commence sectioning the nape hair, by extending the centre crown section down to the nape. Check the width of the centre nape section. The front, crown and nape sections should be the same width from the front of the head down to the nape.

8 Next, secure firmly the sections that are left at either side of the nape. Figure 2.45(a) shows a side view of completed sections and Fig. 2.45(b) shows a back view of completed sections.

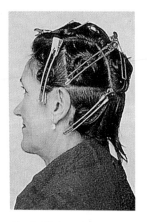
Fig. 2.45(a)

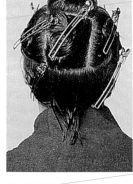
Fig. 2.45(b)

POINTS TO REMEMBER

Always work to the shape of the head. If the hair is extremely short, thick or abundant it may be necessary to add extra sections to hold the hair securely. The sections can be altered slightly as sectioning progresses but remember that the sections should always be the same width as the rods used otherwise problems are created when placing the rods during winding.

Winding a cold permanent wave

Before starting to wind a cold permanent wave, the following points must be taken into consideration as they will determine the size of rod to be used and the amount of curl to be achieved.

- *Texture of hair*: thick hair will require a larger rod than fine hair to achieve the same effect.
- *Type of curl required*: a tight curl requires small rods, a loose curl requires large rods.
- *Type of hair*: i.e. bleached, tinted, porous, resistant, or normal. Bleached, tinted and porous hair will require a special weaker lotion while resistant hair will require a stronger lotion. If in doubt, take a test curl of the hair. Remember that

the condition of the hair after perming is very important – using too strong a lotion for the type of hair will leave the hair in poor condition and could even cause hair breakage.

- *Finished result*: this will also determine the amount of curl required.

Method of winding a basic nine-section cold permanent wave

1 The hair is ready for winding when it has been cut into the desired shape (if necessary), shampooed with soapless shampoo, towel dried and sectioned into nine sections.
2 Commence winding at the centre nape. Using a tail comb divide the hair to produce a sub-section (mesh) which is exactly the same depth as the rod.
3 Apply the lotion, either with a perming brush or piece of cotton wool, approximately 1 cm ($\frac{1}{2}$") from the scalp to prevent the lotion from running on to the skin. This is known as **presaturation**.
4 Comb the mesh out from the head at right angles making sure that the hair is thoroughly combed from the roots to the points. Then comb the mesh upwards towards the crown to allow for the width of the rod when wound.
5 Make sure that the tension is even on both sides of the mesh, otherwise the hair will 'loop' at one end when it is wound, producing an uneven finished curl.

   - When looking down the mesh from the ends (see Fig. 2.46(a)), the points of the hair should be directly in the centre of the mesh at the roots, giving even tension to the hair on both sides of the mesh.
   - If the hair is pulled slightly to one side the tension becomes uneven (see Fig. 2.46(b)).

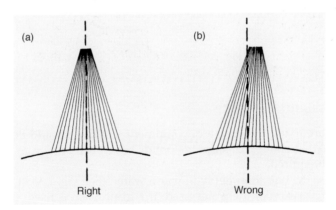

Fig. 2.46

6 Place the end paper over the points of the hair and fold, keeping the tension of the hair even at all times. Note that the end paper is positioned past the end of the hair points (see Fig. 2.47) which helps to avoid the points being bent back when wound (this is known as '**fish-hook**' ends).
7 Carefully wind the end paper and points of hair around the rod and wind down to the root. Winding the hair from the points down to the root is known as **croquignole** winding. Do not pull the hair too tightly when winding as this creates undue tension on the hair and could cause hair breakage, or 'pull-burns' on the skin.
   The hair should be evenly distributed along the length of the rod. 'Bunching' all the hair in the centre of the rod will give an uneven curl.

8 Secure with the rubber band across the top of the rod making sure that it is not twisted or cutting into the hair, otherwise breakage may occur.

9 Proceed down the first major section in the same manner. Keep each mesh the same size as the rod. If the mesh is the correct size each rod will touch the one above, ensuring that there is no root drag on the hair.

10 Continue winding each major section, checking for development at frequent intervals during the wind. A side view of the completed wind is shown in Fig. 2.48.

11 When the whole head is completed, post-damp with lotion, taking care that the lotion does not run onto the skin (see Fig. 2.49).

12 Check the first and last rod wound for development.

13 To contain and utilise the body heat from the scalp, place a disposable polythene cap over the head and await development. Check every three to five minutes.

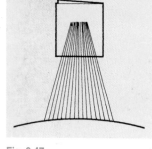

Fig. 2.47

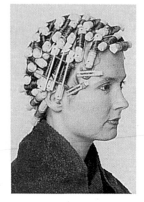
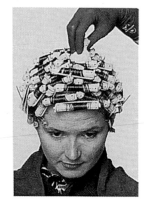

Fig. 2.48 Completed wind   Fig. 2.49 Post-damping

TECHNICAL TIP

Plastic pins can be inserted one at each side of the first two rods to lift the rubber band off the hair and to hold the rod securely in place. Remember to ensure that the pins do not mark hair.

Neutralising the hair

1 Before fixing the curl, a development test curl should be carried out to make sure that enough di-sulphide bonds have been broken to obtain the amount of curl required.

2 Rinse the hair thoroughly in warm water. (See Fig. 2.50.) Check the temperature and pressure of the water used. If a front wash is used, take particular care to avoid water running into the client's eyes and to rinse front rods thoroughly. If a back wash is used (preferred as this reduces the chances of anything washing into the client's eyes) pay particular attention to the rods at the nape.

3 Remove excess water by blotting thoroughly with cotton wool. Leaving the hair too wet will dilute the neutraliser and make it less effective. To check that enough moisture has been removed from the hair, press the palm of the hand onto the rods – if the palm is wet when it is pulled away from the head, the hair requires re-blotting.

4 Apply a strip of cotton wool around the hairline to protect the face and neck.

5 Apply the neutraliser to the wound rods, ensuring each one is completely covered (see Fig. 2.51). Neutralisers are designed by the manufacturer to work with a particular perm lotion, keep them matched. There are a variety of ways of applying the neutraliser, including cream, foam or liquid. These may be

used straight from the container or by using a sponge or brush. It is important to use the neutraliser quickly once it has been mixed or poured otherwise it will lose the oxygen released to the atmosphere.

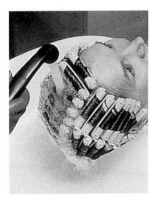

Fig. 2.50 Rinsing the hair in warm water

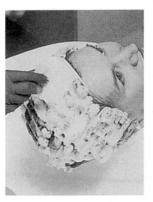

Fig. 2.51 Applying the neutraliser

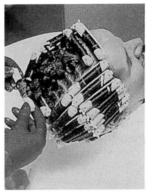

Fig. 2.52 Removing the rods

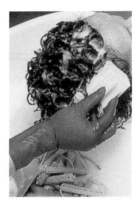

Fig. 2.53 Applying the neutraliser to ends of hair

6 Leave for the time recommended by the manufacturer, usually about five minutes. Cotton wool around the hairline prevents the neutraliser from dripping onto the client's face and neck.

7 Carefully remove the cotton wool and the rods (see Fig. 2.52). The hair should not be pulled or stretched at this stage as the curl is not yet fully 'fixed'.

8 Apply neutraliser gently to the points of the hair as each rod is removed. (See Fig. 2.53.) Do not drag the hair or massage the neutraliser into the hair as this could alter the curl. Check that all the hair has been treated with the neutraliser then leave for a further five minutes.

9 Rinse the hair thoroughly and apply a pH balance conditioner if necessary to remove any traces of alkali that may be left in the hair, and to make sure the perming process has stopped.

10 Always advise the client on the after-care needed for a permanent wave. Clients do not always realise that a perm will dry the hair and make it more porous, therefore the hair will usually need to be conditioned regularly. Other further chemical processes (e.g. bleaching, tinting) should be approached with caution, again because the hair will be more porous and also because the scalp will be more sensitive for a few days after the perm. The hair should be protected from dampness (such as rain or bathing) after a perm as it will revert back to its new alpha stage when wet – that is, it will become curly.

SAFETY TIPS
- Always follow the manufacturer's instructions.
- Cotton wool around the hairline prevents the oxidiser from dripping on face and neck.

POINTS TO REMEMBER

- The sulphur bonds are not completely fixed until the hair is dry. This means that care should be taken when setting or blowdrying after the permanent wave. Stretching or pulling the hair at this point can loosen the curl so if the hair is to be blow dried after the perm (which does involve stretching and moulding the hair) it is often better to allow slightly more curl than required during development to counteract the loosening effect of the blowdry.

- The hair should be thoroughly rinsed in warm water before the neutraliser is applied.
- All excess moisture must be removed after rinsing and before the neutraliser is applied to prevent dilution of the oxidiser.
- The neutraliser must be left in contact with the hair for the correct length of time to ensure adequate fixing of the curl.
- When permanent waving above a graduated neckline, the curl should be large enough to blend into the straight hair at the neckline.

Other basic winding techniques

In addition to the nine-sectioning winding technique there are two other basic winds:

- Directional winding.
- Brickwinding.

Directional winding

Directional winding is used mainly on shorter hair. The hair is wound in the direction of the style, therefore it would be impossible to give any definite method of winding as the variations are limitless. By alternating or mixing the size of the rods a mixed curl strength can also be achieved.

Brickwinding

As the name suggests, this type of wind resembles a brickwork pattern (see Fig. 2.54) and is used to prevent 'tramlines' that may be caused by the sectioning of conventional winding. It is important to start the wind on the top crown area and work outwards and down the head to the nape to allow all the rods to be placed correctly.

> **TECHNICAL TIP**
> When brickwinding, the sides may be wound directionally, either forwards or backwards, according to the finished style.

Record cards

Always complete a client record card when the process is completed. This should contain the following information:

- Date.
- Hair condition.
- Product used, including the strength of the lotion.
- Size of rod used.
- Development time.
- Any precautions necessary.
- Finished result and any comments necessary.
- Recommended after-care treatment.

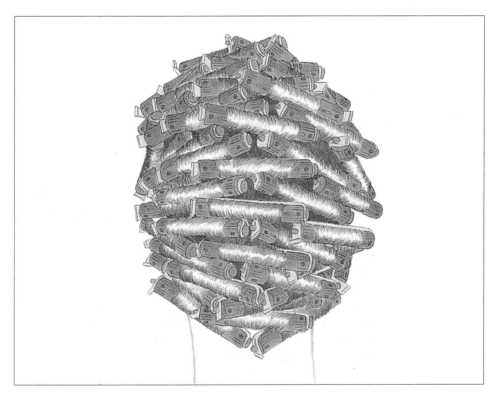

Fig. 2.54 Completed brickwind

Precautions and considerations when permanent waving

1 Always carry out an elasticity, porosity and pre-perm test curl on bleached hair. Bleached hair is in a very porous condition; therefore too strong a lotion can cause irreparable damage.

2 Always use a special or weaker lotion on tinted hair. Tinted hair is also in a porous condition.

3 Test unknown hair for any incompatible chemicals on the hair shaft, e.g. hair colour restorers, with an incompatibility test.

4 Before commencing a permanent wave, check the scalp for cuts and abrasions. If these are minor, cover and protect with petroleum jelly or barrier cream; if major, postpone the treatment.

5 The porosity of the hair must be taken into consideration when selecting the correct strength of lotion. The porosity can, in some instances, vary along the shaft of the hair, in which case a pre-perm treatment may be needed to even out the porosity.

6 Use the correct size rods for the desired result. Hair sections should be the same size as the rod, as too large a section will result in too great a difference between the root and point curl.

7 Partings should be clean and straight, unless 'weave winding' the hair to prevent rod partings on some types of hair.

8 Each section should be combed thoroughly from root to point.

9 The points of the hair should be wound completely round the rod to prevent fish-hook ends.

10 The tension on the wound hair must be even and the hair evenly distributed along the length of the rod. Do not 'bunch' the hair in the middle of the rod.

11   The rubber of the rod should lie flat and untwisted along the top of the wound hair.
12   The perm lotion should not be allowed to come into contact with the skin as it could cause dermatitis.
13   Barrier cream may be used round the hairline to prevent burning of sensitive skin.

TECHNICAL TIP
When leaving hair to develop, remember that heat will speed up the processing time but excessive heat can damage the hair. Therefore always follow the manufacturer's advice regarding development times.

14   Hair should be checked for development during winding, immediately after post damping and every three to five minutes thereafter unless otherwise stated by the manufacturer.
15   Perm lotion should not be allowed to come into contact with anything metallic as this could discolour the hair.
16   If there are any difficulties before, during or after the perming process *always* seek advice from a senior staff member.

Testing hair for perming

Perm lotion can sometimes damage the hair and it is therefore extremely important to test the hair both before and during perming to make sure that the hair is strong enough to withstand the process and also that the condition of the hair is maintained. The tests normally considered when perming are:

- Elasticity test.
- Porosity test.
- Incompatibility test.
- Pre-perm test curl.
- Development test curl.

Some permanent waving faults, causes and remedies are listed in Table 2.9.

Elasticity test

Carried out before perming to determine the general condition and strength of the hair. A few hairs are removed from the front of the head and they are then pulled between the fingers. If the hair is in a weakened, fragile state then it will break. Hair with good elasticity should be capable of stretching up to half its own length when wet and a third of its own length when dry. If the hair breaks or appears weakened, do not proceed with the perm.

Porosity test

This test is used to check the hair cuticle for damage. The cuticle is the protective layer of the hair and, if it is damaged in any way, it will absorb the perm lotion very quickly. If this is the case, it will be necessary to even out the porosity with a pre-perm lotion or restructurant and then use a weaker or specially formulated perm lotion.

Table 2.9 Permanent waving faults, causes and remedies

Fault	Possible cause	Action required
Development time excessively long	Rods too large Use of too few rods Hair meshes too large Wrong strength of reagent Cold salon	Change rods if necessary Redamp with correct strength of lotion and leave until fully developed
Hairline and scalp irritation	Cuts and abrasions on the scalp Reagent running on to scalp Too much reagent applied Cotton wool placed around hairline or between rods when processing	Apply a soothing lotion to the affected areas Use cool water for rinsing and do not massage the scalp
Pull-burn	Rods wound too tightly allowing reagent to penetrate hair follicle	Apply soothing lotion to affected area Refer client to doctors if serious
Hair breakage (within a week or two)	Rods wound too tightly Rubbers too tight or twisted Over-processing Reagent too strong Incompatible reaction	Condition the hair using restructurants and deep penetrating conditioner
Straight finished result (no curl)	Rods too large Insufficient processing Reagent too weak Insufficient oxidation Too few rods used Poor shampooing	Take test curls, if hair is in a good condition, re-perm If hair is in poor condition, treat with conditioning treatments and re-perm with weaker lotion
Discoloration of the hair	Use of metal tools Use of containers used for other purposes Presence of incompatible chemicals on the hair	If incompatible chemicals are present on the hair, rinse off reagent immediately If the hair remains discoloured after rinsing, apply toning or semi-permanent or temporary rinse
Curl weakening	Use of wrong or too weak oxidiser Incorrect timing of oxidiser Insufficient blotting of hair after rinsing Faulty oxidiser Hair pulled excessively when not completely 'fixed'	Take test curls; hair in good condition can be re-permed; hair in poor condition should be treated with deep penetrating conditioners before re-perming
Frizz (curl may appear straight when dry, excessively curly when wet)	Reagent too strong Rod size too small Over-processing Overheating during development	Condition the hair thoroughly using penetrating conditioner and restructurant Cut the hair if possible
Fish hooks on hair points	Points of the hair doubled back while winding	Remove by cutting
Hair too curly	Rod size too small	Hair in good condition can be relaxed by combing through reagent then oxidising Hair in poor condition should be treated with deep penetrating conditioners and restructurants and not subjected to further chemical treatments
Good curl result when wet, poor result when dry	Hair over-stretched when drying Over-processing	Condition the hair thoroughly and cut if possible
Uneven curl along the hair length	Mesh too large for rod size Uneven tension along length of the rod Incorrect use of end papers Hair not combed smoothly from roots to points Hair 'drag' Uneven application of reagent/oxidiser	When hair is in good condition, relax with perm lotion if curl strength is too great; re-perm if curl strength is too weak If hair is in poor condition treat with conditioning agents first

Table 2.9 continued

Fault	Possible cause	Action required
Uneven curl throughout the head	See section above Insufficient mesh for rod length, causing drag at the sides of the section Wind commenced at the more porous area instead of most resistant Reagent insufficient or unevenly applied Lack of control when winding causing 'looping'	When hair is in good condition, relax with perm lotion if curl strength is too great; re-perm if curl strength is too weak If hair is in poor condition treat with conditioning agent first
Straight hair at sides and nape	Incorrect angling or placing of rods Rods too large for length of hair Mesh too large for rod size Wispy hair around the head left out of the rod	If hair is in good condition re-perm the straight hair, making sure that the perm lotion does not come into contact with the curled areas

To determine the hair's porosity, gently slide the fingers down the length of the hair shaft from root to points. Healthy hair feels smooth, whilst the more porous the hair the rougher it will feel.

Previously treated hair such as tinted or highlighted is often damaged (porous) and will therefore require extra care when perming.

Incompatibility test

This test determines whether there are any chemicals on the hair which will react with the perm lotion.

Take small cuttings from various parts of the head and place them in a simple bleach (a mixture of hydrogen peroxide and ammonia). If there are incompatible chemicals on the hair the mixture will foam, get hot and the hair will finally disintegrate. It is therefore important not to carry out the perm if this test is positive.

Pre-perm test curl

Winding a couple of rods with the chosen perm lotion at the back of the head will tell the stylist whether the hair is suitable for perming or not. A pre-perm test curl will also show the strength of lotion to use and how long it should be left in contact with the hair.

Development test curl

This test is carried out during the perming process, once the perm lotion has been applied, to determine how much processing has occurred.

Gently unwind a rod, without removing it completely, then push the hair back gently towards the roots. If the perm is ready the hair will form an 'S' shaped movement, the size of which depends upon the amount of curl required. A large 'S' movement gives a loose curl while a small 'S' shaped movement will give a tight curl. Check different rods at various parts of the head to ensure that there is an even development throughout the whole head. Keep hair points round the rod by holding with the thumbs whilst pushing the hair towards the roots.

Other types of permanent waves

Acid perms

These are believed to be less damaging to the hair than alkaline perms. They are usually supplied with an activator and their own oxidising agent. When the hair has been wound, the lotion is mixed with the activator and applied to the hair making sure, as with all post damping, that each rod is thoroughly dampened with the lotion.

Most acid perms require heat to speed up their development and even then they tend to be slow-acting. When checking the development of an acid perm look at the 'stranding' of the hair mesh as well as the 'S' shape formed. The hair mesh should separate into about seven strands when it has developed.

Foam perm

This requires a special machine which is powered by electricity and has two separate guns, one to pump air into the perm lotion and the other for the neutraliser, making a foam of each. Because of its aerated nature, this perm is applied after the rods are wound and is very comfortable for the client as the lotions do not drip.

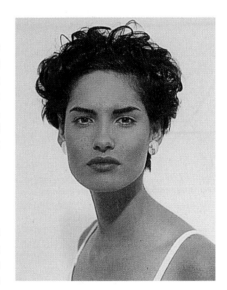

Uni perm

This perm is processed by heat from a machine similar to the old heat perm machine. The machine has heated bars which then heat up the clamps attached to it. The hair is wound taking large sections to accommodate the size of the clamps which are placed over the wound rods and then left to cool. The hair must be pushed to the centre of the rod and the rubber band placed along its top to allow the hair to be properly heated and prevent the rubber band from melting.

Exothermic perming

This type of permanent wave is wound in exactly the same manner as a cold permanent wave except that the lotion is applied after waving instead of during the wind. It is therefore important not to allow the hair to dry out during winding – if it does, re-damp with water. When the wind has been completed, mix the two chemicals together according to the manufacturer's instructions. The mixture will become warm. Apply this warm mixture evenly over the wound rods and await development. When the required amount of curl is achieved, rinse and neutralise according to the manufacturer's instructions and complete a client record card.

You will need:

- Tuition head and clamp.
- Sectioning clips.
- Tail comb.
- Rods of uniform size and end papers.
- Permanent waving lotion and neutraliser for normal hair with applicator bottles.
- Permanent waving lotion and neutraliser for treated hair with applicator bottles.
- Cotton wool and towel.
- Water spray.

1 Wet the tuition head thoroughly with water, remove excess moisture with the towel.

2 Divide the hair into three sections, forehead to crown (the width of a rod), then from ear to ear at either side. Pin the remaining hair out of the way.

3 Wind both the front two sections using the same size rods. When they are wound, place cotton wool around them to protect the other hair.

4 Apply the permanent wave lotion for normal hair to the left side section and apply the lotion for treated hair to the right side section.

5 Leave to develop until an 'S' shape curl is formed.

6 Rinse thoroughly in tepid water, then blot dry and place cotton wool around the rods.

7 Apply the neutraliser and leave for five minutes (or according to the manufacturer's instructions).

8 Remove the rods and apply more neutraliser to the hair ends. Leave for a further five minutes then remove by rinsing the hair thoroughly in warm water.

9 Towel dry the hair and comb through.

Compare the results of both sides of the tuition head. How does the curl strength differ? How does the hair feel on each side?

Level 2 Unit 5A

Name the chemical process occurring during the first, softening stage in cold perming. ☐

What is the main ingredient in cold perms? ☐

What happens in the hair during neutralisation? ☐

What is meant by 'pre-saturation'? ☐

What is meant by post damping? ☐

What can happen if the rod rubbers are twisted on the hair? ☐

How often and how should perming development be checked? ☐

When neutralising, why must the hair be thoroughly blotted after rinsing to remove the excess moisture? ☐

What factors can cause an excessively long processing time? ☐

List three important pieces of advice which can be given on the after-care of permed hair. ☐

PERMING AND RELAXING AFRICAN CARIBBEAN HAIR

There are several key differences between the structure of African Caribbean, Mongoloid and Caucasian hair which influence the products and procedures used when carrying out a perming or straightening process.

Structure of African Caribbean hair

African Caribbean hair has a similar structure to other racial types in that it has a **medulla**, **cuticle** and **cortex**.

The medulla

The medulla is the centre layer of the hair and, unlike Caucasian hair, it often has colour pigment present. Therefore it is often difficult to detect the medulla in African Caribbean hair.

The cuticle

The cuticle of African Caribbean hair has seven to eleven layers, which is more than the four to seven layers of Caucasian hair but less than the eleven plus layers of Mongoloid hair. However, the continual everyday brushing and dressing of the tight curl of African Caribbean hair tends to damage and remove some of the cuticle layers towards the ends of the hair, making them more porous than the root area. The better the hair condition then the more resistant it is to chemical products. However, because of the uneven porosity along the length of the hair shaft, the stylist must be very thorough when analysing the hair to determine the strength of chemicals to use.

The twisting, bending nature of African Caribbean hair also prevents the cuticle layers lying as flat as they do for Caucasian or Mongoloid, preventing light from reflecting as easily and making the hair appear duller. Spray gloss is often used to counteract this and to make the hair more supple and less likely to break.

The cortex

African Caribbean hair is flattened in shape, which means that it has a smaller amount of cortex than the round-shaped Caucasian or Mongoloid hair. Therefore, once chemicals have penetrated into the cortex they react more quickly and great care has to be taken to prevent the hair becoming over-processed or destroyed.

The tight curl of most African Caribbean hair gives two different cortex types within each hair. These types are known as **ortho-cortex** and **para-cortex**. The ortho-cortex contains less sulphur and is on the **outside** of the curl or wave curve whilst the para-cortex is on the **inside** of the curve. This means that the ortho-cortex is stretched more than the para-cortex making it less dense than the compact para-cortex.

The hair's natural colour pigment is deposited mainly in the cortex but, unlike Caucasian hair, a small percentage is also present in both the cuticle and the medulla. The colour pigment (melanin) granules of African Caribbean hair are larger than those in Caucasian hair. The cortex also gives the hair 75 per cent of its strength whilst the cuticle gives it 25 per cent.

The cortex contains the following bonds (see Figs 2.55–2.58):

1 Strong **di-sulphide bonds** which are found between the sulphur atoms. These are the bonds which are broken during perming and relaxing processes.

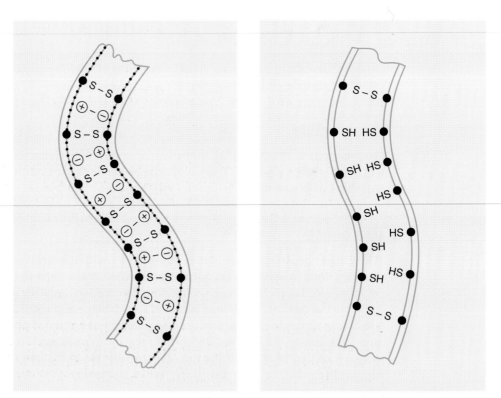

Fig. 2.55 Normal African Caribbean hair which contains di-sulphide bonds (•S—S•), hydrogen bonds (••••) and salt linkages (⊕—⊖)

Fig. 2.56 Ammonium thioglycollate-based straightener is applied to the hair. This gives off hydrogen (H), which reduces cystine (•S—S•) to two cysteines (•SH). Hydrogen bonds and salt linkages are also broken. The curl formation begins to relax

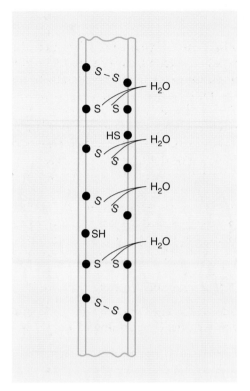

Fig. 2.57 The straightened hair is rinsed to remove the straightener and a neutraliser is applied to the hair. The cysteines are oxidised by the neutraliser and lose their hydrogens to form new cystines. Two hydrogens combine with one oxygen to form water

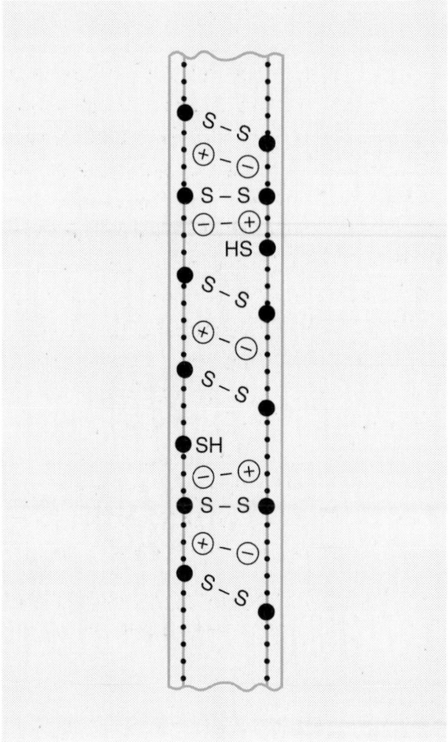

Fig. 2.58 When the neutraliser is rinsed from the hair all three bonds re-form in different positions (compare the original, as shown in Fig. 2.55), which help hold the hair in the new straight form

2 Weaker **hydrogen bonds** which are formed between the hydrogen and oxygen atoms. These bonds are broken by heat and stretching during setting and pressing.

3 **Salt linkages** formed between the negative and positive ions in amino acids. These bonds are found between and within the polypeptide chains, and are easily broken by weak acids and alkalis.

How the natural curl of African Caribbean hair is formed

There are several theories regarding the formation of the distinctive tight curl of African Caribbean hair. The curl formation is believed to be due to the way cell division takes place at the base of the hair in the germinal matrix of the papilla. The cell division here is uneven in that one side divides more quickly than the other. However, to further complicate matters, this additional cell division is not constant on one side but shifts from side to side. The hair bends away from where the cell division is greatest and it is therefore made to bend from side to side which causes it to curl. The process of cell division is known as **mitosis**; therefore the curliness of African Caribbean hair is often said to be caused by uneven rates of mitosis (see Fig. 2.59).

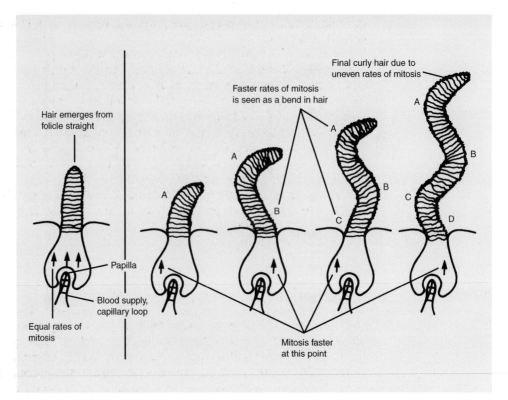

Fig. 2.59 The cyclical theory of hair growth. The first hair on the left has emerged from the follicle as a straight hair because the rates of cell division (mitosis) in the papilla are equal. However, the second hair has emerged curly because the rate of cell division has not been even. The hair bends over to the opposite side from where the cell division is fastest. The arrows in the papilla show where the cell division is fastest. Note that the hair emerging at the skin surface is bending the opposite way each time

Perming African Caribbean hair

Products used when perming African Caribbean hair

Although perming products are similar for Caucasian, Mongoloid and African Caribbean it is always better to use products which have been formulated for the specific hair types. Always make sure that the correct neutraliser is used in conjunction with the perming lotion to ensure a successful result and avoid hair breakage. Types of product used are:

- *Curl rearranger* – ammonium thioglycollate is the active ingredient in these products and it is used in cream or gel form. It is available in three to four strengths, from mild to super or maximum, depending on the manufacturer. Curl rearrangers are used prior to perming to soften and straighten the hair.
- *Curl booster (perm lotion)* – this is often the name given to the perm solution. Ammonium thioglycollate is also the active ingredient in curl boosters although it is in a weaker form than in curl rearrangers. They are used in exactly the same way as a cold perm on Caucasian or Mongoloid hair.
- *Neutraliser* – the main ingredient is either hydrogen peroxide or sodium bromate. Both act as oxidising agents although sodium bromate does not lighten

the hair as much as hydrogen peroxide and tends to be less likely to cause irritation to the scalp.

- *Pre-perm lotion* – this coats the hair with a protective polymer film to even out the porosity. It is left in the hair prior to perming but should be used sparingly otherwise it will prevent penetration of the curl rearranger.
- *Moisturiser* – glycerine is often used as the base for moisturisers. They help to prevent moisture loss from the cortex by coating the hair with oils. Hair needs to be sprayed with moisturisers at least every other day after curly perming to keep the hair and scalp supple. Moisturisers also prolong the life of the perm as they prevent it becoming dry and brittle but care must be taken to use sparingly or they can be difficult to remove when shampooing.
- *Hydrolysed keratin conditioner* – used after a curly perm to minimise chemical damage by helping to replace some of the lost amino acids and maintain the moisture level within the cortex.

Hair structure: perming African Caribbean hair

An African Caribbean perm is usually referred to as a curly perm, or sometimes curl re-director or wet-look perm. Ammonium thioglycollate is the active ingredient in the perm lotion, and it is also used for the process known as **curl rearranging** which is carried out before the perming process to soften and straighten the hair.

The hair structure is altered in exactly the same way as when perming Caucasian hair. The alkalinity of the ammonium thioglycollate swells the hair causing the cuticle scales to lift and open allowing the perm lotion to penetrate into the cortex more easily. A reducing action takes place, breaking the di-sulphide bonds. When enough bonds have been broken, the action is stopped by rinsing the hair thoroughly in warm water. The hair is then permanently 'fixed' in a new position by re-forming the di-sulphide bonds in this new position through the addition of oxygen in the form of a 'neutraliser'. The hydrogen and salt bonds are also re-formed in the new position. This chemical process was explained in greater detail in Unit 5A.

Testing the hair before perming

Tests which can be carried out include; porosity test, elasticity test, incompatibility test and pre-perm test curl. The choice of test will depend on the hair condition and what information the stylist requires. See Unit 5A for details of how these tests are carried out.

Test curl for a curly perm

This is carried out before the perm, using different strengths of lotion to determine the most suitable strength to use and to make sure that the hair can withstand the process.

Method
1 Shampoo the hair and apply pre-perm treatment if necessary (according to manufacturer's instructions).
2 Section off a small section of hair, enough to hold two or three perm rods, at the nape of the neck. If there are any problems, the hair in this area can be more easily covered!

3 Clip the remaining hair out of the way and coat with conditioner to protect.
4 Apply the **curl rearranger** to the nape hair. Straighten the hair with the back of the comb then cover with a cap to retain body heat. When ready, rinse from the hair and blot out excess moisture.
5 Apply **perm lotion** (**curl booster**) then comb hair with a wide-toothed comb. Wind one or two rods, protect surrounding hair from the lotion by placing a strip of damp cotton wool around the wound rods. Cover with a cap then leave to develop, checking every two to three minutes.
6 When developed rinse in warm water. Blot out excess moisture then neutralise.
7 Rinse out neutraliser and apply conditioner. Assess condition, porosity and elasticity of the hair.
8 Record the results.

Curly perming African Caribbean hair

This involves using two lotions, in two stages to alter the hair structure. In the first stage (unless the hair is extremely porous), a curl rearranger is used to soften and break down some of the disulphide bonds. This is then followed by the second, curl booster, stage which moulds the hair into a new curled shape which is softer and less curly than the hair's original state (see Fig. 2.60).

Method

1 Carry out any necessary tests. If they are satisfactory, protect the client with towels and gown and self with tinting apron and gloves.
2 Do not shampoo the hair unless it is heavily coated with oils or gloss. Indeed, it is preferable not to shampoo the hair for at least three days beforehand. However, always follow manufacturer's instructions as this will give specific guidance for their product.

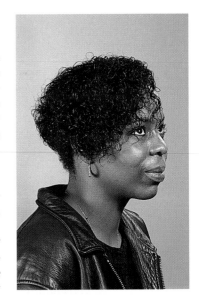

Fig. 2.60 African Caribbean curly perm

3 Apply pre-treatment to the hair if necessary. Blot to remove any excess then place the client under a hairdrier to harden and dry the treatment into the hair.
4 Apply protective cream around the hairline and ears then section the hair into four major sections; forehead to nape then ear to ear across the crown.
5 Starting at the nape, as this is usually the most resistant area, take small subsections of hair approximately 0.6 cm (¼") wide. Apply the correct strength curl rearranger 0.6 cm (¼") from the scalp and along the length of the hair section. Work as quickly as possible, from side to side, up towards the front of the head making sure that the hair is thoroughly coated with the curl rearranger.
6 When application is complete, smooth the hair with the back of the comb or the fingers then cover with a plastic cap to retain the body heat and prevent dry out. Leave to develop following manufacturer's instructions.
7 When the hair is sufficiently softened and straightened, remove the rearranger by rinsing the hair thoroughly in warm water for five minutes.
8 Blot the hair to remove excess moisture. Do not rub the hair as it is now in a fragile state.
9 Resection the head into nine basic sections, or in accordance with the salon's normal practice

10 Commence winding the hair on the correct size rods as for a normal cold perm. The perm lotion (curl booster) may be applied either as each rod is wound (pre-damping) or when the winding is complete (post-damping). Always follow manufacturer's instructions for the best results.

11 Leave to develop. Heat may be applied to quicken the process but, if a drier is used, make sure the head is covered with a plastic cap to prevent the hair drying out. Check for development at the front, nape and sides of the head.

12 When development is complete, rinse the hair thoroughly in warm water for five to ten minutes. Blot carefully to remove excess moisture then place a strip of cotton wool around the hairline to protect the skin.

13 Apply the neutraliser to the rods, pushing it well into the hair. Leave for the time stated by the manufacturer, usually five minutes.

14 Gently unwind the rods then apply additional neutraliser to the ends of the hair where the end papers have been placed. Leave for a further five minutes then rinse thoroughly from the hair.

15 Apply a keratin conditioner to the hair, taking care not to disturb the curl, and leave for three to five minutes. Rinse from the hair and apply an oil-rich 'curl activator' to prevent further moisture loss from the hair. Complete a record of work carried out and advise the client on the after-care of the curly perm.

TECHNICAL TIP
The larger the perm rod, the looser the curl.

Regrowth application of a curly perm

In this case, it is important to apply the curl rearranger to the regrowth area only, but again apply the lotion 0.6 cm away from the scalp. The remaining hair may be coated with conditioner or a protective polymer to help prevent overlapping and possible breakage. When the hair is sufficiently softened and straightened, proceed as for the second stage of a full head curly perm.

If the hair is porous the curl rearranger stage is omitted and the hair is permed using the post-damping technique to prevent over-processing.

SAFETY TIP
Always use the correct neutraliser for the perm lotion. Do not mix different manufacturers' perming and neutralising products. At best the perm may not take; at worst there could be an adverse reaction on the hair.

Precautions and considerations

The same considerations and precautions are necessary for perming African Caribbean hair as for perming Caucasian hair. These have been previously covered in detail in Unit 5A. However, there are also the following additional factors to take into account when carrying out perming processes on this hair type:

1 Do not use curl rearranger or perming products on highly porous or bleached African Caribbean hair.

2 *Always* carry out the necessary tests prior to the treatment to ensure that the hair is strong enough to withstand the double application of ammonium thioglycollate.

3 Use a conditioner or pre-perm lotion on porous hair.

4 Do not curly perm over previously relaxed hair.
5 *Do not* overlap the curl rearranger onto any previously treated hair.
6 Rinse off any of the lotions immediately if irritation occurs.
7 Always use the correct neutralisers for the perm lotion being used.
8 Condition and moisturise the hair before and after the treatment. Always advise the client on the after-care of their hair.

Relaxing hair

Relaxing hair permanently alters its internal structure, reducing any wave or curl movement that the hair may have. For this reason, it is usually better to cut the hair after the relaxing process as it is then more manageable and easier to judge the overall hair length.

Calcium hydroxide, potassium hydroxide and sodium hydroxide are chemicals used to relax the hair. All are extremely alkaline with a pH of between 10 and 14 and if used incorrectly can cause irreparable damage to the hair. Sodium hydroxide, known as caustic soda or lyle, is the most commonly used base for relaxers and, under the 1984 Cosmetic Products (Safety) Regulations, relaxing products in Britain are only allowed to contain 4–5 per cent sodium hydroxide. Relaxers also contain skin coolers and conditioning agents to help lessen skin irritation, replace lost oils and maintain the hair's moisture content. Relaxers can usually be obtained in three strengths: mild, regular and super.

Advantages of using sodium hydroxide relaxers
- They are very quick acting.
- They straighten the hair more effectively than any other straightening agents.
- The hair is less likely to revert back to its previous curly shape after neutralising.

Disadvantages of using sodium hydroxide relaxers
- The hair may become brittle and break off.
- If left longer than ten minutes, the hair may dissolve.
- They can cause severe burning of the skin.
- If sodium hydroxide is left too long the hair may turn red.

How it works

The process of relaxing differs from perming or straightening the hair with ammonium thioglycollate in that the di-sulphide bonds, hydrogen bonds and salt bonds (these are the bonds within the cortex which hold the hair in its natural shape) are broken and rearranged by a chemical reaction known as **hydrolysis**.

This is a very complex process but, put simply, the relaxer (sodium hydroxide) adds water and hydrogen to the di-sulphide bonds (cystine) forming cysteine and sulphenic acid. As the hair straightens, the newly formed cysteine and sulphenic acid react together to form the amino acid, lathionine. Lathionine has only one sulphur atom instead of the two of cystine, therefore the spare sulphur atom attaches itself to the water to form hydrosulphide.

The above process is continuous. The newly formed lathionine is able to hold the hair in a new straightened shape therefore it is not necessary to re-form the sulphur bonds by neutralising as in conventional perming. Instead, the action of the alkaline sodium hydroxide is stopped by rinsing it from the hair and then applying a special **acid** shampoo to neutralise the alkalinity of the relaxer. When the hair is dried, the hydrogen bonds and the salt bonds are reformed in the hair's new position, helping to hold it permanently in its new straightened shape.

A test cutting should be taken before any relaxing process because of the high alkalinity of the relaxer cream.

Pre-testing the hair before the relaxing process

Incorrectly used relaxers can seriously damage the hair. Pre-testing the hair before starting the treatment enables the stylist to select the correct strength of relaxer and will also give an indication of how long the development should be. The relaxer can be tested either on test cuttings of hair or whilst still on the head.

Method 1

Take a few strands of hair from various parts of the head and apply a small amount of the relaxer cream evenly along the lengths. Do not leave the relaxer in contact with the hair longer than recommended by the manufacturer and observe constantly. Shampoo with neutralising shampoo then assess the relaxation of the hair or any damage that may have been sustained. If the test shows any sign of breakage or excessive elasticity, postpone the treatment until the hair has been conditioned and retested at a later date. Record the results of the test.

Method 2

Take a section of hair from the nape area of the head, pull through a piece of aluminium foil with a slit in it, alternatively use an easi-meche packet to hold the hair section. Apply to relaxer and allow to process checking frequently. Rinse the shampoo with neutralising shampoo. Check hair porosity and elasticity. Record findings including the processing time.

Application of sodium hydroxide relaxers

1 Check the client's record card for any previous treatments.
2 Examine the scalp for any cuts, abrasions or inflammation – if any disorders are present postpone the treatment.
3 Examine the hair for:

   - tightness of curl
   - elasticity and tensile strength
   - texture and porosity
   - any breakage.

4 Examine and assess the results of the preliminary pre-perm test.
5 Make sure that the client is adequately protected by a gown and towel. Apply protective cream (petroleum cream or jelly usually) evenly in order to cover the scalp and around the hairline (known as **basing**) to prevent burning or irritation of the skin by the product. Do not shampoo the hair or rub/brush the scalp. Some manufactures only require basing around the hairline and ears.
6 The operator must wear protective gloves.
7 Read the manufacturer's instructions carefully before the treatment commences.
8 Section the hair into six – forehead to nape then ear to ear across the top and ear to ear across the back (see Figs 2.61–2.63).

Perming and Relaxing African Caribbean Hair 153

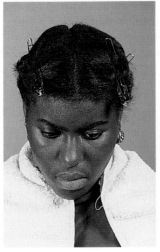

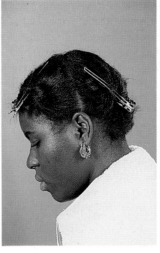

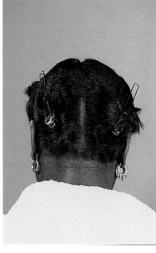

Fig. 2.61 Sectioning the hair for relaxing – front view

Fig. 2.62 Sectioning the hair for relaxing – side view

Fig. 2.63 Sectioning the hair for relaxing – back view

SAFETY TIP
Use specialist African Caribbean products on this hairtype for best results.

9 Start application at the nape area (see Fig. 2.64) and taking small sections, apply sufficient relaxer cream to the hair 0.6 cm ($\frac{1}{4}''$) away from the scalp. Do not allow the relaxer to touch the scalp. Work methodically in small sections towards the front.

10 With previously relaxed hair, apply to the regrowth only.

11 When application is complete (see Fig. 2.65), use a gentle smoothing technique to straighten the hair starting where the cream was first applied. It is important that the hair should not be pulled or stretched during the application.

12 The approximate time for relaxing hair is as follows:

- for fine hair – two to three minutes
- for medium hair – three to five minutes
- for coarse hair – five to seven minutes

The maximum time for even the most resistant hair should not exceed eight minutes.

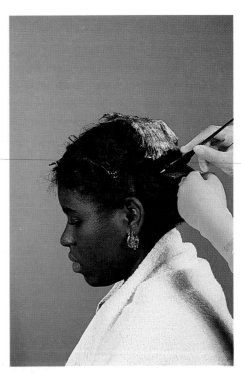

Fig. 2.64 Applying relaxer to sectioned hair

13 Rinse at a backwash with a strong force of warm water. Start at the hairline and hold the hose 10–12.5 cm (4–5") from the head. Do not use hands to remove the cream from the hairline; let the force of the water remove it.

14 Use a neutralising acid shampoo to thoroughly shampoo the hair. On the second shampoo, gently but firmly comb the hair straight and leave for five minutes, then rinse. All relaxers have their own specialist neutralising shampoos. *Always* follow the manufacturer's instructions.

15 Remove excess moisture from the hair by blotting; do not rub the hair. Apply a pH moisturising conditioner as a treatment and leave for at least ten minutes before rinsing thoroughly.

16 Complete a record of work.

17 When styling the hair after relaxing do not use high heated implements, e.g. hot brushes, etc.

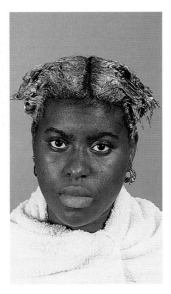
Fig. 2.65 Completed application of relaxer

Contra-indications when relaxing hair

Do not start a relaxing process in any of the following cases:

- Cuts, abrasions or inflammation on the scalp.
- The hair is coated with incompatible chemicals.
- Fragile or broken hair.
- Hair has been chemically damaged, particularly bleached.
- Hair or scalp with an infectious or contagious disease.
- On children under ten years of age.

Precautions and considerations when relaxing hair

1 Always carry out a preliminary pre-perm test.
2 Carry out an incompatibility test if necessary.

> SAFETY TIP
> Apply protective cream to the scalp and skin around the hairline to protect them from the chemicals.

3 Read the manufacturer's instructions very carefully and use only as directed.
4 Examine the hair and scalp carefully to determine the correct strength of relaxer. If in doubt, choose a weaker type.
5 Protect the skin and scalp with a protective cream.
6 The operator must always wear protective gloves.
7 Do not allow the relaxer cream to come into contact with the scalp or any part of the skin.
8 Do not pull or stretch the hair during the application; it could break.
9 Do not use hot brushes, heated curling tongs or any other heated implements on the hair either during or after relaxing.
10 If the cream relaxer enters the eyes, rinse immediately with water and seek medical aid. Sodium hydroxide could cause blindness.

11 If the cream relaxer causes skin irritation, rinse off immediately and shampoo the hair with a non-alkaline shampoo. If irritation persists, seek medical aid.

12 Use a timer when processing to prevent the relaxer being left in contact with the hair too long.

13 Test frequently for development. Do not exceed the maximum time permitted by the manufacturer.

14 When rinsing the relaxer cream from the hair, great care must be taken to see that the chemical does not run into the eyes or ears by careless directing of the water.

15 Use the force of the water to remove the cream. Keep hands protected.

16 Always complete a record card giving full details of the treatment carried out.

17 Advise client on after-care and the importance of conditioning and moisturising treatments after relaxing.

18 Pay attention to health, safety and hygiene at all times.

19 In the event of any unforeseen problems, refer to a senior staff member in charge.

(See Level 3 Unit 8 for problems and causes when relaxing African Caribbean hair.)

Things to do Collect information on the products and techniques for African Caribbean hair. Present this as a report on African Caribbean hairdressing.

What do you know? Level 2 Unit 5B

Name the two different cortex types of African Caribbean hair. ☐

What is mitosis? ☐

What is the main active ingredient in curl rearrangers and curl boosters? ☐

Describe how to carry out a test curl for a curly perm. ☐

Name the main ingredient in hair relaxers. ☐

List the contra-indications to relaxing hair. ☐

Explain what happens to the internal structure of the hair when relaxing it. ☐

What is the purpose of using a neutraliser after curly perming the hair? ☐

What is the purpose of the neutralising shampoo when relaxing the hair? ☐

List the disadvantages of using a sodium hydroxide relaxer. ☐

COLOURING HAIR

Hair colour

Tints are dyes which are used to add colour to the hair. This is the opposite of bleaching, where the aim is to remove the hair colour by decolourising it.

Two major hair pigments are:

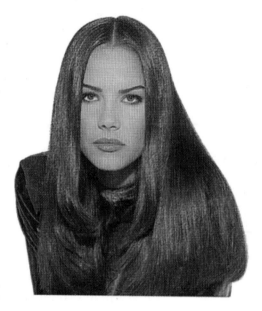

- Black/brown **melanin**
- Red/yellow **pheomelanin**

both of which are found mostly in the cortex, with a small amount in the cuticle. The hair appears to be a certain colour to the eye because the colour pigments in the hair absorb certain colours from the light falling onto it and reflect others. Only those pigments that are reflected reach the eye, so a blue object appears blue because blue light is reflected and the other colours are absorbed. Black objects absorb all the light falling onto them and white objects reflect all the light. In the shades or hues which are visible a mixing of the colours takes place. This mixing of reflected colours is complicated, but depends on the three primary colours from which other colours can be produced. This mixing effect is of great importance in tinting hair because of the way pigments are added to those already present in the hair.

When tinting hair the hairdresser must also take the light quality into account. This can be a problem in that the mix of colours in artificial light is slightly different from that in daylight.

Hair dyes

Hair dyes work by adding coloured pigment molecules to the hair. The pigment molecules are added to the hair in two main ways:

- The pigment coats the cuticle, that is the outside of the hair and does not penetrate into the hair cortex.
- The pigment passes through the cuticle (often aided by making the hair swell using steam or heat and/or an alkali), then into the cortex where it is deposited.

How efficiently this pigmentation happens depends on:

- The size of the pigment molecules.
- The porosity of the hair – often a function of its age, the hair furthest from the scalp being the most porous – and the amount of chemical treatment the hair has received.

Preventing RSI

The operator often keeps shoulders raised because the chair is too high for certain parts of the head. Other parts of the head require bending or angling of the wrist. Over a period of time, these day to day strains accumulate and can result in permanent damage if due care is not taken.

Types of hair dye

There are two main methods of classifying hair dyes, which can be explained in terms of their ingredients and their permanence.

Ingredients

The chemical nature and action of the active ingredients can be subdivided into:

- **Vegetable dyes** – extracted from plants and include camomile and henna. Camomile, for example, is a golden-yellow dye obtained from the flower of the camomile plant. This dye has large molecules which will not penetrate the hair shaft and therefore coat the cuticle. It can be used to add golden tones to faded blondes.
- **Metallic (or inorganic) dyes** – contain the metal salts of metals like lead, copper and iron.
- **Synthetic organic dyes** – 'man-made' substances and the most common ingredient in salon tints. A number of different chemicals come under this heading including the 'para' group.

Permanence

The permanence or length of time the dye will last on the hair can also be subdivided into:

- **Non-permanent dyes** – last until the hair is next wet, e.g. at the next shampoo, and then wash out. Other types last longer (six to eight shampoos) but eventually wash out as well.
- **Permanent dyes** – last until the tinted hair grows out.

Non-permanent dyes

Non-permanent colouring techniques include:

- Temporary rinses.
- Temporary colour sprays and paints.
- Semi-permanent colours.

Temporary rinses

These consist of an acid dye which is rinsed through the hair, then dried on during setting or blowdrying. Acid dyes all share the properties of working at a pH below 7 and will be easy to wash out.

A common acid dye used in temporary tinting is an 'azo' dye (e.g. parahydroxy*azo*benzene). The acid used is an organic acid (citric or tartaric) and has a pH of between 2.5 and 4.0. Acid dyes have large, coloured molecules which do not penetrate the cortex but form a coating around the cuticle. They are soluble in water and are therefore easily removed by shampooing. A temporary rinse adds colour to the hair, but will not lighten the natural colour.

Types of temporary rinses

Temporary rinses may be obtained in the following forms:

- **Coloured setting lotion** – obtained ready mixed, this contains synthetic resin, polyvinylpyrrolidone (PVP) and alcohol to which a suitable acid dye, often an 'azo' dye, is added. On drying, the alcohol evaporates leaving a coloured, plastic film on the hair.
- **Temporary toners** – also obtained ready mixed, these are usually used on bleached hair to correct golden tones. They often contain a mild conditioning agent to which a suitable acid dye is added.
- **Coloured mousse and gel** – normal mousse or setting gel to which a suitable colouring pigment has been added.

Uses of temporary rinses in the salon

1 As an introduction to colour, particularly useful for younger clients.
2 To brighten dull or faded hair. May also be used between permanent dye retouches to counteract any fading.
3 To tone bleached hair or to temporarily rectify a colour fault.
4 To enhance grey hair. It must be remembered, however, that these rinses will not completely cover the grey hairs.
5 To darken natural coloured hair.
6 To add multi or partial colouring to the hair.

Method of application

Temporary rinses are simple to apply. The hair is shampooed then towel dried to remove any excess moisture. The rinse may be applied straight from the bottle by sprinkling on to the roots of the hair (as these are less porous), rubbing through the hair with the fingers and finally combing the hair thoroughly to ensure an even distribution. Coloured mousses and gels are applied to the hair as normal following manufacturer's instructions but extra care must be taken to ensure that the application is even throughout the head.

Porous hair requires extra care as it will absorb the rinse very quickly, causing the resultant colour to be too dark and uneven. Applying the rinse with a tinting brush instead of straight from the bottle allows the operator greater control and enables the rinse to be applied evenly and where necessary, thus reducing the likelihood of a patchy result.

Precautions and considerations

1 Always protect the client's clothing, particularly at the nape, by tucking a dark towel well down over any collars, etc.
2 Assess the texture and porosity of the hair before commencing the application of the temporary rinse.
3 Pre-towel dry the hair thoroughly to prevent dilution of the rinse.

4 Never choose a temporary colour a shade lighter than the natural colour of the hair – it will not have any effect.

SAFETY TIP
Make sure that the client is adequately protected from splashes or spillage.

5 Do not apply strong red shades to hair that contains a degree of white hair, particularly on the front hairline.
6 When applying temporary colours to freshly bleached hair, ensure that an antioxidant cream rinse is applied beforehand. Any hydrogen peroxide left in the hair could cause a bleach-out of the colour rinse.
7 For hair with an uneven or high degree of porosity, either apply a good hair conditioner/restructurant or leave the hair wet, by not towel drying thoroughly prior to the application of the rinse.
8 Do not use cotton wool to apply the rinse. Cotton wool can sometimes absorb certain colour granules, distorting the true colour of the rinse.
9 Use only a fine hairspray when dressing out after a temporary rinse has been used. Heavy lacquering could re-dissolve the colour and give a patchy effect.
10 Do not display temporary coloured setting lotions near sunlight or heat, as either can cause deterioration and colour distortion.

Temporary colour sprays and paints

There are two types of temporary colour sprays. First, a colour in a lacquer-type base (a plastic resin) used in aerosol-can form and second, the puff-on, of a powdery consistency. Both types coat the cuticle.

Hair paints can be obtained in a variety of colours – some extremely bright. The colour is brushed on to dry hair with a painting brush wherever it is required.

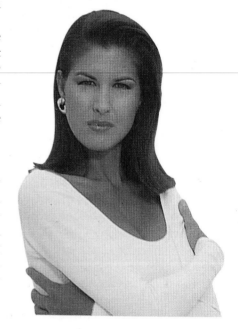

Both hair paints and colour sprays are ideal for special effects. They are the most temporary of the hair colourings and wear off quickly. They can be easily removed by brushing the hair thoroughly (although brightly coloured hair paints usually have to be washed out of the hair).

Precautions

Metallic gold or silver temporary sprays or powder must be completely removed from the hair before perming, tinting or bleaching as these will react with the hydrogen peroxide used in these processes, causing rapid decomposition of the peroxide and, consequently, hair damage. In other words, they are incompatible with the peroxide used in other processes.

Semi-permanent colours

These dyes consist mainly of synthetic, organic dyes known as 'nitro' dyes. Nitro dyes are small coloured molecules which can pass through the cuticle into the cortex. Because they are small they can be gradually washed out.

Nitro dyes do not dissolve easily in water, so benzyl alcohol is used as a solvent to allow the dye to penetrate deeper into the hair cortex. A detergent, such as sodium lauryl sulphate, is also added to the dye to produce a foam and improve the contact between the hair and the dye.

Semi-permanent dyes consist of small coloured molecules which are able to penetrate further into the hair shaft than a temporary rinse. Thus, a semi-permanent dye will usually last through approximately six to eight shampoos.

Diluted 'para'-dyes, which are oxidised to develop their colour either by the air, or more usually, by 10 vol. (3%) hydrogen peroxide are also sometimes used for semi-permanent coloration.

Semi-permanent dyes have a limited colour range and can be subject to colour build-up if used frequently. They will not actually lighten the hair and rely considerably on the base shade of the client. They produce darker tones than a temporary rinse and care should be taken when used on a client with a large percentage of white hair; an auburn colour (red), for example, is totally unsuitable for use on white or greying hair.

Individual heads vary considerably in structure, texture and porosity and these points should be taken into consideration before applying a semi-permanent dye. The larger the volume of hair, the darker and more intense the colour will appear. Porous hair will absorb the dye more readily but will also fade more quickly. If the hair is excessively porous it is often necessary to leave the hair wet, instead of towel drying, prior to the application; alternatively, apply a specially formulated pre-treatment restructurant.

Uses of semi-permanent colours

1 To brighten dull or faded hair.
2 To tone bleached hair.
3 To enhance grey hair (but will not completely cover the white).
4 For use on clients who are allergic to 'para' dyes.
5 To rectify colour faults, e.g. a green discoloration can be rectified by red.
6 For preliminary pigmentation when returning bleached hair to its natural colour.
7 In conjunction with bleach to give subtle or striking effects to the hair (depending upon the colour of the semi-permanent used). For example, streaking or scrunch bleaching the hair, then applying a semi-permanent over the whole head will give lighter and darker tones of the semi-permanent colour.

Method of application

Semi-permanent dyes are applied to damp hair that has been shampooed with a mild shampoo and then towel dried, unless instructed otherwise by the manufacturer.

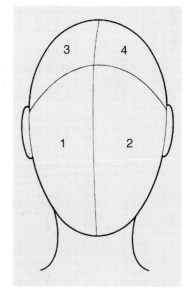

Fig. 2.66

1 Ensure that the client is adequately protected with a tinting gown, dark towel (tucked well down into the nape) and preferably a disposable plastic cape to cover the whole of the client and the chair.

2 The head is sectioned into four main sections (forehead to nape and ear to ear across the crown) (see Fig. 2.66).

3 Apply barrier cream around the hairline to prevent skin from staining. Care must be taken to ensure that it is applied to the skin only.

4 Commence application at the nape and apply semi-permanent with a brush (or sponge or applicator bottle) to the roots and along the hair shaft.

5 Continue application towards the front hairline with the front two sections. Take the sub-sections back and away from the face to prevent the semi-permanent running on to the face.

6 Apply the semi-permanent carefully to the last 1 cm ($\frac{1}{2}$") of the hairline. This is best done with a brush, even when using a sponge or applicator bottle on the remainder of the hair. A brush gives more control and helps to avoid skin staining on the face and neck.

7 Cross-check the application by taking sections across the previous sub-sections. Ensure that the application is thorough and that the semi-permanent dye is evenly distributed along the hair shaft.

8 Comb the hair thoroughly up towards the crown.

9 Remove any staining to the skin with cotton wool.

10 Leave to develop for about 10–20 minutes, or according to the manufacturer's instructions.

11 When developed, add tepid water and massage the head. Rinse thoroughly until the water runs clear.

12 Complete a record of work carried out.

Precautions and considerations for semi-permanent tinting

1 Read manufacturer's instructions carefully *before* application.

SAFETY TIP
Always give a skin test when unsure of the client's skin sensitivity, or when the semi-permanent tint contains a 'para' dye.

2 Some semi-permanent tints will cover up to 50 per cent of white, unpigmented hair, particularly if the pigmented hair is dark. However, they cannot cover white hair where it is concentrated in one area.

3 Extra care should be taken when applying the liquid forms of semi-permanent tints. Although they have better penetration they are more liable to run.

4 Do not use bleach to remove an unwanted semi-permanent – it could cause complications. Instead, apply an alkaline soap shampoo (or toilet soap) which will open the cuticle scales.

Apply a second, soapless shampoo, to remove any soap scum deposit then a conditioner.

5 Poor shampooing, or lacquer left on the hair prior to application, prevents penetration of the colour and gives an unsatisfactory result.

6 Use hot water when shampooing prior to application. This will open and swell the cuticle and allow deeper penetration of the colour.

7 When dealing with extra porous hair, dilute the tint with water or reduce the development time or apply a pre-treatment restructurant.

8 If a regrowth appears on very porous hair, apply semi-permanent to the roots. Leave ten minutes, then apply to the lengths of the hair and comb through, leave for a further five to ten minutes. This will produce an even result.

TECHNICAL TIP
Any stubborn skin stains can be removed by industrial strength methylated spirit (semi-permanent colours are soluble in alcohol).

9 A client requiring a natural brown shade may be better advised to have a permanent tint as the semi-permanent range of browns is limited. Also, a semi-permanent brown colour is difficult to obtain and has to be made up from a mixture of colours.

10 Do not leave the tint on for longer than the recommended time, otherwise the colour result will be too harsh and deep.

11 Permanent wave lotion will remove some of the colour and could cause patchiness. Therefore, when perming and colouring, the perm should be carried out before the semi-permanent tinting.

Tone on tone

This is the term used for non-lightening coloration which adds natural, lasting tones and shine to the hair. It is usually mixed in the ratio 1:2 with a colour releaser (oxidiser) and applied to dry, non-washed hair like a shampoo. It is then left to develop for approximately fifteen minutes or according to the instructions.

When to use tone on tone
- To give shine and lustre.
- To add sheen to newly permed hair.
- To pre-pigment highlighted hair returning to natural colour.
- To correct colour.
- To refresh new and old highlights.
- For men's coloration.

TECHNICAL TIP
When using fashion colour shades on 30–40 per cent white hair, mix with the corresponding natural shade for a natural coverage.

There are three main types of permanent dyes:

- Natural vegetable dyes.
- Metallic dyes.
- Para dyes.

Natural vegetable dyes

Originally, all colouring materials for the hair were obtained from plants, the main one being henna.

Henna is a natural vegetable dye, also known as Lawsone. It is produced from the crushed, dried leaves of the Egyptian privet plant which grows in Iran, Egypt and along the Mediterranean coast. It is a non-toxic dye which is mixed with water and does not require a skin or patch test before application.

Pure henna imparts red pigment to the hair and the shades vary slightly according to the country of origin. The depth of red depends on the length of time that it is left in contact with the hair, i.e. the longer the development time, the more red pigment is imparted to the hair. The shade of red also depends on the base shade of the client, i.e. the lighter the base shade, the lighter the red produced.

Henna colours often have other additives to produce variations. It can now be obtained in powder form or ready mixed, but it should not be used on hair containing over 10 per cent of scattered white hair, nor should it be used on highly bleached hair, as in both these cases the result would be too bright and harsh.

Henna is known as a coating dye, as it does not penetrate the natural pigment. Instead, it stains the hair shaft by adhering to the cuticle.

Metallic dyes

These work by depositing **metal salts** in the hair cortex and on the hair cuticle, which dulls the hair. There are three main types:

- **Sulphide dyes** – here the hair is first coated in sodium sulphide and then with a metallic salt.
- **Reduction dyes** – here a metal salt is converted to just the metal by a reducing agent, e.g. pyragallol. The minute particles of metal are deposited in and on the hair, thus colouring it.
- **'Hair colour restorers'** – these are not usually used in the salon but can be bought by the public from chemists. The idea is to tint the hair in order to darken unpigmented white hair. They contain lead acetate and sodium thiosulphate which react very slowly together and darken the hair by depositing lead sulphide in the cortex and on the cuticle.

> **TECHNICAL TIP**
> To help prevent fading colour, apply an acid balance rinse after removal to close the cuticle scales.

Disadvantages of metallic dyes

- They dull the hair.
- They can colour the skin as well as the hair.

- Some metals used in metallic dyes react with hydrogen peroxide. Therefore the hair cannot be permed, bleached or tinted.

Incompatibility test

Always test hair for the presence of any metallic salts before perming, tinting or bleaching the hair if there is any uncertainty as to what the client has had on their hair. This test is known as an incompatibility test. To carry out the test:

1 Take a small cutting of the hair from the crown area or the front (if the client has been tinting their own hair this will have the highest concentration of tint present).
2 Mix a simple bleach, which is a mixture of hydrogen peroxide and ammonia.
3 Immerse the cutting in the simple bleach.
4 If incompatible chemicals are present on the hair a reaction will occur.
5 Bubbles of gas (oxygen) being given off can be observed. Steam rises and heat is given off. The hair elasticity is increased and breakage occurs until the hair is completely destroyed.

Para dyes (oxidation dyes)

Modern permanent dyes are synthetic organic dyes consisting of solutions of para-phenylenediamine, or similar 'para' compounds, together with other substances, such as conditioners and antioxidants to prolong shelf-life. 'Para' compounds are a derivative of coal tar and can also be called synthetic aniline dyes.

These dyes are used to cover white, grey or most natural hair colour and have a vast colour range. Indeed, it is possible to obtain almost any shade, from natural right through to exotic greens, reds, blues or purples.

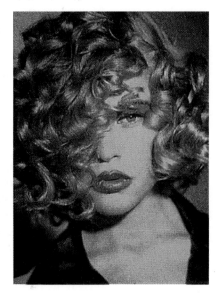

'Para' dyes are manufactured in three forms: cream, liquid and gel. All forms must be mixed with hydrogen peroxide before application. Without the addition of hydrogen peroxide they are completely ineffective.

These dyes are water soluble and have comparatively small molecules (at this point it is often colourless) which will penetrate the cuticle and enter the cortex. When mixed with hydrogen peroxide, the oxygen released makes the small colourless molecules join together to form larger, coloured, insoluble molecules, which are then trapped in the cortex (see Fig. 2.67). They are too large to pass through the cuticle and therefore do not wash out easily. In this way they mimic the natural colouring pigments. For an efficient tint, 20 vol. (6%) hydrogen peroxide is used, unless tints lighter than the natural shade are required, in which case, 30 vol. (9%) is used. Ammonia solution is used in 'para' dyes (as in bleaching) to speed up the breakdown of hydrogen peroxide.

'Para' dyes can be divided into two categories on the basis of how they are used. These are:

- Lightening dyes.
- Covering dyes.

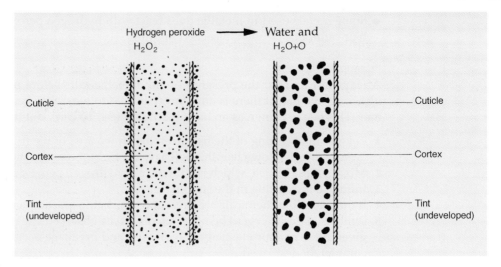

Fig. 2.67 Development of the colour of an oxidation tint

Lightening dyes

This type of dye consists of tinting the base shade of the hair lighter than the original colour.

To obtain a colour lighter than the base shade it is necessary to mix the para dye with hydrogen peroxide of a higher strength than that required to react with the para compounds. This is important because the oxygen from the hydrogen peroxide combines with the para molecules to convert them to large coloured molecules; thus, any additional oxygen attaches itself to the hair's natural colour pigment; making it lighter. The strength of hydrogen peroxide is usually 30 vol. (9%) unless a higher volume is recommended by the manufacturer.

It is useful to note that a higher volume strength of hydrogen peroxide sometimes throws up a golden tone. Therefore, when tinting the hair to pale ash shade (where no gold is required) some manufacturers recommend using 20 vol. (6%) hydrogen peroxide but in a greater proportion when mixing. In other words, the additional oxygen is obtained by adding more hydrogen peroxide. However, these proportions are only for certain tints and all manufacturers' instructions should be followed very carefully. Thus, correct mixing of the tint in relation to the hydrogen peroxide is extremely important to obtain the shade required.

Covering dyes

This type of dye consists of tinting the hair darker or a similar shade to the natural base colour, or matching white hair to the natural base colour.

The para dye is mixed with 20 vol. (6%) hydrogen peroxide as this releases enough oxygen to react with the para compounds without additional oxygen to bleach the natural colour pigment.

Where maximum depth of colour is required, e.g. very dark or black hair or toning after bleaching, 10 vol. (3%) hydrogen peroxide may be used.

To summarise, the base colour of the hair determines the volume strength of the hydrogen peroxide to be used. The lighter the colour required, the stronger the strength (or higher the volume) of hydrogen peroxide. The darker the colour required then the weaker the strength (or lower the volume) of hydrogen peroxide. (See Table 2.10.)

Table 2.10

Volume strength of hydrogen peroxide	Purpose
10 vol. (3%)	Gives maximum depth of colour.
20 vol. (6%)	For normal tinting.
30 vol. (9%) } 40 vol. (12%) }	Lifting peroxides for lightening.

Never use a higher volume of peroxide than necessary, as this causes hair damage and incorrect colour. As a general rule, 30 vol. (9%) hydrogen peroxide is the highest strength that can be safely used on the scalp and 40 vol. (12%) hydrogen peroxide is the highest strength that can be safely used on the hair. Sixty vol. (18%) hydrogen peroxide should only be used with specially designed tints and the manufacturer's instructions should be strictly followed.

Preparation for para tinting: skin testing

Para dyes are toxic dyes in that they can produce para poisoning in some clients. This para poisoning is known as **allergic dermatitis**. The symptoms are unpleasant, with itching and a blotchy appearance on the skin of the face and neck. In severe cases, the face becomes so grotesquely swollen that the eyes cannot be opened and the mouth and lips swell to such an extent that swallowing and speaking become difficult. The skin may erupt and 'weep' over the whole of the body. These symptoms are often accompanied by a violent headache, shivering and a high temperature and it may be many months before a full recovery is made.

It is important, therefore, that the skin is tested for a reaction before each application of a para dye, as even a client who has had regular para dyes can still develop an allergic reaction (often called 'becoming sensitised'). A skin test should be carried out 24–48 hours prior to the tint application and although this may often be inconvenient, to both the client and the hairdresser, it is very much a case of 'better safe than sorry'.

Method of applying a skin test

1 Clean a small area, either behind the ear or in the crook of the arm, with surgical spirit.
2 Mix a small amount of a dark shade of the tint to be used (the darker shades contain more para compound and are, therefore, more likely to produce a reaction) with hydrogen peroxide (as in the manufacturer's instructions).
3 Apply the tint to the clean area, about the size of a one pence piece, and leave it to dry.
4 To protect the area, cover with collodion and leave to dry.
5 Leave for 24–48 hours without disturbing.
6 If no irritation occurs, the test is negative and it is safe to proceed with the tint.
7 If irritation does occur, the test is positive and it is dangerous to proceed with the tint.

Note: A skin test can also be called a patch test, allergy test, hypersensitivity test, predisposition test, idiosyncrasy test or Sabourand-Rousseau test.

Test cuttings

These are taken before a full head tint, complete change of colour or whenever the hairdresser is unsure of the outcome of the tint through hair porosity, base shade, etc. It is simplest to take a small cutting of the client's hair when they book an appointment, so that the hair can be tested before the actual tint application is carried out. In the long term, a strand test can save a lot of unnecessary time and expense through choosing the wrong shade, peroxide strength, etc. It also gives the client a feeling of confidence, knowing that the hairdresser cares about them as an individual.

A test cutting will tell you the:

- Final shade of colour.
- Strength of hydrogen peroxide necessary.
- Approximate development time.
- Durability of the hair, i.e. breakage and tensile strength (stretching or elasticity).
- Whether pre-bleaching or softening of the hair is necessary.

To carry out the test:

1 Take a small cutting of the hair from the front or nape area. (If the hair is white in one area in particular, take a cutting from there also.)
2 Mix a small amount of the tint and peroxide to be used in a bowl.
3 Place the cutting in the tint. To keep the cutting together, bind the ends with a small piece of sellotape.
4 Await development.
5 When the tint has developed, rinse the hair and test for durability by pulling between the fingers.
6 Dry and assess the results.
7 Record the results, together with the test cutting on the client's record card as follows:

- tint and shade used
- strength of peroxide
- durability of the hair
- development time

8 Discuss the effect and final result with the client.

> **TECHNICAL TIP**
> The development time of the test cutting should only be used as a rough guide, as warmth or heat will make the tint act more quickly. Therefore, even the temperature in the salon can have an effect on the length of the development time when actually carrying out the tint application.

Colour selection

Human hair consists of two major groups of pigment which are deposited in the hair as it grows: melanin (brown or black) and pheomelanin (reddish-yellow).

Each head of hair has a different distribution of these pigments and depending on the reflection of light and the density of the hair, the base shades of the hair will be different on each head. If the hair is in good condition, i.e. has a smooth cuticle, it will reflect more light and will, therefore, appear lighter. If the hair is thick and abundant, it will be more dense and the colour will appear darker. This phenomenon can be easily shown by the black lines in Fig. 2.68, where diagram (a) appears darker than diagram (b).

The colour of the hair also reflects onto the face of the client and this too should be taken into consideration when choosing a colour.

Colouring preparations can be divided into two groups:

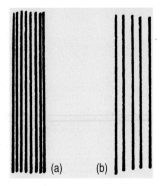

Fig. 2.68

- **Cold shades** – all ashen and matt shades (blues, greens, etc.).
- **Warm shades** – all red or golden shades.

The cold shades will give the illusion of a darker colour, while warm shades will give the illusion of a lighter colour.

A shade chart should be used when selecting a colour. A particular shade of colour is very difficult to describe and the use of a shade chart prevents unnecessary mistakes by allowing the client to show the hairdresser exactly the shade or colour that they require.

Once the shade of colour has been chosen, the hairdresser must then take into consideration the base shade of the client's hair as this will determine the strength of hydrogen peroxide to be used. The porosity of the hair is also an important factor. If the hair is excessively porous it is often advisable to choose a shade lighter to counteract the darkening tendency of this type of hair. The amount of white hair present on the head often creates a problem. It is sometimes necessary to use two different shades or two different peroxide strengths on one head to achieve a uniform shade, e.g. when hair is white at the front of the head and dark at the back.

In brief, the points to consider when selecting a colour are:

- Client's requirements, i.e. warm or cold colour (most clients require a subtle colour change only).
- Complexion, skin colouring and age of client.
- Lightening or covering.
- Base shade of the client.
- Texture and density of the hair.
- Tensile strength of the hair.
- Condition and porosity of the hair.
- Amount of white hair present.

Always remember that each client is an individual and if in any doubt, you should take a test cutting.

Matching a regrowth

It is sometimes necessary to match a regrowth to previously tinted hair without having any record of the previous treatment, e.g. for a new client who has had their hair tinted at a different salon. The procedure for matching a regrowth is as follows:

1 Ensure non–allergy to 'para' by skin test.
2 Take incompatibility test to determine whether any metallic salts are present on the hair (particularly important if the client has been tinting their own hair).
3 Check base shade of the regrowth against natural shades in the shade chart.
4 Check base shade of the remaining, tinted hair.
5 Check the percentage of grey.
6 Choose the shade nearest to the tinted hair, deciding if the tone is lighter, darker, warmer or cooler than the regrowth base shade.
7 Choose correct volume strength of hydrogen peroxide. Normal rules:

- 30 vol. strength when lifting more than two shades if there is not much grey to be covered
- 20 vol. for the average tint, i.e. the same or similar tone, slightly lighter or slightly darker, with or without grey
- 10–15 vol. for maximum coverage with no warmth or lift, e.g. black tints

8 If undecided between two shades of colour, always choose the lighter as it is far easier to apply a darker shade afterwards than to strip out unwanted colour.
9 If in doubt as to which volume of peroxide to use, always choose 20 vol. for safety.

Permanent tinting process

Preparation of the operator

A tinting apron should be worn over the overall to prevent staining. Rubber gloves should be worn to protect the hands, not only from unsightly stains but also to prevent dermatitis, which can be caused by constant contact with para.

Preparation of the client (gowning)

It is very important to protect the client's clothing at all times during the tinting process. Any stains to the clothing can be difficult to remove and the hairdresser may have to replace a spoilt garment which could cause embarrassment to all concerned. A tinting gown should be placed around the client to cover all their clothing and, preferably, it should be large enough to cover the chair also. This will prevent any tint from splashing onto the chair and perhaps staining another client's clothing later. Dark towels should be used, for obvious reasons, and these should be tucked down firmly at the nape to prevent them from slipping. A neck strip or strip of cotton wool placed around the nape is also a precautionary measure. Special plastic, disposable capes can also be placed at the back, over the gown and the towel to help to protect the towels and chair, etc.

To prevent staining of the skin, barrier cream should be applied around the hairline, but care must be taken not to allow the cream to coat the hair. If the tint application is carried out carefully and controlled, there should never be any risk of skin staining, but sometimes with the darker, particularly blue-black shades, it is very difficult not to stain the skin.

Preparation of materials and equipment

All necessary equipment and materials should be assembled before commencement of the application, to prevent rushing backwards and forwards across the salon during and after the application. A competent trainee can assemble all materials and equipment ready for the stylist, thus aiding the efficiency of the salon and freeing the stylist for the more skilful tasks.

The equipment should be assembled on the flat top of a trolley that can be easily wiped clean afterwards.

Preparation of a para dye

Para dyes are usually mixed with an equal quantity of hydrogen peroxide, in the ratio 1:1. This is a simple procedure with liquid and semi-viscous forms, but with the cream form of tint, the manufacturers clearly state the amount of hydrogen peroxide to be used. There are one or two exceptions to the 1:1 ratio, but again, these are clearly stated in the manufacturer's instructions.

To mix the tint, squeeze the tube (from the bottom and roll up to prevent oxidation, by the air, of the remaining tint if only using part of the tube) or empty the contents of the bottle into a non-metallic bowl. If more than one colour is used to produce a particular shade they should be thoroughly mixed together in the bowl before adding the peroxide. Next, mix the correct amount of hydrogen peroxide with the tint, adding it very slowly to form a thick, creamy mixture. If the peroxide is added too quickly, the mixture becomes lumpy and the resultant coloration will be uneven.

Application of a para dye regrowth

The application of para should always be done methodically, carefully and as quickly as possible. The method of applying a para dye can be varied, depending upon the porosity of the hair and the degree of white hair present. It must be remembered that the more resistant the hair, the longer it will take for the colour molecules to penetrate into the cortex; therefore, resistant areas should be treated first. Generally, the nape area is the most resistant as it does not get the same 'weathering' as the front area and is therefore not usually as porous.

Method of application

1 Assemble equipment and materials, then check that the client's skin test is negative.
2 Protect the client's clothing with dark gown, towels, etc. Ensure that the towel is tucked firmly down into the nape.
3 Disentangle the hair and check the scalp for cuts and abrasions. If minor, protect with petroleum jelly, if major, postpone the treatment.
4 Divide the head into six major sections, forehead to nape, ear to ear across the top of the head and ear to ear across the back. If the hair is excessively greasy, wash with a mild, soapless shampoo, then thoroughly dry before sectioning. This is to prevent the excess sebum from forming a barrier on the hair shaft.
5 Apply barrier cream around the hairline, ensuring that it is applied to the skin only.
6 Mix the tint according to the manufacturer's instructions, then commence application at the nape, unless more resistant elsewhere. Apply the tint evenly with the tinting brush to the regrowth area around the outline of the first major nape section.

7 The size of the regrowth determines the size of the sub-sections: for small regrowth – small sub-section; large regrowth – large sub-section. However, sub-sections should not normally exceed 1 cm ($\frac{1}{2}''$). To ensure a thorough application, the tint should penetrate through to the next sub-section, but make sure you do not overlap onto the previously tinted hair. The brush is stroked in the direction of the hair.

8 Then stroke up and across the sub-section.

9 Continue to apply the tint until the front sections are reached. Tint around the outline of the front section, ensuring that all wispy hairline hairs are covered.

10 The front sub-sections may be taken towards the front hairline or down from the centre parting.

11 Check the application by cross-checking across the sub-sections to ensure that the application is even and thorough.

12 Remove any stains to the skin carefully with cotton wool.

13 Lift the hair away from the scalp carefully with the tail end of the tinting brush to allow the air (and oxygen in the air) to circulate freely.

14 Cotton wool may be placed behind and above the ears to prevent the tinted hair from falling back and staining them.

15 Await tint development. Heat may be applied to quicken the process either with the aid of a steamer or an accelerator.

16 Check the development frequently by removing the tint from a small section of hair with a piece of damp cotton wool. Dry the section with another, dry, piece of cotton wool. The development is complete when there is no line of demarcation between the regrowth and the previously tinted hair. This is known as a strand test.

17 When developed, add a small amount of water to loosen colour and massage the head. Rinse off the tint thoroughly with tepid water until the water runs clear. Apply a cream or acid balance shampoo, massage gently, then rinse. Apply a second shampoo if necessary.

18 Apply an acid or pH balance conditioner, rinse, then thoroughly towel dry.

19 Complete a record of work carried out.

Combing through

It is not necessary to comb through the lengths of the hair for every tint retouch. Tints do tend to fade and lighten slightly due to the ultraviolet rays present in the sunlight. However, if the undiluted tint is repeatedly combed through the hair it will damage the cuticle scales, making it more porous at each successive treatment. A vicious circle is produced, whereby the more porous the hair becomes, the more quickly it fades! Acid balance shampoos and conditioners help to counteract fading by tightening the cuticle layers. If fading does occur, the tint should be diluted with water or a liquid shampoo before applying to the lengths of the hair. Combing through undiluted tint is used only very occasionally or when the client has a colour change.

It is important when combing through either undiluted or diluted tint to ensure that the tint is applied to each strand of hair, otherwise the result will be very patchy. When the tint has been applied to the lengths of the hair, rub the hair gently between the fingers to distribute the tint evenly. Do not remove the tint from the roots by dragging it down the lengths of the hair to the points, this again can produce an uneven result.

Full head application of a para dye

Clients are often reluctant to say if they have used any products on their hair, so before carrying out a full head application it is wise to take an incompatibility test (see Level 2 Unit 5A) to ensure that there are no metallic salts present on the hair shaft. The client should be tested for any allergy to para by giving them a skin test and once the colour has been selected, a test cutting should be taken and the resultant colour of the hair cuttings shown to the client. This enables any adjustments to be made before the application. Remember that the test cuttings will appear slightly lighter than the finished colour because of the density of the hair on the head. When all the tests are found to be satisfactory it is safe to proceed with the application.

The first-time application of a covering, darkening dye is quite straightforward. Section the head as for a retouch and commence application at the most resistant area. Apply the tint carefully to the roots and lengths of the hair shaft. The application must be thorough to ensure that every hair is evenly coated throughout its entire length. If the points of the hair are very porous, apply the tint to the roots and mid-lengths first and the points of the hair last.

The full head application of strong reds, purples, light reds and lightening dyes must take into account the effect of body heat. The roots of the hair are closest to the scalp and the heat from the scalp activates the tint more quickly in this area; therefore, the application to the section begins approximately 10 mm ($\frac{1}{2}''$) from the scalp. When application to all mid-lengths and points of the hair has been completed, the tint is left to develop approximately to the half-way stage or over. In the case of high lift tinting it is sometimes beneficial to protect the root area with strips of cotton wool placed along the sub-sections; this prevents the tinted hair from accidentally touching the roots. Fresh tint is then mixed and applied to the root area and left to develop until the colour is even from root to point.

When tinting long hair, allowance must be made for not only the effect of body heat, but also for the varying degree of porosity throughout the hair length. The hair points are the most porous due to wear and weather, while the mid-lengths are usually the most resistant and will absorb the tint more slowly. Application should, therefore, be made first to the mid-lengths, then the points and finally to the roots. (See Figs 2.69–2.71.)

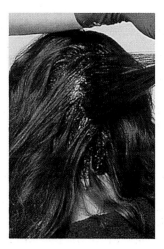
Fig. 2.69 Application to the roots

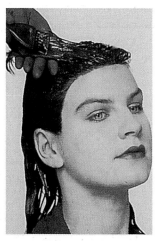
Fig. 2.70 Application along the hair shaft if necessary

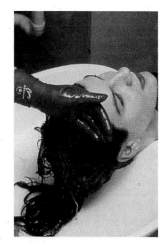
Fig. 2.71 Rinsing

Record cards

It is essential to complete a record of work done for each client after every application of tint. The professional hair colourist may find it necessary to mix any number of colours to produce a certain shade of colour and it is very difficult, if not impossible, to remember exactly what has been used on every head. A record card should record the colour/s used and in what quantity, the strength of hydrogen peroxide, the date of each skin test and the result, the development time and any remarks concerning the finished colour result. Any faults should also be recorded for further reference (see Fig. 2.72 for an example of a typical record card).

Name:	Base shade: ....
Address:	% white: ....
....	Hair texture: ....
Tel No:	Hair condition: ....

Date	Skin test	Tint Strength	Development peroxide	Remarks

Fig. 2.72 Sample record card

Contra-indications for permanent para tinting

Do not proceed with the tinting when:

1 The client suffers from a contagious disease of the hair and/or scalp, e.g. ringworm.
2 Incompatible chemicals are present on the hair shaft as shown by an incompatibility test.
3 You get a positive reaction to a skin test.
4 A lighter shade of tint is to be applied over a dark dye. The previous dye should first be removed or lightened, otherwise the new lighter shade will not show.
5 Hair is very weak and fragile. This type of hair should always be tested for tensile strength (see test cutting page 169) particularly if a full head tint lightener is required. Only if these tests prove satisfactory should the tint lightener be attempted.

SAFETY TIP
Always check the scalp for cuts and abrasions. If minor, protect with petroleum jelly. If major, postpone treatment.

Precautions and considerations for para tinting

1 Take a skin test before each para application.
2 If in doubt, always take tests of the hair to ensure that it can be tinted satisfactorily. This is called a **strand** test.
3 Regrowth should not be allowed to exceed 1 cm ($\frac{1}{2}$").
4 Ensure adequate protection of the client and the operator.
5 Check carefully that the correct shade of tint is mixed with the correct volume strength of hydrogen peroxide. In a busy salon it is an easy mistake to put a tube or bottle of tint back in the wrong box, with disastrous results.
6 Mix the correct amount of hydrogen peroxide with the tint, usually a 1:1 ratio.
7 Never use a higher strength of hydrogen peroxide than necessary.
8 Only mix the tint when ready to apply, otherwise the colour molecules will become too large to enter the cortex and result in poor coverage.
9 Commence application at the most resistant area.

> **TECHNICAL TIP**
> Grease or heavy lacquer on the hair can form a barrier and prevent satisfactory penetration of the tint. If this is the case, shampoo, then dry under a warm drier before commencing the application.

10 Always work as quickly as possible. Remember that the colour molecules are being oxidised as soon as the tint is mixed.
11 When a regrowth is too wide, in excess of 1 cm ($\frac{1}{2}$"), and the hair is being lightened, it may be necessary to pre-soften the middle band of untreated hair with 20 or 30 vol. hydrogen peroxide, then dry under a warm hairdryer. Proceed with the root application as normal, overlapping the middle band. This will counteract the effect of body heat on the 1 cm ($\frac{1}{2}$") nearest to the scalp. Be careful: this is a difficult procedure and should only be attempted by experienced operators.
12 Always check the application by cross-checking, to ensure that no area is inadvertently missed and that the application is even throughout the whole of the head.
13 Remove any stains to the skin after the application and before development. They are much easier to remove at this stage.
14 Lift the hair away from the scalp when the application is complete. This allows the air to circulate more freely.
15 Do not remove the tint before it is fully developed. All the colour molecules should be completely oxidised to give a satisfactory result.
16 Never repeatedly comb through undiluted tint, it can make the ends of the hair very porous and cause colour fade.
17 Give attention to the health and safety of yourself and the client at all times.
18 Always advise the client on the after-care of tinted hair. Explain the importance of regular retouching of the regrowth and the use of conditioning treatments.

Rectifying colour faults

Several unsatisfactory outcomes can result from hair colouring. Table 2.11 is a summary of the main ones with their causes and remedies.

Table 2.11

Fault	Possible cause	Action required
Patchy and uneven colour after tint application	Insufficient application or covering of tint Overlapping, causing colour build-up in parts Under-processing, i.e. not allowing full colour to develop Use of spirit setting lotions which may remove colour Regrowth too wide – average length of regrowth should be 10 mm ($\frac{1}{2}$") or 4–6 weeks' growth Uneven damage to the hair (uneven porosity) Colours not blended when mixing	Correct by spot tinting, applied to light areas
Colour too light	Too light or insufficient colour in the shade chosen Hydrogen peroxide strength too low to allow full colour molecule development Hydrogen peroxide strength too high for degree of lift required Under-processing or hair too porous to hold the colour	Retint, using the correct shade of colour with the correct volume strength of hydrogen peroxide for the correct length of time
Colour fades after two or three shampoos	Under-processing, i.e. colour molecules not fully developed Poor condition, hair too porous Unnecessary combing through of undiluted tint Wrong shampoo used after application	Retint, mixing the tint as a semi-permanent colour bath to add colour only. Watch development carefully. If the hair is highly porous use a special restructurant before tinting
Colour too dark after application	Colour choice too dark Poor condition – porous hair will sometimes take up too much colour Possibly incompatible chemicals present, e.g. metallic dyes	Test the hair for incompatible chemicals. If test is positive do not treat hair with other chemicals. If negative condition, then correct by using a colour reducer, following the manufacturer's instructions, or use a mild bleach to lighten the colour. Always test tinted hair before using either a reducer or bleach
Hair too red or brassy	Peroxide stength too high Insufficient development, not all colour molecules have developed Natural colour base too warm for chosen colour If pre-bleached, wrong choice of neutralising colour or not bleached light enough	Apply a matt or green colour to mask the unwanted red or a purple/mauve to mask the yellow, brassy tones
Unexpected discoloration of the hair	Poor condition, too porous to hold the colour Repeated combing of undiluted tint through the hair Possible reaction to incompatible chemicals	Test the hair for incompatible chemicals. Recondition and restructure porous hair if test is negative. Counteract any unwanted discoloration with a contrasting colour or remove colour with colour reducers or a mild bleach.
Colour build-up	Overlapping during application Combing undiluted tint through the hair unnecessarily	Apply a simple bleach or colour reducer, then condition the hair thoroughly
Roots too light	Failure to allow for body heat when lightening Strength of hydrogen peroxide too high Wrong colour choice when matching a regrowth Check carefully for development	Retint the roots using a mixture of tint and 10 vol. (3%) strength of hydrogen peroxide or one shade darker tint.
Hair resistant to tint or poor coverage	Closely packed cuticle scales – often strong white hairs are resistant to tint Tint and hydrogen peroxide mixed too soon before application, thus colour molecules have become too large to enter the cortex Wrong product or colour shade used Incorrect application Not enough product used Insufficient development	Retint, using correct shade of tint with 20 vol. (6%) hydrogen peroxide for coverage. If the hair is resistant, because of first cause given on left, then correct by pre-bleaching to open the cuticle scales, lengthen the development time and use a darker shade of tint. Moist heat will also help to swell the cuticle scales.

Table 2.11 continued

Fault	Possible cause	Action required
	Too weak peroxide strength to oxidise fully the the colour molecules	
Insufficient lift	Wrong strength of hydrogen peroxide used Wrong quantities of tint and hydgrogen peroxide mixed Insufficient product used Insufficient development Natural base shade too dark for chosen colour	Retint with correct colour and volume strength of hydrogen peroxide. Allow sufficient development. Pre-bleaching may be required if the natural base shade is too dark

Bleaching

Bleaching is a process which lightens the shade of the hair by lightening or decolorising the colouring pigments in the hair shaft. The two main pigments are melanin and pheomelanin, which are found as tiny granules, mostly in the hair cortex, but some are in the outer hair cuticle. The bleaching process is a permanent lightening of these natural pigments and cannot be removed by shampooing .

In bleaches of all types the oxidising agent is the active ingredient in the bleach and it is the hair pigments which are oxidised. The bleaching process in chemical terms is summarised as:

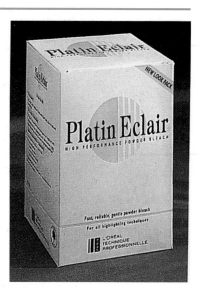

- The oxidising agent(s) in the bleach break down, releasing oxygen.
- This oxygen penetrates the hair shaft and decolorises the pigments This decolorisation can be seen when bleaching black hair, as a series of colour changes as the pigment is increasingly oxidised. These are:

Black → Brown → Red → Orange → Yellow → Pale yellow → White

The main oxidising agent used in bleaches is hydrogen peroxide (formula: H_2O_2), which can break down (or decompose) to release oxygen.

Hydrogen peroxide (H_2O_2)

This is an effective bleaching agent which releases oxygen and can then bind to the hair pigments and lighten their colour. This ability to act as an oxidising agent is also used in:

- 'Neutralising' perms, where the oxygen rebuilds the di-sulphide linkages in the hair, thus 'fixing' the perm.
- Developing oxidation tints, where the oxygen converts the small, colourless tint molecules into larger, coloured ones.

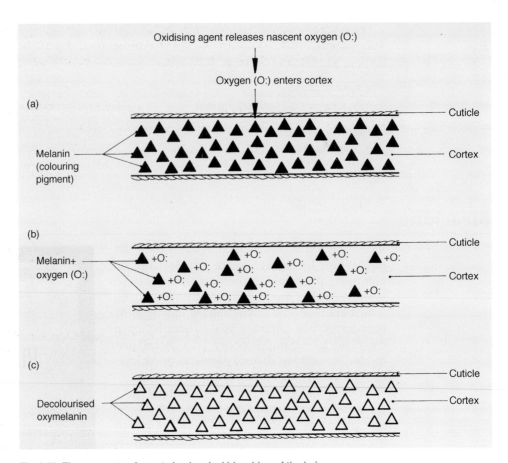

Fig. 2.73 The sequence of events in chemical bleaching of the hair

Hydrogen peroxide is colourless and odourless and looks very much like its close relative, water (H_2O). The difference is that hydrogen peroxide has an 'extra' atom of oxygen in its molecule making it H_2O_2, compared with water which is H_2O. Because of this 'extra' atom of oxygen, the hydrogen peroxide molecule is unstable and will easily break down or decompose and release the 'extra' oxygen atom as follows:

Hydrogen peroxide $\rightarrow$ Water + Oxygen
H_2O_2 $\rightarrow$ H_2O + O:

Strength or concentration of hydrogen peroxide

There are two alternative methods of expressing the strength, or more properly, the concentration of hydrogen peroxide solutions. These are:

- Volume strength (or vol. strength); the units are vols.
- Percentage strength expressed as a '% solution'.

Volume strength

This refers to the amount or volume of oxygen gas which will be released if a particular amount of hydrogen peroxide is completely broken down to oxygen and water. The stronger the solution the more oxygen it can release, so the higher the vol.

strength. This method of expressing the concentration is closely linked to the use of hydrogen peroxide as an oxidising agent because the higher the vol. strength the more oxygen it can release, so the faster and more complete the oxidation.

Percentage strength

This refers to the quantity of hydrogen peroxide as a percentage (%) of the total volume of the solution, the rest being water. There is a relationship between 'volume' and percentage strength as laid out in Table 2.12.

Table 2.12

Volume strength (vol.)	Percentage strength (%)
100	30
60	18
40	12
20	6
10	3

If one of these can be remembered, perhaps that 10 vol. = 3%, then the others can be calculated from this reference. For example, 60 vol. is six times stronger than 10. 10 vol. = 3%, therefore 60 vol. = $6 \times 3 = 18\%$.

Peroxometer

This is used to measure directly the strength of a peroxide solution (but cannot be used for cream peroxide) if there are doubts as to its actual strength, e.g. after a long period of storage. The peroxometer consists of a weighted float with the strength of peroxide marked on it as a scale. The stronger the peroxide the higher the float rises, because the density of the liquid is higher.

Types of bleach

Bleaches can be divided into two categories:

- Brighteners or brightening shampoos.
- Alkaline bleaches, which include:
  - simple bleach
  - oil bleach
  - powder bleach
  - emulsion or gel bleach

Boosters or activators

These can be used with emulsion bleaches. They increase the speed of the bleaching as they are oxidising agents which can release extra oxygen which adds to that being produced by the hydrogen peroxide. Chemically, the active ingredients are usually a mixture of ammonium and potassium persulphate. Ammonium persulphate breaks down rapidly releasing its oxygen and is therefore fast acting. Potassium persulphate breaks down more slowly and therefore acts more slowly.

Boosters or activators can only be used with hydrogen peroxide because they cannot physically break up the pigment granules in the hair. Hydrogen peroxide can do this and the boosters then speed the **decolorisation** of the pigment once the granules break up.

Brighteners or brightening shampoos

These will lighten the hair a few shades only and are used to:

- Lighten blond hair that has grown darker with age.
- Brighten 'mousy' hair.
- Make resistant hair more likely to tint.

Brighteners are applied over the whole head and the rate of lightening is sensitive to body heat, that is, the nearer the scalp, the warmer the conditions, so the faster the bleaching action. Consequently, it must be removed before any appreciable lift of colour is obtained, otherwise the hair nearest the scalp will be lighter than that further away. The bleaching action takes place mostly in the cuticle, where there are relatively few pigment granules (most being in the cortex), so the amount of lightening is relatively small. A typical list of ingredients is:

- 20 ml of 20 vol. (6%) hydrogen peroxide.
- 20 ml of hot or warm water.
- 10 ml of shampoo.

The shampoo is added to improve the contact by breaking the surface tension between the solution and the hair.

Commercially produced lighteners contain an organic acid (e.g. tartaric acid) which stabilises the preparation and gives a pH of 4.0 to 4.5.

Method of application

1 Shampoo the hair as normal.
2 Apply the solution as a second shampoo. Lather up and leave for approximately ten minutes.
3 Rinse thoroughly.

Alkaline bleaches

These are usually made up immediately before use, the alkali used being **ammonium hydroxide**.

Ammonium hydroxide (ammonia solution)

This is supplied to salons in a concentration of 35 per cent (that is, 35 parts of ammonia in 100 parts of the solution). This is often expressed as the density of the liquid and this solution has a density value of 0.880 – this is described as 'eight-eighty ammonia.'

Precautions

- Ammonia solution, especially when heated, will give off large amounts of choking ammonia fumes.

- If 0.880 ammonia solution is mixed with 100 vol. (30%) hydrogen peroxide, oxygen is given off explosively quickly.

- Excess ammonia creates too much swelling of the hair shaft, leaving it in a porous, weakened state.
- Traces of the alkali left in the hair cortex may result in a continued bleaching action which lasts for 3–4 months, with a continual deterioration in the hair strength and condition. This process, called **creeping oxidation**, can eventually result in a large amount of hair breakage. It can be rectified by applying a mild acid cream conditioning rinse, where the acid penetrates into the cortex and neutralises the remaining alkali.

Action of the alkalis used in bleaching

The alkaline pH produced by mixing the alkali with the oxidising agent has two main effects:

1 It causes the hair to swell which helps the oxygen released by the oxidising agent to penetrate the cortex and decolorise the melanin granules.
2 It neutralises the acids added to hydrogen peroxide which makes this chemical break down rapidly, releasing oxygen. In addition, ammonium hydroxide acts as a catalyst and therefore accelerates further the breakdown of hydrogen peroxide.

Preventing RSI
Keep your elbows down and close to your body whenever you can and remember to adjust the chair to a comfortable height for you. Always remember to bend your knees – not your back.

Types of alkaline bleaches

Simple bleach

A simple bleach consists of 20 vol. (6%) hydrogen peroxide mixed with a few drops of 0.880 ammonia solution. It will lighten the hair a few shades but tends to leave the hair appearing 'brassy', the final colour being dependent on the amount of the red/yellow natural pigment, pheomelanin, in the hair. Care must be taken when mixing because, if mixed incorrectly, the high pH value can cause hair breakage and burns. This type of bleach was originally used for pre-bleaching prior to tinting as it does not leave a chemical deposit on the hair, so the tint could be applied without first removing the bleach.

Modern tint lighteners have almost eliminated the need for pre-bleaching, except in the case of very resistant hair.

Oil bleach

This is produced as a liquid, and really the name is inaccurate because modern 'oil' bleaches contain no oil or bleach. Originally, an oil called 'Turkey red oil' was used, but this has been replaced by a **thickener** which has the ability to form a viscous gel when mixed with hydrogen peroxide (which actually does the bleaching). This can then change into a mobile liquid during brushing on to the hair and then change back into the viscous gel to prevent dripping once applied to the hair (this is the same principle as used in 'non-drip' paints). Despite these changes, these bleaches may run down the hair shaft during the application and make overlapping when carrying out a retouch almost inevitable. In addition to the thickener, an ammonia solution is present in an oil bleach.

Oil bleaches lift the hair colour by relatively few shades and tend to produce 'golden' tones in the hair.

Powder bleach

This consists of two powders, one being **magnesium carbonate**, which forms the paste but does not take part in the bleaching process; the other being **ammonium carbonate** or **sodium acetate** which makes the pH slightly alkaline at a value of 8.5. The powder is mixed with hydrogen peroxide to form a creamy 'pastelike' mixture. If the mixture is too thick, however, it will not coat the hair evenly and will not penetrate the hair meshes. While the mixture is developing, a crust is formed on the bleach which slows down evaporation and allows more action of natural heat from the scalp.

Modern powder bleaches are now mainly used for bleached streaks and highlights as they have a high degree of lift and will usually lighten dark hair to blonde.

Emulsion bleach

This is used in conjunction with boosters/activators and also has a high degree of 'lift'. When mixed, the emulsion bleach has a gel-like consistency which makes it easier to apply for a full-head bleach. The emulsion itself contains an alkali, a thickening agent, conditioners and modifiers.

Table 2.13 gives a summary of the different types of bleach.

Table 2.13

Bleach type	Ingredients	Degree of lift
Simple bleach	Hydrogen peroxide + ammonia 0.880	1–3 shades
Brightener shampoo	20 vol. (6%) hydrogen peroxide + water + liquid shampoo	1–2 shades
Oil bleach	Ammonium hydroxide + thickener (mixed with hydrogen peroxide)	2–4 shades
Powder bleach	Magnesium carbonate + ammonium carbonate (or sodium acetate) mixed with hydrogen peroxide	Will usually lighten from dark to blond
Emulsion/gel bleach	Alkali + thickeners + conditioners + modifiers, used in conjunction with activators (mixed with hygrogen peroxide)	Will usually lighten from dark to blond

Uses of bleaching

1 To lighten previously unbleached hair.
2 To pre-lighten prior to tinting.
3 To lighten or remove tint from hair.
4 To lift the cuticle scales slightly and make the hair more porous – therefore, resistant hair becomes more susceptible to tinting as it can penetrate into the cortex more easily.
5 To break down any resistant patches before a tint is applied.
6 To give highlights and streaks to the hair.
7 In conjunction with tint to produce extra hair colouring techniques.

Preparation for bleaching

Before commencing a full-head bleach it is often wiser and safer to take a test cutting of the hair when the client books the appointment, particularly if it is a new client whose hair is unfamiliar to the operator. A test cutting taken and completed before the commencement of the bleach application can divert many disasters and also gives the client confidence in the operator's professionalism.

Hair cuttings are taken from the front, crown and nape areas, as these areas can vary in porosity. If the client has been treating their own hair with chemicals, these may not have been evenly applied to the hair or may be incompatible with the bleaching agent to be used.

A skin test is not required before bleaching unless the client has an extremely sensitive skin (strong bleach mixtures can burn sensitive skin), or in rare cases, the client may have an allergy to ammonia. If in any doubt, apply a skin test as for tinting, but using bleach instead of tint.

Preparation of operator and client

Bleaching agents will remove colour from clothing so adequate measures must be taken to protect both the operator and the client.

The operator should wear rubber gloves to protect the hands and a tinting apron to protect the salon dress or overall.

The client's clothing should be protected in the same manner as for tinting, with a tinting gown to cover the clothing and preferably the chair also. The towel should be tucked firmly into the nape to protect collars, and also to prevent the towel from slipping during the bleaching process. A cotton wool strip or neck strip placed at the nape is an added protection. A disposable plastic cape to cover the gown, towel and back of the chair prevents any bleach splashing onto these areas, removing the colour and rotting the material.

Preparation of materials and equipment

All materials and equipment should be assembled, prior to the bleaching application, on the flat top of a trolley that can easily be wiped clean afterwards.

Preparation of the bleach

Bleach is usually mixed with hydrogen peroxide in a 2:1 ratio, i.e. 2 parts hydrogen peroxide to 1 part bleach, unless otherwise stated by the manufacturer. Measure out the required amount of bleach into a non-metallic bowl then add the hydrogen peroxide slowly while mixing. Always follow the manufacturer's instructions.

Application of a full-head bleach

1 Assemble equipment and materials.
2 Protect the client's clothing with tinting gown, towels, etc. Ensure that the towel is tucked firmly into the nape.
3 Disentangle the hair and check scalp for cuts and abrasions.

4 Ensure that the client's hair is free from grease or heavy lacquer. If this is so, shampoo gently with a mild soapless (or lacquer removing) shampoo, then dry.
5 Divide the head into six major sections (forehead to nape, ear to ear across the top and ear to ear across the back).
6 Apply barrier cream around the hairline, ensuring that it is applied to the skin only.
7 Mix the bleach with the hydrogen peroxide, according to the manufacturer's instructions.
8 Commence application at the nape (unless more resistant elsewhere) and apply the bleach mixture evenly to the mid-lengths and points, if the hair is short, mid-lengths only if the hair is long (see Fig. 2.74). Allow approximately 10 mm ($\frac{1}{2}$") untreated hair at the roots to counteract the body heat which will develop the bleach more quickly. In the case of long hair, the points are usually more porous and will therefore develop more quickly.

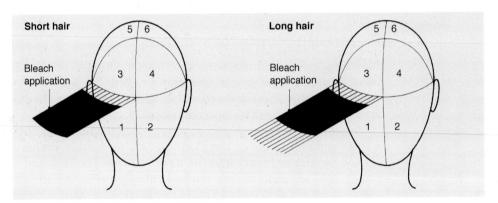

Fig. 2.74

9 Continue applying the bleach in this manner through from sections 1 to 6, in the correct order. Care must be taken to prevent the bleached areas touching the roots, otherwise the result will be patchy. To avoid this, strips of cotton wool may be placed between the sub-sections.
10 When the application is complete, gently work the bleach into the hair with the fingers to ensure that the bleach has penetrated each section. Extreme care must be taken at this stage to prevent the bleach touching the root area. In the case of long hair the bleach is now applied to the points of the hair in the same order as before, i.e. commencing at the nape through to the front area, unless the hair is more resistant elsewhere.
11 Check through the application to ensure that all sections are evenly and thoroughly covered.
12 Await bleach development, checking frequently taking a strand test. If the hair is not the correct shade, re-apply bleach to the strand of hair that has been checked. When the desired shade has almost been reached, mix up a fresh bleach and apply to the root areas as quickly as possible (work in the same order as previously).
13 Check that all the hair has been completely and evenly covered by cross-checking across the sections. Gently lift the hair out from the head to allow the air to circulate.

TECHNICAL TIP
Remember that the scalp may be very tender at the rinsing stage and excessive massage will cause discomfort to the client.

14 Await development, checking frequently using a strand test.
15 When the hair is an even shade throughout the entire length of the hair shaft, remove the bleach by rinsing thoroughly in tepid water. It is very important that all the bleach is completely removed from the hair.
16 Apply a mild acid balance or cream shampoo and massage the head gently. Rinse the hair thoroughly and repeat.
17 Apply a mild acid balance conditioner to counteract the alkalinity of the bleach and prevent creeping oxidation. Rinse the hair thoroughly using warm water.
18 Towel dry the hair and disentangle.
19 Apply a temporary rinse or toner to neutralise any unwanted golden or brassy tones. If a toner containing a 'para' compound is used the client must have had a skin test 24–48 hours previously to ensure that there is no allergy to this type of tint.
20 Complete a record of work carried out and advise the client on after-care.

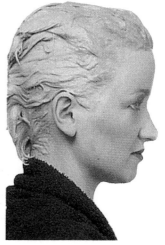

SAFETY TIP
Treat the hair carefully because of its increased porosity and elasticity.

Bleaching a regrowth

The bleaching of a regrowth requires far more skill and attention than the colouring of a regrowth because of the excessive damage that can be caused to the hair by bleaching agents incorrectly applied.

When carrying out a bleach retouch, the operator must take extra care not to overlap the bleach onto the previously treated hair as this could, at best, give a striped effect, and at worst could cause breakage of the hair.

The bleach must be applied quickly and evenly if an even result is to be achieved and must be forced well down to the scalp to prevent the appearance of tiny black pin-pricks at the roots. Each hair must be thoroughly covered with the bleach as any areas that are missed or overlooked will be clearly visible on the finished result.

Body heat has the effect of increasing the chemical activity close to the scalp; therefore the regrowth should not be allowed to exceed 1 cm ($\frac{1}{2}$"). This means that the client will require a retouch every three to four weeks, depending on the rate of hair growth. If the regrowth is greater than 1 cm ($\frac{1}{2}$") it is very difficult to achieve an even shade throughout the length of the hair shaft and it often results in a striped effect which is difficult to rectify.

Method of application for a bleach retouch

Proceed as for a full-head bleach application, but apply the bleach to the regrowth area only. Do not overlap onto the previously bleached hair. When application is complete, check carefully across the sections to ensure an even coverage. Await development (this is complete when there is no demarcation line between the regrowth and the remaining hair). When the hair is the same shade throughout the length of the hair shaft, remove the bleach by rinsing thoroughly in warm water and applying a mild acid balance shampoo then a mild acid balance conditioner. Complete a record of the work carried out.

> **TECHNICAL TIP**
> Bleaching colour out is sometimes referred to as a 'cleanse'.

Special attention must be paid at all times to the sensitivity of the scalp, the porosity and elasticity of the hair both during and after bleaching. The application of heat to shorten the development time should be approached with caution as it could cause extra damage to the hair and scalp by opening the skin pores and swelling the hair too much.

Contra-indications when bleaching

Do not proceed with the bleaching process in the following cases:

1 When the hair has been coated with a metallic substance, e.g. hair colour restorers.
2 If hair is over-processed or excessively damaged, e.g. after over-perming.
3 If the hair is extremely fine or fragile – use a very mild bleach only and test hair carefully beforehand.
4 When any contagious or infectious diseases are present on the hair or scalp.
5 When there are any severe cuts or abrasions on the scalp.

Precautions and considerations when bleaching

1 Always take into consideration the porosity and tensile strength of the hair before bleaching. Bleaching agents are strong chemicals that can damage the hair if used incorrectly, and the hair must be strong enough to withstand the treatment. If in doubt do a test cutting.
2 Never use too high a volume strength of hydrogen peroxide on the hair, it can cause unnecessary damage.
3 Do not allow the regrowth to exceed 1 cm ($\frac{1}{2}$"), otherwise the result could be 'stripy', because of the effect of body heat at the scalp.
4 Use barrier cream around the hairline if the skin appears sensitive.
5 Remember to allow for the effect of body heat at the roots when commencing a full-head bleach application.
6 Work quickly and methodically when bleaching the hair – the quicker the application the more even the result (providing that the application is thorough and even).
7 The application of a steamer during processing should be approached with caution as it can make the bleach 'runny' and it could run down the hair shaft on to previously bleached hair.
8 Remove all the bleach when fully developed. Any traces of the bleach (an alkali) left on the hair could cause creeping oxidation.

9   Bleached hair is less elastic and more porous than untreated hair; therefore, it will require far more attention when conditioning, perming or tinting.
10 Give attention to the health and safety of yourself and the client at all times.

Bleaching faults and corrections

Even if you follow all the precautions before and during bleaching, there are still some faults that could occur. These are listed in Table 2.14.

Table 2.14

Fault	Cause	Remedies
Hair breakage	Use of too strong a bleach mixture Overlapping when retouching the roots Incompatible chemicals present on the hair prior to bleaching, e.g. metallic dyes Bleaching of hair that is already in a porous and weakened state Over-processing Use of other strong chemicals over the bleached hair, e.g. permanent wave lotion Unnecessary application of heat during processing	Condition the hair and apply restructurant
Scalp irritation or inflammation	Sensitive skin Use of too strong a bleach mixture Cuts and abrasions present on the scalp prior to bleaching	Seek medical aid
Hair feels slimy and slippery when wet and takes a long time to dry	Hair in a highly porous state Use of too strong a bleach mixture Over-processing Use of other strong chemicals over the bleached hair	Condition the hair and use restructurant
Tiny dark pin-pricks at the root of the hair	Bleach not pressed into the root area firmly enough	Leave, but the client will require a retouch application sooner than normal
Uneven colour along the length of the hair shaft	Under-processed retouch Over-processed retouch No allowance made for the effect of body heat on a full-head application Uneven application Overlapping Regrowth allowed to exceed 1.25 cm ($\frac{1}{2}$")	Spot bleach darker areas. Rebleach if under-processed. Tone lighter areas if over-processed
Uneven colour throughout the whole head	Commencing application at the most porous area instead of the most resistant – this causes hair to be lighter in some areas than others Uneven application Application too slow Sections too large	Spot bleach or rebleach darker areas
Finished result has an orangy-red cast	Base colour too dark for strength of bleach mixture used Excessive amount of red pigment present in the hair shaft Use of too weak a bleach mixture Too much ammonia present in the bleach mixture	Test hair for strength and porosity. If satisfactory, rebleach; if unsatisfactory, apply a green or matt toner

Table 2.14 continued

Fault	Cause	Remedies
Hair too yellow or brassy	Under-processed Incorrect choice of bleach for the base shade Incorrect choice of volume strength of hydrogen peroxide	Apply a violent/mauve corrective toner

Bleaching techniques

Hair is naturally bleached by the effects of the sun's rays and it is possible to recreate this subtle effect through **highlighting** (the lightening of limited strands of hair). When more dramatic effects are required, it may be necessary to bleach the full head or partial 'blocks' of hair.

However, highlighting is far kinder to the hair than a full-head bleach and is therefore usually more popular. The method chosen to achieve this natural effect will depend on the base shade, length of hair and the hairstyle. Bleach can be streaked or merely painted onto the hair wherever a lighter effect is needed but some of the more popular techniques include:

- Traditional cap.
- Weaving.
- Scrunching.

Traditional cap method

Although this method does not have the accuracy of the weaving method, it has the advantage of being less time consuming and is therefore a popular method with busy salons. However, it is not recommended for use on long hair.

Method of application

1 Assemble equipment and materials.
2 Comb hair into the position it is normally worn (if the hair is excessively greasy or heavily lacquered, shampoo it then dry thoroughly).
3 Fix the highlighting cap firmly over the head by pulling it over the head from the front. (See Fig 2.75.)
4 Pull fine strands of hair through the holes in the cap with a crochet hook, starting at the front hairline and working through to the nape.
5 When enough strands of hair have been pulled through, comb the strands gently with a wide-toothed comb to ensure that no hair is tangled or overlaps another.
6 Mix the bleach with the hydrogen peroxide to form a stiff paste to prevent the bleach from running down through the holes and causing 'spotting' at the roots.
7 Apply generously and evenly to the hair, but do not press the bleach onto the cap – it could be forced through the holes.
8 Cover with a plastic, disposable cap to retain the body heat and await development. Apply heat if necessary to decrease the development time.
9 When the desired degree of lift is obtained, rinse thoroughly. Apply a small amount of conditioner to the highlights as this will allow the highlighting cap to be removed more easily.

10 Remove the highlighting cap. Shampoo the hair, rinse thoroughly and apply a mild acid balance conditioner.

11 Complete a record of the work carried out.

Precautions when highlighting with a cap

1 It is usual to pull only fine strands of hair through the cap. If the strands are too thick, it can give a striped effect, or alternatively the finished result can be too light, causing a definite regrowth to be seen within a few weeks.

2 Sprinkle talcum powder inside the cap before placing it over the client's head. It prevents the hair from sticking to the rubber of the cap and allows the strands of hair to be pulled through more easily.

3 Think carefully about the final desired result before commencing the application. It is possible to use bleach in conjunction with tint lighteners, e.g. the strands may be treated with bleach at the front of the head and a tint lightener used on the strands of hair at the back of the head to give a more subtle, shaded effect.

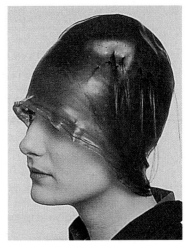

Fig. 2.75 Bleaching with a cap

SAFETY TIP

Be aware of the health and safety of yourself and your client at all times.

4 Do not highlight or streak the hair along any definite partings in the hairstyle. If the client does wear their hair with a parting, take a fine mesh of hair along this parting and section this area off before placing the cap over the head.

5 After pulling the strands of hair through the cap, comb the strands carefully to ensure that the hair is not tangled or bent at the roots.

6 A stronger solution of hydrogen peroxide can be used for highlighting as the bleach does not come into contact with the scalp. The highest volume that can be safely used on the hair is 40 vol. (12%), unless otherwise stated by the manufacturer.

7 Do not use a 'runny' bleach for highlighting as it can seep through the holes in the cap and cause 'spotting' at the roots.

TECHNICAL TIP

Always discard any highlighting cap that has become perished, or when the holes become too large, otherwise the bleach will seep through the holes.

8 Stroke the bleach onto the strands of hair, do not dab or force the bleach down onto the cap – the bleach could be forced through the holes.

9 Always ensure that all the bleach is removed from the hair to prevent creeping oxidation. An acid balance conditioner used after rinsing helps to neutralise any traces of alkali that may be left on the hair.

10 Advise the client on the after-care of the highlights. The bleached strands of hair will be drier and more porous than the untreated hair; this must be allowed for if the client requires other chemical processes on the hair, e.g. perming.

Weaving with easi-meche or foil

This method requires more time and effort, but the finished result is far more subtle than the cap method. The whole head can be woven, or just certain areas (partial weaving) to accentuate and lighten specific parts of the head, e.g. crown or front areas.

The work should be completed as quickly as possible to prevent the first sections woven from becoming lighter than the other sections. If this should happen, remove the foil or easi-meche from the sections that are developed sufficiently and remove the bleach with water. The use of tint lighteners in place of bleach often gives a more subtle result – they do not lighten as quickly, nor do they take the hair as light as bleach (see Fig. 2.76).

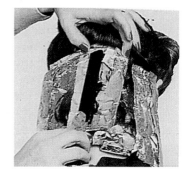

Fig. 2.76 Weaving with foil

Sectioning the hair

Sectioning the hair prior to the application is very important as it allows the operator to work quickly and methodically through the head in the correct order. The hair is usually divided into six sections but this depends on individual preference.

Method of application for full-head highlights

1 Assess hair and scalp. Protect the client's clothing and assemble equipment and materials.
2 Section the hair, making sure the partings are clean and accurate.
3 Mix the hydrogen peroxide with the bleach to form a stiff paste.
4 Starting at the nape, weave in and out of a fine mesh of hair with the tail end of the tail comb or pin-tail comb.
5 Place a strip of aluminium foil, non-shiny side next to and beneath the woven hair.
6 Brush the bleach evenly on to the woven hair, making sure that all the strands are completely covered (see Fig. 2.77).
7 Using the tail end of the tail comb, crease the foil then fold it over towards the root hair.
8 Fold both sides of the foil in towards the centre, creasing the foil with the tail comb first, making a parcel.

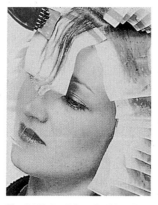

Fig. 2.77 Applying the bleach using easi-meche

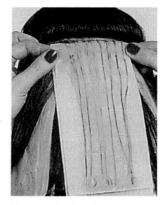

Fig. 2.78 Sealing the easi-meche packet

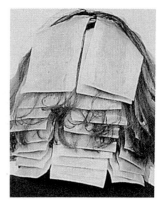

Fig. 2.79 Completed weave

9 If necessary, fold another piece of foil into a long strip and wrap around the base of the parcel to prevent it slipping. Alternatively, easi-meche can also be used in place of the foil (see Fig 2.78).

10 Continue weaving and wrapping up from the nape to the front of the hair frequently checking the first wrapped parcel for development.

11 The number of parcels depends on the thickness of the hair and the effect required. For the best results, the woven strands of hair should be very fine; if they are too thick it will give a striped effect.

12 When weaving the front sections take a fine section of hair at the hairline, then weave the hair *behind* this section. If the actual hairline is woven the effect could be striped and there will be an obvious growth to be seen almost immediately.

13 When the weaving and wrapping are complete (see Fig 2.79), check the first parcel wrapped, and depending upon the length of time taken to wrap the rest of the head, this should now be lightened sufficiently.

14 Remove the parcels in the same order as they were placed on the head.

15 Rinse the hair thoroughly, removing every trace of the bleach.

16 Shampoo with a mild acid balance shampoo and apply mild acid balance conditioner.

17 Complete a record of work carried out.

POINTS TO REMEMBER

Retouching should only be required after three months and then only at the crown, front hairline and any partings. After a further three months, highlighting should be repeated on the roots of the entire head. Avoid the ends of the hair if it is already highlighted by blocking them in a suitable barrier, otherwise the effect will be an overall bleached look.

Lowlights

In this case, a number of lighter and/or darker colours than the natural base shade are used on fine streaks of hair to produce a natural colour movement. It is particularly useful on grey hair as an alternative to a full-head permanent tint. Lowlights blend the white hairs with the natural coloured hair and eliminate the need to retouch the roots every four weeks as with permanent tints, it is also much easier to return the client to their natural colour if they so wish.

Lowlighting can also produce good results on bleached or very light hair using toning colours to put darker toning lights in the hair. One to three colours can be used and they are applied either using a streaking cap, easi-meche, spatula, or tin foil in the same manner as for highlighting (see Fig. 2.80).

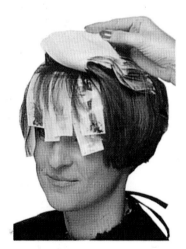

Fig. 2.80 Application of lowlights

POINTS TO REMEMBER

When highlighting/lowlighting with easi-meshe/foil/spatula

1 The tint should be at least two shades lighter than the natural base shade when a lighter result is required.

2 Two shades of tint may be used instead of one, in which case the colours are alternated up the sections.

3 For subtle effects, the colours should tone and complement each other.

4 Faded red hair is given new vibrancy if gold and bright red shades (mixed as tint lighteners) are used to lowlight the hair. The colours may appear extremely bright on the shade chart, but as they are only applied to fine strands of hair they blend with the natural hair colour to give a brighter but subtle effect.

5 The easi-meche/foil/plastic method of highlighting/lowlighting is more time consuming but it gives a far superior result on long hair.

When highlighting/lowlighting with the cap

1 Remember to comb the hair in the direction of the finished hairstyle before placing the cap on the head.

2 Take only fine strands of hair, otherwise the final result could be striped.

3 Check that there is no seepage of bleach (or tint) through the holes of the cap onto the scalp, otherwise the result will be patchy.

Precautions for highlights and lowlights

1 Introduce the client to colour with subtle coloration. Once they have gained confidence they will become more aware of what the salon has to offer and be willing to be more adventurous.

2 Use colour as an extension of the client's personality, but do not use too bright or very dark colours on older clients, it can be ageing.

3 When a subtle effect is required always look at the natural base shade carefully, there are usually golden or reddish glints to be seen that can be emphasised and highlighted. When using two or more colours on the hair try to keep within the same colour tones, and use different depths of these tones, e.g. red tones, gold tones, beige tones, etc. This will produce a more natural effect.

4 Do not be afraid to experiment with more than one technique on one head. With confidence, the operator will develop his/her own personal techniques.

5 When using tin foil to add lights to the hair, ensure that there is no seepage at the roots by wrapping a doubled strip of tin foil around the packet at the root.

6 Always discard rubber streaking caps when holes become too large. The bleach or tint can seep through these holes onto the scalp and hair with disastrous results.

7 Some of the tinting techniques are so quick that it is a great temptation to tint more of the hair than necessary. Remember that it is better to apply to too few areas than too many. More highlights can be added but they could prove time consuming to remove.

8 The main mistake when highlighting hair is to weave or pull the meshes of hair too thickly. This can give an unsightly striped effect and make the hair so light overall that a regrowth can soon be seen.

9 Always advise the client on the after-care of their coloration. The condition of the hair is of prime importance, as tinted hair only looks good when it is healthy. The client will also need advice on the upkeep of their colour and on how often salon visits will be necessary.

10 Be aware of the health and safety of the client and yourself at all times.

Things to do

The aim of this assignment is to help you to understand how bleaching and/or tinting the hair can improve the client's hairstyle by accentuating the shapes and lines within the style. It may help you to remember that where you lighten the hair it will appear finer and less dense while where you darken the hair it will appear thicker and more solid.

1 Analyse the hairstyles shown in Figs 2.81–2.83 then decide how you would accentuate the shape of each style using bleach or a combination of bleach and colour (tint).

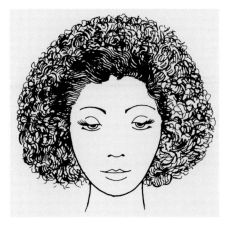

Fig. 2.81

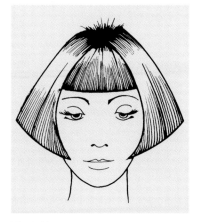

Fig. 2.82

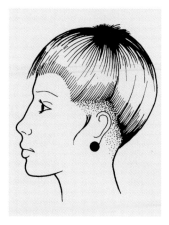

Fig. 2.83

2 Using whatever medium you consider suitable, e.g. crayon, paint, pastel, etc., colour the hairstyles to show the finished effect that you wish to create.

3 Take cuttings of hair for each style (these can be obtained from either your workplace or tuition head) and use these cuttings to illustrate:

   ● the base shade of the hair (give the number and letter, which you can find by matching it to the hair swatches in the tint shade chart)
   ● the type of bleach and/or tint you would use
   ● the strength of hydrogen peroxide required for each
   ● the approximate development time
   ● the elasticity and porosity of the hair both before and after the process.
   ● the finished effect

4 Write out a detailed report for each style. Include the following information in your report:

   ● the effect you hope to achieve
   ● reasons for your choice of tint, bleach and hydrogen peroxide strength
   ● a comparison of the elasticity and porosity of the hair before and after the chemical processes
   ● approximate development times

5 Design a folio of fashion bleaching and colouring techniques using the above information. Include any other interesting techniques that you may find in trade journals, etc.

What do you know?

Level 2 Unit 6

*Name **two** natural vegetable dyes. What advantages do these dyes have over other types of hair dye?* ☐

*List **two** methods used to allow dyes to penetrate more rapidly into the hair cortex.* ☐

Why is the hair porosity an important factor when using a colour rinse? ☐

What is meant by a dye being 'incompatible' with hydrogen peroxide? ☐

Why is it inadvisable to use either a semi-permanent or temporary rinse that is lighter in colour than the client's natural base shade? ☐

If a client requires both a perm and a semi-permanent tint why is it necessary to perm the hair before carrying out the tint? ☐

What is henna? ☐

What is the sequence of colour changes as hair pigments are bleached? ☐

What is the per cent equivalent of 20 vol. hydrogen peroxide? ☐

What substance is given off as hydrogen peroxide breaks down? ☐

When mixing bleach, what is the usual ratio of bleach to hydrogen peroxide? ☐

When bleaching a full head of natural hair, why is it necessary to apply the bleach mixture to the root area last? ☐

What is the desired maximum length of a regrowth for bleaching? ☐

What is a 'test cutting'? Why may it be used before bleaching? ☐

Describe a 'strand test'. For what purpose may this be carried out when bleaching? ☐

What is the correct term for the process of bleaching? ☐

How can 'creeping oxidation' be prevented? ☐

What are the two techniques for highlighting? ☐

Why is lowlighting useful on grey hair? ☐

SALON RECEPTION

Background information

Clients are fundamental for a salon to succeed and to stay in business. How a client is treated and the quality of the service they receive will determine:

- Whether they return.
- Whether they recommend the salon to others.

'First impressions count' is very true in these situations so all clients should be greeted politely and welcomed to the salon.

Attitude of staff to clients

The attitude of the staff towards the client and their work is very important. All members of staff should be pleasant, polite and helpful and show enthusiasm for their career. A sulky, sullen stylist makes the client feel unwelcome, uncomfortable and disinclined to return to the salon. Instead, it should be the aim of all staff members to give the client the best possible service and to ensure that a visit to the salon is an enjoyable experience.

Listed below are a few simple guidelines to maintain a good client/assistant relationship.

- Good manners. This involves showing respect to the client. Be polite at all times and always make them feel welcome. Never be too familiar, nor too distant, as both of these attitudes can make the client feel uncomfortable.
- Do not talk to other members of staff while dealing with the client, unless they are included and involved in the conversation.
- Confidentiality is very important in the salon. Reasons for this and the possible consequences of breaking the rules governing confidential information are covered in detail in Level 1 Unit 4, page 27, and Level 2 Unit 1, page 52.
- Make sure that the client is comfortable at all times, particularly if they have to wait for their appointment.
- Never sit down, comb your own hair or apply make-up in the salon; it gives an unprofessional impression. Use the staff-room for this purpose instead.
- Never eat, smoke or drink in the salon. Again, use the staff-room.
- Remember that every client is paying for a service. They are entitled to courtesy and respect as well as the best possible service you can give them.

Note: Never discuss or gossip about other people with the client.

Communicating with the client

Effective communication with the client is essential to clarify the service they require and ensure they fully understand the time, cost and processes involved. Misunderstandings, even little ones, are very bad for the salon's reputation.

Effective communication involves:

- Active listening.
- Questioning.
- Non-verbal behaviour – involved in both listening and questioning, which are covered in detail in Level 1 Unit 4 and Level 2 Unit 1.

Always discuss fully the client's requirements. Apart from the obvious fact that you need to know this information before beginning any hairdressing service, it also helps to build up a strong client/stylist relationship which strengthens the trust that a client must have in the person who is dealing with their hair.

Never argue with other members of staff while working in the salon and never argue with the client; it is most unprofessional. Beware of argumentative subjects, e.g. politics and religion, as some people have very strong opinions and it is very easy to offend them, even unintentionally.

Posture

Correct posture is an imporant issue for any hairdresser. Incorrect posture can lead to tiredness, inefficiency and physical strain, all of which will mean that the client is not receiving the best service and could lead to long-term problems for the hairdresser. Posture is discussed in more detail in Level 1 Unit 6 (see page 40).

Appointments

A booking should be entered in the appointment book in pencil so that it can be easily removed if the client cancels. The name of the client and the service required must be written **clearly** so that it can be easily read by all the staff; it is very embarrassing to call the client by the wrong name. If your handwriting is poor the information should be printed instead.

When booking an appointment, enough time must be allocated to each service otherwise the stylists become overbooked and clients have to wait, neither of which gives a good impression of the salon and causes frustration to all concerned. Different salons operate different systems and some salons employ staff as specialists to carry out certain tasks such as perming or tinting. In this case, a client booking an appointment for a permanent wave followed by a semi-permanent colour and cut and blowdry may have more than three people working on their hair at separate times, and this has to be organised correctly in the appointment book. Thus, it is very important that all the staff know exactly what system is in operation in their own salon and how to dovetail bookings so that the salon runs smoothly and efficiently.

Timing of salon services

Knowing how long a process takes is essential for phasing appointments correctly. Table 2.15 lists some common services and the times they may take.

Record keeping

A detailed record should be kept of all hairdressing treatments, particularly those that will be carried out over a period of weeks. This builds up a very clear picture of how the hair is reacting and progressing with the treatment and any modifications made. A typical 'record card' of hair/scalp treatment is shown in Fig. 2.84.

Client records may be kept on paper and filed or they may be kept as computer information on disk.

Table 2.15

Service	Approximate time needed in minutes
Shampoo	5
Cutting	30–40
Blowdry	20–45
Setting	60–90 (including drying time)
Perms	90 (virgin hair) 75 (treated)
Colouring	Varies, up to 60
Bleaching	Varies, up to 60
Plaiting	Varies, up to 90

Use of the telephone

The telephone is a vital link with the client and it is crucial that they hear only a voice which is always pleasant and helpful, no matter how busy the salon may be. Time must always be found to answer the phone – if staff are too busy to book an appointment at that particular point in time, the name of the salon should be stated and then, if necessary, the client could be asked to hold on for a moment. All staff must be trained to answer the telephone and to book appointments, even if the salon employs a receptionist. Bad telephone technique such as an abrupt reply or an unhelpful manner could lose many potential or regular clients.

In some salons, incoming telephone calls for members of staff are not allowed. Therefore, any rules regarding the receiving or ringing out of calls should be clearly indicated to all staff to prevent any unnecessary friction in the salon.

RECORD CARD
HAIR/SCALP TREATMENT

Name: .... Tel No: ....

Address: ....

....

Hair assessment	Type	Porosity	Diseases/abnormalities

Scalp assessment	Skin type		Diseases/abnormalities

Cause of damage						
Date	Conditioner/ lotion	Type of massage	Time	Source of heat	Time	Result

Fig. 2.84 Sample record card for hairdressing treatments

Telephone services

There are now many operator services available for business use although not all are suitable for the smaller hairdressing salon. New technology has meant that all communication services, including the telephone, are being expanded and updated at a bewildering speed. Consequently, it is often a useful exercise to become reacquainted with the facilities that are available approximately every twelve months or so.

The telephone is a vital link between the salon and the client so any faults should be rectified as quickly as possible to prevent loss of business. If the telephone is completely out of order then the fault should be reported immediately from elsewhere on a 'live' telephone.

Use of the telephone directory

All the information needed for using the telephone is contained in the *phone book*. This is issued by the telephone provider to all their subscribers free of charge and is written specifically for the area in which the subscriber lives.

The phone book contains far more information than just the names, addresses and telephone numbers of its subscribers. It also gives information on what services are available, how to use those services, the procedure for emergency calls, reporting faults, and how to handle nuisance calls. It provides information on places of interest, call charges and useful numbers within the subscribers' locality. It also gives guidance on how to find the number required and how to make local, national and international calls.

If using British Telecom, some useful numbers to remember are:

100 **Operator services** (including alarm calls, credit card calls, fixed time calls, freefone calls, personal calls, transferred charge and advice of duration and charge (ADC) calls).

151 **Faults** – telephone lines or equipment.
192 **Directory enquiries**.
999 **Emergency services**.

Using the emergency services

There are three main telephone emergency services: Fire, Police, Ambulance (with Coastguard and Mountain Rescue depending on the location), each of which consists of a highly skilled team used to dealing with all types of disasters.

An emergency usually involves an unusual or frightening situation so the most important thing to remember is to keep calm even though this may be difficult in the circumstances.

The correct procedure for contacting the emergency services is as follows:

1 Dial **999** or the emergency number shown on the number label.
2 When the **operator** answers, give the telephone number shown on the telephone.
3 Ask for the **service** you require.
4 When the service answers give the **address** where help is needed.
5 Supply any other **information** which may be of use.

Note: Always try to speak **clearly** to prevent any misunderstandings and to enable the services to react immediately and bring help as quickly as possible.

Taking messages

Always **write down** a verbal message as it is often difficult to remember the correct information, particularly if the person who is to receive the message is not available at that precise moment. Writing down a message also has the added advantage of acting as a **reminder** to pass on the message at a later time.

The following facts should be included when writing down messages:

- Date and time of message.
- Name of the person giving the message.
- Name of the person to receive the message.
- Exact details of the message.
- Name of the person taking the message.

When these details have been recorded, repeat the message back to the caller to make sure that it has been written down correctly.

Processing cash and non-cash payments

Most salons will have their own system for keeping records of daily transactions. Computerised cash tills are now commonly used to balance stock control by allowing a constant and immediate check on any items that require reordering. Electronic cash registers (tills) have what are called 'clerk keys' which will keep each stylist's takings, and any other sundries such as sales, separate on the till roll which makes the totalling at the end of the day much easier. However, salons without either of these systems have their own individual procedures which usually involve the checking of daily totals against the cash till receipts, client dockets, sales receipts and appointment book to ensure that there are no discrepancies.

Salons also have to have some form of **petty cash** to deal with any small items that may have to be purchased during the working day such as coffee, sugar, etc. This may be in the form of a petty cash box or a book which lists any items purchased with a total at the end of each day. Whatever type of system is operated it is essential to keep a precise record, together with any receipts, of any cash used during the day, otherwise time can be wasted wondering why the day's takings do not add up correctly.

At the beginning of the day a set amount of small change and notes, known as a **float**, is put in the cash till. This is to make sure that there is enough change in the till should the client not give the exact amount for their service. The float must be subtracted from the day's takings when 'cashing up' at the end of the day.

Remember that the handling of cash is always open to abuse by both staff and clients; therefore an efficient and effective system of cash control is essential to maintain a successful business.

Cash transactions

All members of staff must be competent in operating the cash till, receiving cash, giving change and calculating any relevant VAT. It is also essential that staff are familiar with the varying procedures necessary to ensure the validity of client payments made by cheque, credit card, account card or gift voucher as errors in these areas can be extremely costly to the salon.

Accepting cash payments

Great care must be taken when accepting cash from a client as mistakes can easily happen, particularly during busy periods. The short-changing of a client can cause ill-feeling and loss of future custom.

Procedure for accepting cash payments

1 Inform the client of the charge for the service(s) they have received.
2 Check that the cash received is in the correct currency.
3 Ring up the correct amount on the cash till or computer. If the client requires change, place any paper money on the top before removing the change from the cash till to prevent any misunderstanding as to the amount given.

Non-cash payments

Non-cash payments include cheques, credit cards and gift vouchers which are all legal tender but must be processed correctly to ensure that the salon receives payment for their services.

Cheques

A cheque is paid directly into a bank account.

The writing on any cheque should be legible and must contain the following information, in ink, if it is to be accepted by the bank:

- Correct date.
- Name of the person or salon to whom the cheque is to be paid.
- Amount to be paid in words as well as numbers.
- Signature of the person writing the cheque.

Procedure for receiving a cheque

1 Ensure that the cheque contains the information listed above.
2 Ask to see the client's **cheque guarantee card**. This is a card issued by the bank which, when used with a cheque, ensures that the bank will honour payment up to a certain amount even if the client does not have that amount in their bank account at that particular time.
3 Check that the signature on the cheque matches the signature on the guarantee card and that it is not past the expiry date.
4 Ensure that the bank name, bank code and account number are the same on both the cheque and guarantee card.
5 Write the guarantee card number on the back of the cheque.
6 Return the guarantee card to the client then place the cheque in the cash till.

Precautions and considerations

Make sure that:

- The writing on the cheque is in ink.
- The writing is legible.
- Any alterations are signed or initialled by the client.
- The correct date has been entered.
- The amount is made out in sterling, i.e. UK currency.
- It is not an 'open' cheque, i.e. it has the name of the person to whom it is payable written on it, otherwise it could be misused by someone else.
- There are no spaces where other words could be added or altered.
- The date on the cheque guarantee card is valid.

Credit cards

Some clients prefer to use this method of payment, particularly for large bills, as it allows them to spread payment over a period of time. However, not all salons accept credit cards, particularly smaller establishments, as a charge is made by the bank to the salon for the use of the facility. However, as with a cheque, the bank will honour the payment even if the client has insufficient funds in their account to cover the debt.

Procedure

1 Use the imprinter and relevant voucher to duplicate the credit card details.
2 Using a pen, write in the date, description of goods, amount in words and numbers, your signature and the authorisation code.
3 The client must then sign the form in the space provided.
4 Check that the signature is the same on both the form and the credit card.

5 Check that the date on the credit card is valid.

6 Tear out the carbons then give the top copy to the client for their records and keep the remaining copies in a safe place.

Electronic funds transfer (EFT) cards

These are the latest credit cards to come onto the market and fulfil the roles of both bank guarantee card and service card. The current account is debited electronically without the client having to write a cheque.

The card is drawn through a special terminal which then stores the details of the transaction. A two-part voucher is supplied which the client has to sign. One part is kept by the client as a record of the transaction and the other is retained by the salon. *Always* check that the signature on the voucher is the same as that on the EFT card.

Note: Due to the high level of theft and fraud linked to credit cards of all types it is likely that all cards will soon have to include the card-holder's photograph. When this becomes common, checks will need to be made on:

● The match between photo and person with the card.
● Any tampering with the photograph.

Gift vouchers

These are usually in multiples of pounds and are at their most popular during the Christmas season. Each salon will have its own system for processing gift vouchers but usually it is easier to deal with them if they are thought of as paper currency and treated as such. Change is not usually given however.

Travellers' cheques

These are another method of non-cash payment. Rather like gift vouchers, if the salon accepts them they can be treated as cash. Check the signature on the cheque with that on the traveller's folder.

Value added tax (VAT)

Any salon with a yearly turnover of more than £45,000 must charge the client a tax, known as VAT, on all of its services (this does not include any sales, as retail items have any necessary VAT included in the price). This tax is then collected by the salon and returned, through certain procedures, to Government funds.

VAT can be included within the price of the service or may be added onto the bill at the end. At present, VAT is charged at 17.5 per cent of the service. Therefore, a service costing £10.00 would incur £1.75 VAT, and so the client would pay a total of £11.75 for the service they had received.

Things to do

1 To help you to gain a greater understanding of the services which your salon has to offer, make a chart in the format set out below. You can obtain the information by reading the information contained in the packaging and instruction leaflets of the products, by asking the people who work with you and by watching the various services being carried out in the salon.

When it is complete ask if the chart can be put up in your staff-room at work as a reminder while you are learning your reception duties.

Service	Timing stylists	Timing client	Benefits and effects	Cost to client
(a)	(b)	(c)	(d)	(e)

In column (a) list all the services that your salon has to offer – you may be surprised at how long this list will be! Any large services, such as perming, should be subdivided into the different types as their benefits and costs will be different even if the timing is very similar.

In column (b) give the timings for the separate stages, particularly large tasks. This will help you to dovetail appointments in the future

In column (c) find out the total time that the client will be in the salon.

In column (d) write down the benefits and effects of each service and look at the finished results in the salon. Why and how do you think their hair has been improved?

Use your own experience as well as other resources to complete this column. For example, if you have had your own hair permed or coloured, why do you think that it is better than before and why did you have it done?

Fill in column (e) by looking at the salon price list.

2   Make a list of the terms used in a salon to cover all the aspects of non-cash payments.

  ● Explain how each is used.
  ● Explain how non-cash payments are recorded. What is the documentation involved?

What do you know?

Level 2 Unit 7

List the main areas involved in dealing with clients. ☐

Why should bookings be entered in the appointment book in pencil? ☐

Why is a good telephone manner important? ☐

What telephone number would you dial to report a telephone fault? ☐

What action should be taken if a client has to wait? ☐

What are the main areas to consider when communicating with a client? ☐

What is the procedure for contacting the emergency services by telephone? ☐

When writing down a verbal message, what facts should be included? ☐

What is the procedure for accepting cash payments? ☐

Give **eight** precautions/considerations when receiving a cheque from a client. ☐

EFFECTIVE TEAMWORK

A good salon has a good atmosphere of co-operation between staff, staff being interested and motivated in their work and keen to offer a top quality service to the salon's clients. People can sense this atmosphere when they enter the premises. What produces this atmosphere? Key factors are the hairdresser:

- Working as an individual – the best team is still made up of a number of individuals.
- Working a a team member – supporting others.
- Feeling positive about their job role in the salon – feeling that they are valued by the organisation and that a reasonable level of interest is taken in their development.

These areas will now be considered in more detail.

Working as an individual

This involves a number of key activities which are:

- Organising own work – using the appointments system.
- Adapt to changing circumstances – such as clients being late, or unexpected clients turning up.
- Making best use of time in the salon.
- Preparation and clearing up of work areas.
- Resolving problems as an individual when possible, but also knowing who to refer a problem to at other times.
- Provide information on matters important to the salon (health and safety for example) promptly and accurately when asked.

Organising own work

This is based on the appointments that have been made. A consideration of the types of appointments booked will produce a plan for activities based on:

- **What** needs to be done/organised for the procedures requested.
- **When** the client is booked in.
- **How** the services will be carried out.
- **Where** they will need to be carried out.
- **How long** the service or services to the client will take.

This should allow a plan that makes best use of the salon's resources and provides a good efficient service to the client. Unfortunately the best plans go wrong when the *unexpected* happens. There are events not anticipated in the planning which can upset the whole thing if allowed. What are these events and what action can the hairdresser take?

Adapting to circumstances

Basically the salon staff need to be able to *adapt*. Some examples of unexpected events and the possible strategies for the hairdresser are summarised below.

Client is late

The question is 'how late'? If only a little late there is usually a little 'slack' in the appointments schedule which can allow for this. Use the time productively while waiting. There is always something worth doing, or if not sure, *ask*. If the client is **very** late their appointment is probably gone and other clients are being processed. Offer the client another appointment as soon as possible, e.g. later the same day or with another stylist or look to rearranging later appointments (perhaps use more of the salon junior's time for some basic processes?).

Unscheduled client

Make sure they feel welcome and not a liability. Proceed as above by rescheduling, offering a later appointment, etc.

Overbooking

This really should **not** happen! The major cause is someone not writing the appointment down in the appointment book or keying it in. If it does, carry on as you would for an unscheduled client.

Changing client requirements

This is where a client has booked in for one thing and then either with or without consultation with the hairdresser decides they want another salon service. This may require some:

● Rescheduling.
● More use of junior staff.

Services taking longer than planned

This one is not uncommon and contingencies like having a little slack time built into appointments can help here. If very prolonged then schedules can be replanned and more use made of junior staff.

Staff absence

In this case then clients can be fitted into other stylists' appointments. Junior staff can be used for some basic operations, e.g. blowdrying, to free up stylist time. As a *last resort* clients can be telephoned, the position explained and their appointments rebooked.

Preparation of work areas

This requires that the work areas are clean and tidy, that equipment and products are ready for the next client, and that they are left in good order at the end of the salon service. Routine hygiene practices should be automatic (these are listed in Level 1 Unit 6, page 45.

Problems and what to do

There are a whole host of problems that can occur in the salon, these may be:

- Technical.
- Personal.
- To do with colleagues.

As experience and skills develop, a hairdresser can manage an increasingly wide range of problems but there will always be some instances where it is sensible to ask for help and advice. In general, if in doubt do ask for help from you supervisor, but remember it is important to learn from the advice and experience of others.

Providing information when requested

Effective management is about many things but a key process is **communication** between supervisors/managers and their salon teams. There is a variety of information that may be requested in order to monitor and improve salon procedures and processes. These include:

- **Provision of services** – how many of which type, any problems?
- **Personnel** – is the team working effectively? Can there be improvements? Staff appraisal.
- **Health and safety** – are policies known and understood? Are procedures being followed? Are there any problems? Are these sorted out in a reasonable timescale? Are channels of communication open?

The important thing with requests for information is to be:

- **Prompt** – provide the information quickly.
- **Accurate** – bad information causes bad decisions to be made for the best of motives.

Working as a member of the salon team

Always remember that all members make a significant contribution to the effectiveness of the team both in terms of their varying personalities and in their various skills and experience. Good teams work together well. There has been a mass of research into what makes this happen or hinders it. Here is a summary of some key things about effective teams:

- **Interpersonal skills** – treating others with courtesy and respect. Managing disputes well. Trusting each other.
- **Shared skills and experiences, aims and objectives** – this comes out of good interpersonal skills. Requests for assistance are responded to positively and the help given is encouraging and within the competence of the helper.
- **Supportive supervisor manager** – good teams need to develop good interpersonal skills and the sharing of skills and experience needs to be fostered, encouraged and reinforced. Team members need to be encouraged to promote good relations in the team. Development of team members needs to be given a high priority; to enable the team members, and therefore the team as a whole, to be more effective in their **job role**.

Self-improvement within the job role

Many salons operate an **appraisal review** system. There is a detailed account of this in Level 1 Unit 4, page 33. Here is a summary:

1 Strengths as well as weaknesses need to be identified and recorded.
2 Improvements need to be agreed, not imposed, and the action plan for the person's development needs to be:
   - realistic
   - constructive/developmental
   - subject to a review after a fixed time period
3 It is important to be **positive** about the appraisal/review. It is an opportunity to tell your supervisor/manager about what you do. Particularly what you feel you do well and those areas you would like to develop. The appraisal process **makes** them listen!

Think of reviews or appraisals as a **positive** experience. It should support you and the team. It should form part of a general ongoing awareness of opportunities for improvement and it should be supported and encouraged by salon management.
   Areas where there are constant developments are in:

- Fashion trends.
- Technology (products, tools and equipment).

The hairdresser needs to keep abreast of these changes. Information about these areas can be found through sales reps or in:

- Trade journals.
- Exhibitions/presentations/demonstrations.
- Training/update sessions organised in the salon or elsewhere (local FE College for example).

In this, as in so many areas, a good team works together by sharing ideas, things they have seen, and the skills/techniques they have picked up from the sources listed above.

Things to do

1 Get together with other staff members. Have a 'brain-storming' session on 'what makes a good team.' Any and all contributions should be recorded (where people can see them if possible, e.g. on a flip-chart sheet). Next discuss how many points on your list fit a team known to you and how many do not. Then have another session on discussing/planning how a particular team could be made better. Write these down. If appropriate show your points to a manager/supervisor/tutor and ask for their comments.

2 Make a list of problems you feel could sort out yourself if they occurred in the salon and those you would need help with. Store this and discuss it with your supervisor/manager/tutor and ask for their comments.

3 As a group consider how hairdressers can update themselves on fashion trends, techniques, products, tools and equipment. Which would be the most cost effective? Which would be the most time effective?

What do you know?

Level 2 Unit 8

What are the main problems that can occur in the organisation of work in the salon? What should be done if these problems occur? ☐

What type of information may be requested by management? ☐

What are the key aspects of an effective team? ☐

What are the main features of an appraisal/review system? ☐

List the main sources of information that can be used by hairdressers to update and improve their expertise. ☐

SALON RESOURCES

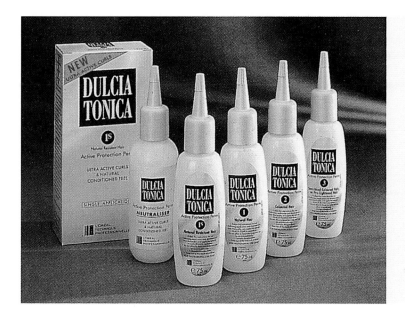

Use of resources in the salon is introduced in Level 1 Unit 5, page 35. This section takes a more detailed look at this topic. Good stock control procedures are essential to ensure a profitable, professional business. There should be a system in place which is relevant to both internal and external auditing procedures. Also take into account the need for good security and the relevant health and safety requirements.

Organising and monitoring stock taking procedures

The first priority is to actually organise and then put into practice a system of stock control to suit the needs of the organisation. Consider the following:

● Documentation.
● Security and safe handling of stock.
● Stock taking procedures.

Documentation

This does not have to be complicated but it does have to be accurate. Indeed, if the system is too complex staff will be less likely to complete the documentation and keep it up to date.

All stock that is for use or sale within the salon, including tools, equipment and products containing chemicals, should be entered in some type of **stock book** or **computerised system**. It is usually convenient to divide the stock into broad categories which makes the checking of stock levels far easier. If anyone needs to know the current stock level of a certain shampoo type they have to be able to find it easily and quickly. Time wasting is expensive for any business!

The documentation should be designed to accommodate the monitoring of day-to-day usage and also the retail sales of stock within the salon. However, the system is only as good as those who use it, therefore to be effective all staff must be made aware, both verbally and in writing, of how the system operates and why it is important to keep regular and accurate records.

Security and safe handling of stock

Part of the reason for having a well-controlled stock system is to help prevent pilfering. It is a sad fact that some people will be tempted to take what is not theirs given the opportunity. Although a tight stock control system will not totally prevent this from happening, it will act as a strong deterrent and if a stock check is carried out daily it gives some indication of when the stock went missing and may therefore help to identify what has happened to it.

Staff should also be made aware of the need for correct, safe handling of stock in accordance with the Health and Safety at Work and COSHH (Control of Substances Hazardous to Health) regulations to ensure the protection of themselves and others at work.

Stock taking procedures

The purpose of stock taking is twofold. Firstly, as an **internal audit** to ensure that stock levels are maintained and to aid the internal security system, and secondly to provide documentation for **external audit** requirements.

It is up to each organisation to determine how often they will require the stock to be checked. However, it is of the utmost importance to keep an up-to-date record of stock levels which means that as stock is used it should be entered as such in the records. Taking regular, random stock checks is usually a means of ensuring that this is the case. A full stock take of **all** stock and equipment must be carried out at least once a year to comply with external audit requirements and the specifications of the Inland Revenue when completing 'year end' account books for audit.

Stock rotation, replacement and safety

Good stock keeping involves checking that the products are in supply when needed and that they are easily located in the stock room. Running out of stock is unprofessional and gives a very bad impression of the salon. There is nothing more irritating to a client than to arrive for a treatment only to find that the colour/perm, for example, is out of stock. To help prevent this happening, it is important to have a system of stock control which carefully monitors stock levels so that materials can be ordered in plenty of time. Remember that when stock is ordered through the post there will be a lapse of several days before the order is received. If stock is required immediately then it has to be obtained from a cash and carry store.

Unforeseen circumstances and abnormal situations can arise from time to time. For example, the salon could have a sudden surge of clients requiring perms or the suppliers themselves could be out of the particular stock item that the salon needs. These problems, although unforeseen, still reflect badly on the organisation of the salon if they cause inconvenience to the client. Planning ahead and having a system of stock control which has back-up supplies, particularly of popular items, can prevent a crisis occurring.

Hairdressers work with many hazardous substances and it is therefore extremely important that all staff members are aware of the ingredients and potential dangers of all substances used in the salon. They should be given training in what to do in an emergency and, indeed, it is now a requirement of law that all salons carry out an assessment of the substances used in the workplace. This legislation is referred to as **COSHH Regulations** and is intended as a safety measure to protect both staff and clients.

To ensure that stock is maintained in optimum condition and is safely stored away to avoid risking the health and safety of both staff and clients, check the storage instructions and shelf-life of all stock **each** time that it is delivered. These instructions should include specific guidance and will influence positioning of stock regarding:

- Safe storage.
- Rotation.

Safe storage

Stock should be stored with due regard to product size and accessibility. For safety reasons, large, heavy items such as gallon containers, etc., must be stored at ground level whilst smaller, lighter items, such as cotton wool, should be stored at higher levels. Products which have a quick turnover, such as tints and perms, should be placed at eye level for ease of access and help prevent strain to the back.

A recommendation that the product be stored in a cool, dark place means exactly that. If it is stored on a window ledge or over a radiator the product will deteriorate very rapidly whilst in some instances it could become unstable, as may be the case with hydrogen peroxide, and explode.

When staff are dealing with stock and equipment, there are certain laws of the land (legislation) which ought to be noted. **The Health and Safety at Work Act (HASAWA) 1974** which gives guidance regarding the safe handling of tools, equipment and substances is very important. All staff members should be aware of the content of this Act and there are many leaflets produced by a variety of organisations for this purpose. Relevant literature should be available for staff perusal at all times and can usually be obtained from the local environmental health officer or the regional office of the Health and Safety Executive. Both are listed in the phone book.

Rotation

Products with a limited shelf-life should be sold or used in rotation to ensure that they do not go over their sell-by date and become ineffective. Always place new stock behind or underneath the old to try to alleviate this problem.

Stock that has been stored incorrectly (in the wrong place or with the cap left off, for example) can become useless before the stated sell-by date. Items which have been dropped or where the packaging has become damaged may affect the product's effectiveness when used. For this reason, regular spot checks of both the storage arrangements and also the condition of the products is advisable. Products for retail also need to be regularly checked to ensure that clients are not sold goods which are damaged or have an exhausted shelf-life.

Product deterioration

Product deterioration can be either the fault of the salon or the supplier. If a product has deteriorated through bad salon practices such as incorrect storage or non-rotation of products then it should be disposed of in an appropriate manner with the consent of the employer. A note must be made in the stock documents regarding any stock which has to be discarded, to ensure that records are correct and stock is not just presumed to be missing. Hairdressing products are expensive and, if any have to be discarded in this way, perhaps new methods of stock organisation and staff training need to be considered.

Always check the soundness of stock when it is received. If goods purchased from the supplier are damaged or faulty they should be returned immediately with a letter stating why they are being returned. No payment should be made until you are entirely satisfied with the standard of the product. Remember that the ineffectiveness of any item used or sold in the salon reflects on you as the practitioner/retailer!

Supervising incoming delivery of stock

All stock must be **carefully** checked as soon as it is received to ensure that any shortages, discrepancies, damaged or inferior goods within the order are quickly identified and dealt with. All goods either used or sold by the salon must be of high quality as there is legislation which protects the client (consumer). They are entitled, by law, to receive what they have paid for. For example, if a particular permanent wave claims to have certain properties or give a certain result then this is what the client is entitled to and if the salon fails to supply this then they are obliged, by law, to reimburse the client. All staff should be aware of their responsibilities regarding the relevant sections of the **Consumer Protection Act** so that any problems are dealt with professionally and within the requirements of the law.

When stock is ordered and delivered through the post, the following overall system usually operates.

1 New stock is ordered. A copy of this order must be kept for future reference.
2 The new stock is delivered. It is usual for the driver of the delivery van to ask for a signature to prove that the stock has been delivered safely. Before signing make sure that the merchandise is in good condition with no breakages. If there are any defects, send the whole order back and refuse to sign.
3 A **delivery note** will be found with the order when it is delivered. The contents of this must be checked against both the **original order** and the **actual** stock delivered. This is to check that what was originally ordered has in fact been delivered.
4 An **invoice** may also be included inside the order or it may be sent through the post separately. This document lists the various products contained in the order, gives their price and also shows the amount of value added tax (VAT)

payable. The invoice should be checked against the delivery note to make sure that the correct products are being charged for. Once checked the invoice must be kept in a safe place as it will be required when paying for the goods and also as proof of purchase within the yearly business accounts.

5 A **statement** will be received separately and does not itemise the stock delivered: instead it simply gives the date and number of the invoice(s).

Once a statement has been received – and there are no discrepancies between the stock ordered and the stock received – then the stock must be paid for.

The cross checking of the order in this manner is very important as mistakes can often be made somewhere between the placing of the order and its actual delivery. If such a mistake should occur, immediately notify the supplier (and employer if appropriate) otherwise all types of problems can arise over payment or deliveries, etc.

Things to do

Task 1

Carry out research into the different methods of computerised and manual stock control systems. Trade journals will usually have contact addresses to enable you to obtain information regarding the different computer programs which can be used for controlling and monitoring stock.

Write a short summary of your findings under the following headings:

- Methods.
- Advantages and disadvantages of each.
- Comparison and evaluation of the methods.

Task 2

The following case study has been devised to give you an opportunity to formulate 'proposals' which could improve the effectiveness of the organisation. If a proposal is well researched and produced in a logical, coherent manner the senior manager is more likely to take your suggestions seriously.

Read the case study carefully then carry out the tasks indicated. Evaluating and discussing your ideas with others is a useful exercise as it will enable you to identify any perceived difficulties and will also allow you to see another viewpoint.

The manager of your salon is very concerned that junior staff are not exercising enough care and attention when they are dealing with stock and equipment. The manager discusses the problem with you and asks if you will come up with some ideas for the next meeting.

1 Draft out a list of simple and realistic guidelines regarding security and safe handling of stock.

2 List any other additional ideas you may have.

3 Present your proposals to your manager (or other members of your group).

4 Discuss and evaluate the proposals. Are they realistic? Would they be easily implemented? Are they cost effective?

5 Amend your proposals, if necessary.

6 Keep a copy of your amended proposals in an Evidence File or your Portfolio.

What do you know?

Level 2 Unit 9

What should be taken into account to ensure a satisfactory stock control system? ☐

What is the difference between an external and an internal audit? ☐

Why is it necessary to keep accurate and up-to-date records of stock levels? ☐

How can you ease the problem of unforeseen circumstances with regard to stock? ☐

What do the initials COSHH stand for? ☐

Why should stock be used in rotation? ☐

Why is it necessary to store the stock with due regard for product size and accessibility? ☐

Why should new stock be checked immediately that it is received? ☐

What is the purpose of an invoice? ☐

Give a brief summary of the procedure for the receipt of incoming stock deliveries at your salon. ☐

SALON HEALTH AND SAFETY

Everyone working in the salon has a responsibility both for their own health, safety and security and for that of the salon's clients. A well-run salon is efficient and safe.

Personal health, hygiene and appearance

This topic is covered in Level 1 Unit 6 page 40. It concerns standards in:

- Personal appearance.
- Personal hygiene.
- Taking care to maintain good posture.

For details of the importance of these areas and the consequence see page 40. In addition there are two other important areas of responsibility. These are:

- When the hairdresser has a potentially infectious condition.
- Personal protective equipment.

Infectious condition of salon staff

If someone has a potentially infectious condition such as a cut or graze on their hands or fingers, then it is important that they report this to their supervisor. Small cuts and nicks are not uncommon in hairdressers, especially when training. These are a potential source of infection to others, i.e. they can cause **cross-infection** and should be:

- Cleaned.
- Covered with a sterile dressing.

Expert advice on whether the infection (or potential infection) could be a hazard in the salon can be obtained from health clinics or general practitioners.

Personal protective equipment

There is legislation regulating a variety of health and safety matters which is of importance in hairdressing. An introduction to these can be found in Level 1 Unit 6, page 42 and a more detailed treatment in Level 3 Unit 6, page 330. The Personal Protective Equipment at Work Regulations (1982) requires employers to provide 'suitable and sufficient' protective clothing/equipment as and when it is needed. In hairdressing there is the supply of:

- **Rubber gloves** – to protect the hands during hairdressing operations.
- **Overalls/aprons** – to protect the hairdresser from spills, client's hair fragments, which can cause infection.

There is sometimes a tendency not to wear rubber gloves, especially if there is a cut or graze on the hands or the early stages of dermatitis. The close-fitting gloves trap sweat and heat and can irritate these conditions. A light dusting with talc can help this and it is worth remembering that exposing sensitive skin to more water, shampoo or other chemicals will in the long run lead to a worse situation than the short-term discomfort of wearing gloves.

Many hairdressing products are hazardous – bleaches, perm lotions and permanent tint, for example – and it is very important not to expose the skin to these. Even low-hazard products like shampoos can cause problems due to the long-term repeated exposure to skin contact that shampooing without protective gloves, or at least a barrier cream, produces.

General salon safety

It is good practice to make many health and safety practices automatic. This would include ensuring that

- Work areas are kept clean and tidy and other general hygiene practices are maintained.
- Hairdressing products are used and stored properly.
- Tools and equipment are checked over before use.
- Tools and equipment are kept and used properly.

A good source of help and information on Health and Safety are local Environmental Health Departments. Good hygiene practices are covered in Level 1 Unit 6, page 45.

Hairdressing products

The storage and use of hairdressing products is covered by a number of pieces of health and safety legislation (see Level 3 Unit 6, page 45). The main point is that the products are handled, used and stored in a safe manner following:

- Manufacturer's instructions.
- Requirement of legislation – a good example is the responsibility the hairdresser has to the client and the Control of Substances Hazardous to Health Regulations 1992.

Safety tools and equipment

Tools and equipment should be kept clean and in good order. It should be routine to give them a quick check before use. Electrical equipment poses a particular hazard due to the possibility of it becoming damp or wet during hairdressing operations and consequently giving someone an electric shock. Cables to electrical equipment also tend to tub or fray and sometimes are jerked, and this tends to pull the flex out of the equipment and/or the plug. This can expose the bare cable with again the possibility of someone receiving an electric shock or a burn should the cable short out with an electric spark.

As with products the care, maintenance and use of salon tools and equipment is covered by a number of regulations. Particularly important is the Provision and Use of Work Equipment Regulations 1992 – see Level 3 Unit 6, page 331.

Hazards in the salon

In addition to products, processes, tools and equipment covered earlier in this Unit, other potential hazards include:

- Spillages.
- Slippery floors.
- Obstructions preventing easy access or escape to parts of the salon and/or exits.

In most cases these can be dealt with by the hairdresser by cleaning up spills, washing floors made slippery by shampoos or water and moving obstructions, etc. Sometimes there are recurrent hazards where something keeps happening. Report these to your supervisor, in writing if necessary.

Waste disposal

A number of potentially hazardous waste materials are produced by a hairdressing salon, these include:

- Tissues/swabs, etc., used in chemical treatments.
- Neck strips.
- Hair clippings.
- Sharps.

These need to be disposed of safely. All sharps, such as razor blades, must be disposed of safely in accordance with the salon's procedures. All other waste needs to be sealed into plastic bags and not left where the bags may become damaged and allow the contents to spill out.

Emergencies in the salon

Some hairdressers never encounter emergency situations, but salons must be organised on the assumption that an emergency can occur at any time. Emergency procedures are introduced in Level 1 Unit 6, page 46, and detailed in Level 3 Unit 6, page 338.

In summary, it is in everyone's interests to know:

- What to do (and what **not** to do).
- Salon procedures.
- Basic first aid.

Salon security

For details about this topic see Level 1 Unit 5, page 38 and Level 3 Unit 10, page 340.

Things to do

1 List routine hygiene practices in the salon. Explain how each helps protect staff and clients.

2 Carry out a **safety audit** on a salon. Look around carefully for potential problems. Design a poster encouraging safety in the salon.

3 Find out and list a salon's emergency procedures for:

- accidents – to staff and/or client
- emergencies – such as fire or a bomb alert

What do you know?

Level 2 Unit 10

Why is personal appearance and hygiene important in the salon?

Where can a hairdresser get advice about

- *Infectious conditions?*
- *Health and safety legislation?*

*List some possible **hazards** in the salon. What can be done to reduce these?*

*List some possible salon **emergencies**. Explain what procedures should be followed in each case.*

Unit 11

SETTING AND DRESSING HAIR

Setting

Setting is carried out using either dry methods or a wet technique. This will be covered in two sections:

1 What happens to the hair during setting.
2 Basic techniques for producing hairstyles using these methods.

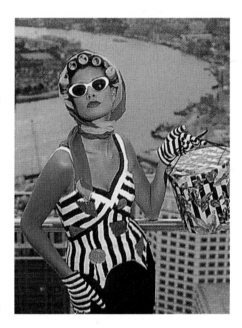

What happens to the hair during setting

The most important aspect of hair structure to do with setting is the way the minute chains of molecules making up hair are held on to some of their neighbouring chains, or to explain it technically, the way the amino acids making up the **polypeptide chains** or **keratin** are able to make **cross-linkages** between the chains. This is shown in Fig. 2.85.

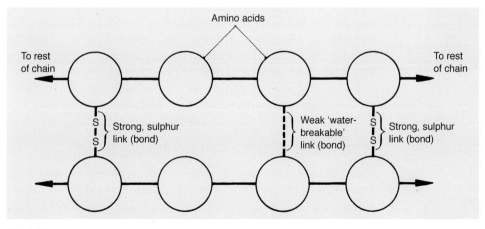

Fig. 2.85

There are two types of cross-linkage:

1 Types that can be broken by water (known as **water-breakable** cross-linkages).
2 A stronger type of linkage that cannot be broken by water (these involve atoms of sulphur and are known as **sulphur bonds**).

At a first stage, dry and wet sets involve breaking some of the weaker water-breakable cross-linkages. At a second stage, setting involves making the polypeptide chains change their position (which is possible when the cross-linkages are broken) and at a third stage the chains are fixed in their new position by re-forming the cross-linkages so that at the end the hair is styled.

Why sets are not permanent

The air around us usually contains some water molecules that make up an invisible gas, called water vapour.

This water taken in from the air breaks some of the water-breakable cross-linkages which have been fixed in their positions during the setting process. When these are broken, the polypeptide chains slip back into their original positions and the style disappears or 'drops out'. How quickly this happens depends on air humidity, so set hair drops out more quickly when exposed to damp (humid) air. When the style is 'washed out', a large amount of water is put directly on the hair either deliberately, in shampooing, or accidentally, for example when caught in a rain shower.

What happens to the hair during wet setting

When hair is wet, most of the water is on the outside. For example, in a shampoo, the hair is wet in order to wash away oil and dirt which have collected on and between the cuticle scales on the surface of the hair shaft. As the cuticle is wet, some of the water penetrates into the hair which breaks some of the water-breakable cross-linkages between the polypeptide chains of the hair (see Fig 2.85). When some of the cross-linkages are broken, the polypeptide chains can be moved past each other very slightly, which over the length of the whole hair adds up to waving or curling the hair. The hair is then fixed in position when removing the water by drying it. This wet, move and fix by drying sequence is the basis of wet or what is known as a cohesive set. When hair is in its natural, unstretched state it is referred to as **alpha keratin** and when stretched it is known as **beta keratin**. Therefore, when the hair is wet, stretched and then dried during setting or blowdrying it changes from alpha to beta keratin (i.e. it goes from A to B) and it will remain in beta keratin until the cross-linkages revert back to their previous positions.

What happens to the hair during dry setting

Here the hair is not wet. In other words, no extra water is added but some of the natural moisture in the hair is driven out by heat. Much heat is supplied by the techniques used in dry setting, for example, heated rollers. The heat is in direct contact with the hair which means it is carried into the hair with less being lost into the atmosphere.

Some of the water is turned into hot water vapour (steam), some is lost through the cuticle and the rest breaks some of the water-breakable cross-linkages, which allows the polypeptide chains to be moved, for example, by stretching the hair around a heated roller. Next the cross-linkages re-form, fixing the chains in their new positions as the hair cools. Because some of the water vapour usually present in the hair has been lost during dry setting, the hair ends up with less moisture inside after dry setting, compared to wet setting. The hair will therefore quickly absorb any water vapour from the air around it as soon as any is available. The equipment used when dry setting includes heated curling tongs, crimping irons, straightening irons, hot brushes, marcel waving irons and heated rollers, etc., all of which involve the use of heat very close to the skin of the face and scalp. Extreme care must therefore be taken to prevent skin burns.

TECHNICAL TIP

To make both wet and dry sets last longer, use a setting lotion.

With a wet set, it is mostly the water added during 'wetting' that is driven off, so the hair at the end of this process contains only a little less, or the same amount, of water than at the beginning. Thus, it does not usually absorb water as quickly as a dry set and, therefore, lasts longer.

Setting aids

Setting aids coat the hair shaft with a barrier to prevent the absorption of atmospheric moisture which has the effect of making the 'set' last longer. The main types of setting aids are:

- Setting 'lotions'.
- Gels.
- Mousses.

Which one is used depends on the type of finished style. Gels, for example, have the greatest moulding facility.

All setting aids contain weak glues which hold the hair in place. Glues are not necessarily 'sticky'; some work by bonding together and these can be used in setting aids.

Setting lotions are the most 'runny' of the setting aids. This may cause problems with application due to dripping and running.

Gels contain chemicals which 'stiffen' the material but which do become much less viscous when rubbed on the hairdresser's hands and then the client's hair. Materials which are viscous until brushed or rubbed and then become more liquid are called **thixotropic**. They have the advantage of giving a 'non-drip' application of a relatively large amount of setting agent and give a good moulding ability to the stylist.

Mousses are foams which contain very small bubbles. The smaller the bubbles the denser the foam. The bubbles are produced by the **propellent** in the pressurised container when it is released. Mousses are often used for scrunch and natural drying.

The active ingredients of setting aids depend on the type being used. Some use natural gums, for example, **tragacanth** and **karaya**. Many use an artificial gum or plastic called **polyvinylacetate** (PVA) which coats the hair. In practice, PVA is often mixed with **polyvinyl pyrrolidone** (PVP) to make it stick to the hair better. The mixture is often 60 per cent PVP and 40 per cent PVA.

As well as gluing the set hair to some extent, some setting lotions and mousses also contain a dye used to temporarily colour the hair.

Setting tools

These include:

- Combs.
- Brushes.

Combs

There are a variety of combs that have been engineered to aid the dressing, disentangling or setting of hair. Whichever type of comb is used it should be made of a sturdy, durable material which will not create static electricity and which must also be easy to sterilise after it is used. Vulcanite is the material used in the manufacturing of most hairdressing combs as it fits all these requirements.

The teeth of the comb should have rounded points with a fine taper and there should be adequate space between them where they join the base.

> **SAFETY TIP**
> Combs with broken or irregular teeth should not be used as they may scratch the scalp or tear the hair.

Types of combs

Combs can be obtained in many shapes and sizes, the most common of which are:

Tail comb

This comb has fine teeth. The tail part of the comb can be made of the same material as the teeth or it can have a thin metal, stiletto tail (known as a pin-tail comb). Care must be taken when using a pin-tail comb as the tail is almost like a fine knitting needle and if used carelessly it can stab either the client or the operator.

Tail combs are for sectioning, lifting or weaving the hair. Never use the tail comb for disentangling the hair as the teeth are too fine.

Dressing comb

Dressing combs have a fine end and a rake end and can be obtained in various sizes according to individual preference. They are used for disentangling and dressing of hair.

The wide teeth of a dressing comb are usually used to smooth and mould the hair into the desired shape. There are many sizes of dressing combs to choose from and the stylist should choose whichever is the most comfortable to handle. Very large dressing combs are more difficult to use but are ideal when there is a lot of volume and for backcombing the hair as it smooths the hair into shape very quickly and easily without flattening or removing too much of the backcombing.

There are various other dressing combs available; some are specially adapted to incorporate larger teeth at one end to smooth the hair, and prongs at the other end to lift the hair if necessary, thus incorporating the duties of both dressing comb and tail comb. Other combs have been designed to aid backcombing by having alternate long and short teeth.

Setting comb

This comb also has a fine and a rake end, usually smaller than a dressing comb and can also be used by the stylist when finger waving.

Afro comb

These combs are very thick with large teeth which are ideal for creating volume without frizz on extremely curly or African Caribbean hair when the curl needs to be sustained throughout the style.

Brushes

There are many different brushes and the choice depends upon the task the brush is used for and also upon general preference. The one most commonly used to dress out a set is called a general-purpose brush. These are made in various shapes and sizes and can be half, three-quarters or full round. Natural bristle is recommended because of its more gentle action on the hair.

Practical methods of setting hair

The main methods used are:

- Rollers.
- Pincurls.
- Finger waving.

Rollers (roller setting)

Rollers are used in setting to give lift, height and volume to a hairstyle. To produce a successful style that is durable and lasts well, careful planning is needed. The planning can be divided into two areas:

- Natural hair direction.
- The size of rollers.

> **Preventing RSI**
> Adjust the chair height to avoid bending and to avoid holding the arms up – both great strains on the arms and shoulders. Headaches are a common result of straining the shoulder muscles – as they are attached to the skull at the back and sides of the neck. Change your position by using a stool to sit on. Turn the chair for further flexibility. Avoid bending your back; bend your knees to keep your spine in its proper position.

Natural hair direction and setting

The rollers should be placed in the hair in the direction of the finished style; therefore, it is very important to decide beforehand the movements of the finished style. Before placing any rollers in the hair, always comb the hair thoroughly to see which way the hair falls naturally. The growth direction of the hair is known as the hair growth pattern. This growth direction of the hair is 'built into' the hair due to the distribution and angle of the hair follicles in the skin.

Setting the hair against the hair growth pattern may produce a good result when it is combed out initially, but the style will not last very long and will tend to 'stick out' at odd angles to the scalp the following day. As most clients expect their sets to last from one shampoo to the next, it is important to make full use of any natural features like hair growth patterns and incorporate them into the style.

Different results can be achieved depending on how the roller section and rollers are angled from the scalp. Remember that the hair will dry where it is placed and it is therefore important to angle the roller and roller section correctly to achieve the desired result.

Figure 2.86 shows how: (a) hair is wound at right angles to the scalp; (b) the roller should be placed exactly in the centre of its own section; and (c) the setting gives a normal root lift.

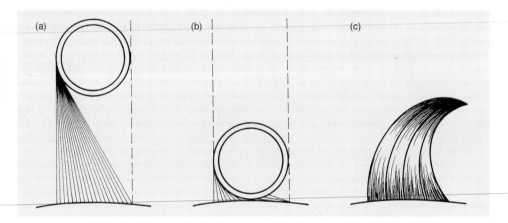

Fig. 2.86

Figure 2.87 shows how: (a) the hair is dragged forward at an obtuse angle from the scalp; and (b) the setting gives more lift and volume.

Figure 2.88 shows how: (a) the hair is dragged back at an acute angle from the scalp; and (b) the setting produces dragged roots and less lift and volume.

The placing of rollers in straight, ladder-like rows, particularly at the hairline, should be avoided if possible as it causes breaks in the hairstyle and makes dressing out more difficult. Any wispy hair at the nape of the neck should not be dragged as this will not curl it tightly enough. If the hair has been correctly set there should be little need for much backcombing when dressing out as the hairstyle should fall into place when it is brushed.

The size of rollers

After planning the direction of the set (pli), the next step is to choose the size of the roller to use in order to achieve the required result. Various factors will influence the size of curler to use:

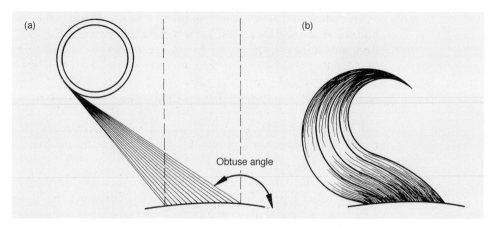

Fig. 2.87

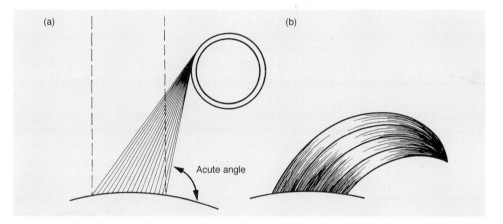

Fig. 2.88

- The texture and density of the hair.
- The length of the hair.
- The amount of curl already present.
- The required result.

The texture and density of the hair

It is important to check carefully not only the texture of the hair, but also the density, before selecting the roller size to use.

The texture of the hair refers to its diameter; a large diameter applies to thick hair and a small diameter to fine hair.

The density refers to the amount of hair on the head. It is possible to have fine textured hair that it very abundant (i.e. a lot of hairs per square inch on the scalp); likewise, it is possible to have thick textured hair that is very sparse (i.e. few hairs per square inch on the scalp).

Fine textured hair usually requires a smaller roller than thick textured hair to produce the same amount of curl because there are fewer water-breakable cross-linkages in fine hair, although if the hair is very abundant (or dense) this can create too much curl because of the amount of hair present.

Thick textured hair usually requires a larger roller, but again the density of the hair must also be taken into consideration because if the hair is very sparse this does not always apply.

TECHNICAL TIP
The more times the hair is wound round the roller, the more polypeptide chains are moved when the cross-linkages are broken – so when they are fixed in their new positions by drying, a tighter curl is produced.

The length of the hair

The longer the hair, the heavier it becomes, therefore very long hair may require a smaller roller than is usually necessary to counteract the 'dragging effect' of this length of hair, particularly if a curly style is required. However, the size of roller is very dependent upon the amount of curl that is required in the finished style.

Long hairstyles that are very smooth require extremely large diameter rollers and in this case the use of too small a roller would result in too much wave and curl movement which would be difficult to eliminate when dressing the hair.

The amount of curl already present

Naturally curly hair and permed hair may require a larger roller than straight hair because of the amount of curl and body already present in the hair.

The required result

The final decision depends on the type of style the client requires, i.e. whether the finished dressing is to be smooth, curly, wavy or a combination of any of these.

The main rule to remember is that a small roller will produce a small curl with a lot of bounce, while a large roller will produce a large curl with less bounce.

Method of placing a roller in the hair for normal root lift

1 Divide off a section of hair the same size as the roller. This should be the same length and the same width as the roller.
2 Comb the hair thoroughly from the roots through to the points at a right or obtuse angle from the scalp,
3 Place the points of the hair in the centre of the roller, making sure that the tension is even on either side of the section. Then turn the roller, using the thumbs to hold the points in position until they are locked round the roller.
4 Wind the hair and roller evenly down to the scalp. The wound roller should be in the centre of the section when wound.

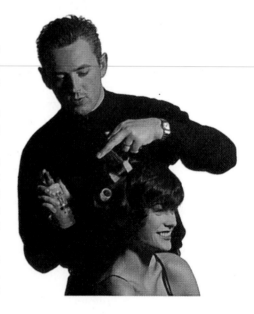

Note the position of the securing pin. It should hold the roller firmly in position without marking the hair and it should never be secured in such a way as to mark the client's scalp or cause discomfort.

Once the skill of correctly placing a roller in the hair has been mastered, it is possible to experiment with different roller positions to create different effects. Combing the wet hair into the direction of the finished style before setting, then placing the rollers in the required direction leads to more interesting styling and also produces a more durable hairstyle for the client.

Mistakes and precautions when roller setting

1 Hair section too wide – this causes drag at the roots, either in front of the roller or behind the roller.

2 Hair section too narrow – the roller will overlap onto the next hair mesh so that the root hair of this section will be dried completely flat to the head. (See Fig. 2.89.) If all the hair sections are too narrow, the root lift will be uneven throughout the head and there will be difficulty in placing the rollers.

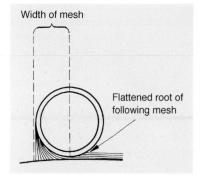

Fig. 2.89

3 Hair section too long – the hair has to be dragged at the sides of the section causing loose hair at each end of the roller when winding (see Fig 2.90).

4 Hair section too short – creates the same problem as the hair sections which are too narrow, i.e. the roller will overlap and flatten the hair at the sides of the roller and can also cause difficulties when placing the other rollers.

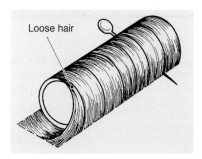

Fig. 2.90

5 Roller pin pressing onto the scalp – will leave marks on the skin and will cause the client discomfort.

6 Roller pin not securing the roller properly – the roller will drop or become displaced while drying, which will spoil the finished style.

7 Roller pin marking the hair – can create 'kinks' in the hair when dry.

8 Hair points bent back or not wound completely round the roller when winding will create 'fish-hook' ends, which when dressed make the hair appear frizzy on the ends.

9 Uneven tension or winding – leads to uneven movements in the hair.

10 Avoid placing the rollers in straight, ladder-like rows as this can cause breaks in the style and creates difficulties when dressing the hair.

11 Wispy nape hairs should be wound correctly. If they are dragged the napeline of the finished style will be uneven.

12 Never underestimate the importance of good use of the natural direction of hair growth. A well-placed set, skilfully carried out, not only helps the dressing of hair but is also the basis of a long-lasting style.

Pincurls

To style the hair with pincurls the hair should be thoroughly wet to enable the operator to mould the hair correctly. It is important to use and incorporate any natural hair growth patterns and movements that may be present in the hair to give durability to the style. As with roller setting, the hair should be combed in the direction of the finished style and the pincurls placed in that direction. A pincurl is usually taken from a square section and the curl must be kept as round at the points of the hair as it is at the roots. The durability of the pincurl depends on the perfect roundness and how smoothly it is wound from the roots. Twisting or buckling the hair either at the roots or along its length will not give a satisfactory result as the hair will dry where it is placed.

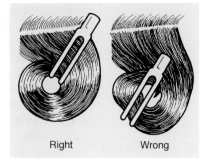

Right   Wrong

Fig. 2.91

Pincurls may be secured with either one-pronged or two-pronged clips, depending upon personal preference, but these should be inserted in such a way that the ends of the clip secure the points of the hair firmly in position while the head of the clip rests on the stem of the curl so that the clip does not hinder the formation of the next pincurl. (See Fig. 2.91.)

Special care should be taken when securing hair that is either fine, bleached or highly porous as this type of hair marks easily.

Pincurls are best suited to medium textured hair with a slight natural movement. Very thick or extremely curly hair is difficult to pincurl and buckles easily while very fine, straight hair usually requires extra lift and body.

The size of the pincurl is determined by the hair texture and the required result. Thick hair usually requires a larger pincurl than fine hair to achieve the same result. The diameter of the pincurl will determine the amount of curl in the finished movement, but the set will loosen and drop slightly when it is dressed, so allowance should be made for this by making the diameter of the pincurl slightly smaller than the required result.

Types of pincurl

There are several types of pincurls to produce various results:

- Clockspring.
- Flat barrel spring.
- Barrel spring or stand-up.
- Stem curls.
- Sculptured curls.
- Reverse pincurls.

Clockspring (see Fig. 2.92)

This type of pincurl is small and tight with a closed centre which produces a tight curl on the ends and a looser wave at the root. A clockspring pincurl is usually used at the nape of the neck when a curly effect is required.

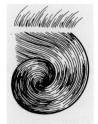

Flat barrel spring (see Fig. 2.93)

An open-centred curl which is formed flat to the head. This is the most common type of pincurl and is also used when reverse pincurling to form wave movements.

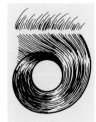

Fig. 2.92   Fig. 2.93

Barrel spring or stand-up (see Fig. 2.94)

This type of pincurl also has an open centre and is formed so as stand up from the head. It is secured by passing a clip through the curl at the base. The stem direction of a stand-up pincurl is directed up and away from the direction of the finished dressing, thus creating lift and volume in the same manner as a roller. If it is used in conjunction with rollers, the pincurl must be the same diameter as the rollers used.

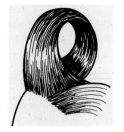

Fig. 2.94

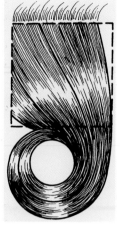

Stem curls (see Fig. 2.95)

Stem curls are open-centred pincurls with a long stem. A section of hair is taken from a square base and wound either from root or point. The curl is then placed above, below or to either side of the base, depending on the direction of the finished style; this produces a long stem to the pincurl and can be used to accentuate hair growth direction at the nape or sides of the head.

Fig. 2.95

Sculptured curls (see Fig. 2.96)

The hair is combed thoroughly and moulded in the exact position in which it is going to be dressed and is then secured by either tape or clips. Tape is usually used in preference to clips as it does not mark the hair and it holds the moulded hair more securely in position. A sculptured curl produces a soft effect at the nape, sides or fringe area, especially on very short hair.

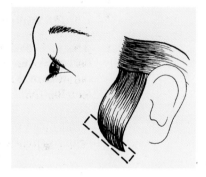

Fig. 2.96

Reverse pincurls (see Fig. 2.97)

Reverse pincurls are, as the name suggests, curls that are formed in one direction and then reversed back around the head in the opposite direction. On looking closely at a wave movement, it can be seen that it is an 'S' shape, which bends in one direction and then bends back in the opposite direction. By reversing the pincurls one way and then another it is, therefore, possible to achieve wave movements in the hair.

Precautions and considerations when pincurling

1 Hair should always be thoroughly wet when pincurling.
2 Consider the hair and hair growth patterns carefully before starting to pincurl the hair.
3 Use and incorporate any natural wave movements into the style.
4 Always work to the shape of the head, i.e. in curved movements, not straight lines.
5 The durability of the curl is maintained by its perfect roundness, therefore a pincurl should be as round at the points as it is at the roots.

6 Do not twist or buckle the hair, either when forming the pincurl or when securing it.

7 Special consideration should be given to permed, tinted, bleached or highly porous hair, as these hair types are often more difficult to pincurl and can mark or buckle more easily.

8 The hair should be kept flat when forming the pincurl unless it is a stand-up pincurl.

9 The diameter of the pincurl determines the size of the final curl; therefore, care must be taken to wind the correct size of pincurl for the desired effect – bearing in mind that the set will drop slightly when dry.

10 When reverse pincurling, the pincurls along each row should be wound in the same direction but in the opposite direction to the previous row. The curls should be a uniform size and arranged in a brickwork pattern to eliminate unwanted partings.

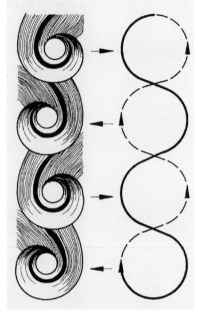

Fig. 2.97

Finger waving

Also known as 'flat waving' or 'water waving', this is a method of moulding the hair into 'S' shaped movements with the fingers and comb, producing a wave movement. The point at which the hair changes direction is known as the crest (see Fig. 2.98(a)) and the height of the crest and, therefore, the depth of the wave depends on the amount of moulding with the fingers. Finger waving (see Fig. 2.98(b)) can be achieved on straight or wavy hair but naturally tight curls, coarse or permanently waved hair will not usually wave successfully.

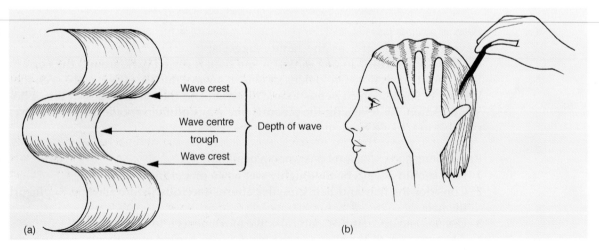

Fig. 2.98

Precautions and considerations when finger waving

1 The hair should be clean and thoroughly wet. A thick gel setting lotion will help to keep waves in position.

2 The hair should be well tapered and of reasonable length, particularly on the crown.
3 Utilise any natural wave movement in the hair – do not fight against the natural growth. To find the natural wave, comb all hair back from the client's face, then push forward. The hair will fall in its natural line.
4 Do not use clips, grips or wave claws unless absolutely necessary as they mark the hair and flatten the wave centres.
5 Use the coarse end of the comb and avoid scratching the scalp by leaning the comb slightly towards you.
6 All waves should be the same width and slightly smaller than the required result to allow for slight loosening.
7 Always wave towards the parting and never wave in straight lines.
8 Ensure that the underneath hair is waved. 'Lifting' the hair into place when finger waving can distort the roots.

Things to do

This task has been devised to help you to understand the effects of different roller sizes on the hair.

Divide your tuition head into six sections. Wind a different size roller onto each section. Dry the hair and remove the rollers. Examine the result then write your findings in the form of a table as shown.

	Size of roller	*Result*
Section 1		
Section 2		
Section 3		
Section 4		
Section 5		
Section 6		

Dressing hair

Dressing the hair is of equal importance to either setting or blowdrying for, although good setting or blowdrying will make the style durable and easier to dress, the actual dressing of the hair will give the final image, and it is this final image which will either please or displease the client and will also serve as advertisement for the salon.

Dressing the hair requires plenty of practice to gain the confidence to work quickly and efficiently and to know when enough work has been carried out on the head. It is almost like putting the finishing touches to a painting. A good artist will know almost instinctively when the picture looks 'right' and therefore stop working on it. By dabbling about too much after this stage the image can be completely ruined!

The following considerations should be addressed when dressing hair:

● Use of tools.
● Amount of dressing creams, shine enhancers and waxes.
● Amount of volume required.
● Line and balance.
● Final image.

Use of tools

Dressing the hair can be made much easier and simpler by using the correct tools for the effect required.

Use of dressing creams, shine enhancers and waxes

These are used to reduce static electricity and to replace any natural oil that may have been removed when shampooing. They will also add a shine or gloss to dull, dry hair.

Most of these products are made from mineral oil with perfume added. Mineral oil is used in preference to vegetable oil because it does not go rancid and does not penetrate the hair shaft but remains on the surface only, so giving a better shine than vegetable oil. This also helps to protect the hair from dampness.

Dressing creams

Dressing creams do not need to be used on every head of hair but only if the hair is dry or very 'fly-away'. Do not use them on hair which tends to be greasy as they will encourage this condition.

Method of applying dressing creams

After brushing the hair thoroughly apply a small amount of the cream to the palm of the hand (about the size of a pea). Rub the hands together then gently stroke the hair with the hands making sure that the cream is also applied to the underneath layers. Care must be taken to avoid applying too much cream as this will make the hair too greasy and lank. When the cream has been applied, re-brush the hair thoroughly to distribute the cream evenly throughout the whole head.

Shine enhancers

Dressing oils or shine enhancers as opposed to creams can be obtained in spray or aerosol can form and are known as spray on shine or hair gloss. They are usually applied after completion of the dressing to add shine and lustre to the hair. Hold the can or spray about 30 cm (12") away from the scalp and direct the spray just above the head to prevent the oil being concentrated in one area. The oil will then drop onto the hair and will coat it more evenly if applied in this manner. It is very important to use this type of dressing oil sparingly – too much will make the hair appear greasy and lank.

Waxes

Waxes are used to give texture to the hair. A small amount is rubbed quickly between the hands. The friction of the rubbing movement creates heat which melts the wax. The wax is then quickly applied to the hair before it cools. Once cool it becomes more solid again which helps to hold the hair in position in addition to giving it a more textured look. Do not use on fine, lank hair.

Amount of volume required

Some hairstyles require very little volume while others need more than can be created by either the amount of hair itself or by the way that it is set/blowdried. There are two methods of creating extra volume when dressing the hair:

- Backcombing.
- Backbrushing.

Backcombing

This is pushing the hair back on itself at the root to give a lifted full effect using a comb. Tapered hair is easier to backcomb than clubbed hair as the finer ends are more easily pushed back on themselves. Backcombing is also sometimes used to temporarily straighten over-curly hair.

Backcombing the hair at the roots underneath the hair section will give volume, while backcombing on top of the section will help to blend the hair together and will give an even spread of hair; this is often called **teasing**.

When backcombing hair

1 Brush the hair into the shape and direction of the style then decide which area of the head requires extra volume; usually this is on top of the head and crown area but sometimes the whole head will require extra volume.
2 Start at the top or front of the head and take a narrow section of hair in the direction of the style.
3 Lift out from the scalp at right angles. Holding the hair section firmly in one hand and the comb in the other, insert the comb into the section approximately 2–3 cm ($\frac{3}{4}$–$1\frac{1}{8}$″) away from the scalp.
4 Push back the hair to the root repeatedly until enough hair has been pushed back to form a padding at the root. The more the hair is pushed back the greater will be the lift.
5 Continue in this manner until the areas which require extra volume are completed.
6 Always remember to hold the hair firmly while backcombing. Allowing the hair section to sag while the comb is pushing back the hair to the roots prevents the hair from being pushed back correctly and will make the style flop.
7 The size of the section depends upon the density and thickness of the hair and the amount of volume required, but the finished backcombing should not be visible at the front of the section as this creates difficulties when smoothing the hair over the backcombing.
8 If the backcombing does penetrate through to the front of the section then the section is too fine.

It is usually only necessary to backcomb the hair at the root area as this is where the lift is needed. Only if extreme height is required by the hairstyle is it usually necessary to backcomb the hair past the mid-lengths towards the points.

A common fault when backcombing is not pushing the hair right back to the scalp thus creating a padded effect at the mid-lengths instead of the roots. When the hair is smoothed over, the root area remains 'floppy' resulting in no lift whatsoever!

The teasing method

Teasing does not give the same lift to the hair but is used to blend the hair together, thus giving an even spread of hair and a smoother finish to the dressing. It can be used in conjunction with backcombing or on its own.

Larger sections of hair are taken where required and held between the fingers and thumb. The hair is then pushed back on itself on top of the hair section while the hair between the fingers is pulled in the direction of the style. When smoothing the hair after teasing, care must be taken to smooth the hair gently so as not to remove all the backcombing.

Backbrushing

This is pushing the hair back on itself either under or on top of the hair section to give a lifted effect using the brush.

Backbrushing gives a softer effect than backcombing and is useful for longer hair; backcombing long hair tends to create too much lift and there is the danger of the hair becoming too entangled.

Removal of all backcombing and backbrushing

Clients should always be advised as to how to remove backcombing, or backbrushing from their hair correctly. Incorrect removal can be very painful for the client and damaging to the hair.

Commence removal at the nape of the neck, with the wide spaced teeth of a dressing comb. Always start at the points of the hair and work down towards the roots.

Line and balance

Balance refers to the shape of the dressing in relation to the client's face, head and neck. The lines of the hairstyle should complement the wearer and each movement should flow naturally into or complement the next. Judging when the finished style is 'balanced' requires practice and that indefinable something – instinct or flair perhaps – that tells the stylist that the dressing looks right on the client.

The use of the mirror while dressing the hair helps to keep a check on the balance of the hairstyle by putting the style in perspective. Dressing the hair at close quarters limits the vision of the stylist to one area only; so by frequently checking the outline and shape of the dressing in the mirror the stylist can see at a glance where and if the shape needs to be altered.

When the dressing is complete, stand away from the head and check the line and balance of the style at the front, sides and back of the head. First look at the silhouette of the hairstyle; this will help to show up any defects in the balance of the dressing, then check that the movements and/or smoothness within the silhouette are correct. Next check that the edges along the hairline are even and that the lines blend into each other and complement the face and neck.

Final image

It is the final image on which the client, to a great extent, will judge the salon. It is worth a few extra seconds therefore to check that nothing mars the line of the hairstyle.

Remove any stray, wispy neck hairs with the scissors, and when completely satisfied with the result show the client the finished style from all angles in a hand mirror.

Do not apply any lacquer before making sure that the client is pleased with the result – the style may have to be changed slightly and this is difficult after the lacquer has been applied.

How to apply the lacquer

1 Protect the client's eyes and face with a face shield or with the free hand.
2 Aim the spray just above the dressing to allow the lacquer to drop onto the hair. While lacquering the hair, the spray should be moved in the direction of the hairstyle so that any movement of air does not disturb the dressing.
3 Spray the lacquer from a distance of 30 cm (12″) so that a fine even spray coats the hair. Spraying the hair too near to the head will saturate only one area and

this could wet the hair too much causing it to drop. Alternatively, the lacquer may form 'blobs' on the hair which, when dry, will look like white nodules sticking to the hair.

4 When enough lacquer has been applied to the hair, re-check the dressing carefully and smooth any fly-away hairs with the flat of the hands or the back of the comb.

Manufacture and design of hair fixing sprays

Hair fixing sprays are developed from synthetic plastic polymers dissolved in alcohol which coat the hair with a clear plastic film. A mixture of two plastic film-formers is often used. For example: polyvinyl pyrrolidone (PVP) and polyvinyl acetate (PVA) in the ratios of PVP–PVA:

- 60–40 per cent for general use.
- 70–30 per cent for hard holding.

When lacquer is sprayed onto the hair the alcohol evaporates leaving the resin or plastic coating on the hair. This tends to stick or mildly glue the hair in place when the alcohol solvent evaporates. Hair lacquers can be sprayed onto the hair using either a hand-pumped spray or a pressurised aerosol spray can. Public concern for the environment has made manufacturers more aware of the need to produce aerosol spray cans which are 'ozone friendly', i.e. they do not contain ozone destructive gases – **chlorofluorocarbons**.

> **SAFETY TIP**
> Because the contents are often **flammable** do not allow a client to smoke when lacquering their hair. As the contents are under pressure, heat will increase the pressure and may cause the can to burst. Do not store on heaters or in direct sunlight. Do not puncture or burn, even when empty.

Procedure for dressing a basic set

1 Gown the client to ensure that any loose hairs or flakes of skin do not fall onto the clothing.
2 Check that the hair is completely dry by removing one of the rollers (usually where the hair is thickest or longest) and test the ends of the hair. If the hair is damp it will lose its springiness and will not comb out into shape.
3 Remove the rollers and clips from the hair gently without tugging, then allow the hair to cool for a few minutes.
4 Loosen the set and help eradicate any roller partings by double brushing or using the brush and comb to brush the hair thoroughly from root to point in all directions over the head.
5 Apply a small amount of dressing cream if the hair appears dry or fly-away. If an aerosol or spray type is used this may be applied when the dressing is complete.
6 Brush the hair into shape using one brush and following each stroke with the other hand to smooth and shape the hair. Stroke the brush in the planned direction of the set taking into consideration any wave or curl movements.
7 Backcomb or backbrush any areas of the hairstyle that require extra volume or lift – but remember, not all styles require backcombing.
8 Lightly comb the surface of the hair to shape and smooth into position, the free hand can also be used to follow the comb to help to smooth the hair. It may be necessary to tease certain areas at this stage so that the lines and movements blend into the shape.

9 Check the line and balance of the hairstyle from all angles to ensure that it is the correct shape and suits the client. Remove any wispy neck hairs.

10 Show the client the finished result in the hand mirror and if they are satisfied with the style apply a light spray of lacquer, remembering to use a face shield or the hand to protect the face and eyes.

Precautions and considerations when dressing hair

1 Make sure that the hair is completely dry before combing or dressing the hair. Straighter hair will drop it it is damp, while permed or naturally curly hair will frizz and in either case the correct shape will not be achieved.

2 Use the correct tools for the effect required. For example do not use a tail comb for disentangling or smoothing the hair, the teeth are too fine and it can be painful for the client.

3 Fine hair should not be brushed as vigorously as normal or thick hair as it loses its springiness more easily.

4 Always work in the direction of the set when brushing, backcombing or smoothing the hair.

5 Use dressing creams and oils sparingly. Using too much may result in the hair having to be shampooed again to remove the excess grease.

6 Only backcomb or backbrush the hair where necessary. Putting too much backcombing into the hair is time wasting and not particularly beneficial to the hair as it can damage the cuticle scales.

7 Take hair sections of the correct size when backcombing: too fine and the backcombing will be visible at the front of the mesh; too thick and the backcombing will not penetrate into the mesh far enough and it will be 'floppy'.

8 Do not backcomb right to the points of the hair, it will destroy any curl at the ends of the hair.

9 Make sure that the backcombing is at the root of the hair to give the necessary lift – if it is only present at the mid-lengths the hair will flop.

10 Do not let the comb penetrate too deeply through the meshes when smoothing backcombed hair as this can remove too much backcombing.

11 Any areas that still require lifting even after backcombing can be done so by inserting the tail end of a tail comb at the roots and gently lifting the hair.

12 Check regularly in the mirror when dressing the hair – it helps the stylist create the correct shape and balance.

13 Make sure that the movements within the style complement each other and that the hair is sufficiently blended.

14 The final dressing should be balanced from all angles, so check the style at the front, sides and back.

15 It is sometimes a good idea to check the finished dressing in relation to the client's body proportions by asking the client to stand.

16 When the dressing is complete remove any fallen hairs, etc., from the client's neck and shoulders with a neck brush.

17 Only use the lacquer after the client has been shown the finished style, then if the style needs to be altered slightly it can be done with the minimum of fuss.

18 Do not spray the lacquer too close to the head as this concentrates the lacquer into one area of the head and can wet the hair causing it to drop.

19 Use only a fine spray of lacquer. Using too much can cause 'beading' of the lacquer and when dry it will look like white nodules on the hair.

20 Finally, do not 'over-work' the hair. When the balance, shape and smoothness are correct – leave it!

Dressing long hair into a vertical roll pleat

The finished style can be seen in Fig. 2.99.

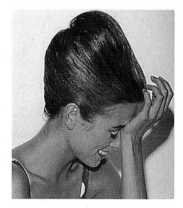

Fig. 2.99

1 Backcomb or backbrush the hair if necessary to give volume and hold the hair together (see Fig. 2.100). The backcombing/backbrushing is usually done underneath the hair section at the roots and possibly mid-lengths. If the whole hair length is done then it can be very difficult to smooth over.

2 Leave out the top sections and take one side of the back section just past the centre back (see Fig. 2.101). Secure firmly with hair grips positioned alternately up and down next to one another to prevent any hair from slipping through.

3 Brush the hair from the other side of the back section and brush towards the centre. Fold this hair under and secure firmly with hair grips making sure that they are positioned not to show (see Fig. 2.102).

4 Smooth the top hair and blend it in with the pleated back hair either by twisting it round into a curl, as shown in Fig. 2.103 or under like an envelope. Secure firmly with hair grips.

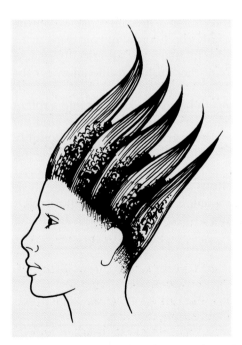

Fig. 2.100

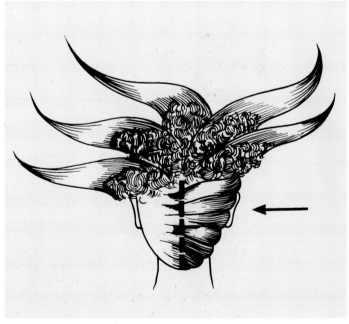

Fig. 2.101

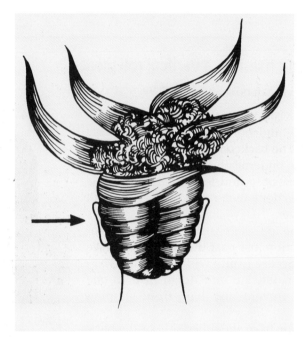

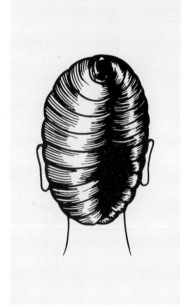

Fig. 2.102

Fig .2.103

Dressing long hair into a horizontal roll

1 Backcomb or backbrush the hair, if necessary, to give volume and hold the hair together (see Fig. 2.104). Initially, the backbrushing should be placed underneath the direction in which the hair is to be dressed.

2 Smooth the top hair in the direction of the finished dressing, decide on the height at which to place the roll, then carefully place a row of hair grips in an arc around the sides and back of the head. The hairgrips are usually placed approximately 2.5 cm (1") below the height of the finished roll to allow for the actual rolling of the hair (see Fig. 2.105).

3 Starting at one side of the head, the underneath hair is folded over into a roll in the direction indicated by the arrows in Fig. 2.106. Work in sections round the head, securing each rolled section with a hair grip when it is thoroughly smoothed and in the correct position. Care should be taken to avoid showing any hair grips in the final dressing.

4 Figure 2.107 shows the finished dressing. Rolls can be varied by making them fuller or tighter, higher or lower. When dressing long layered hair into a roll it may be easier to brush the lower sections into a roll first, then smooth and blend in the top layers afterwards.

Plaiting the hair

A plait is a method of weaving strands of hair together. The techniques are the same for both European and African Caribbean hair. Any number of hair strands from two to sometimes more than seven may be used to create various effects.

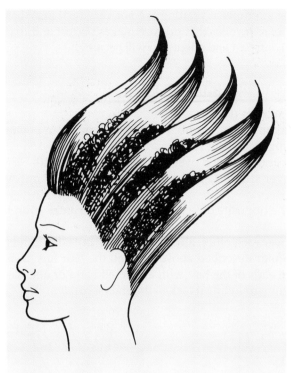

Fig. 2.104

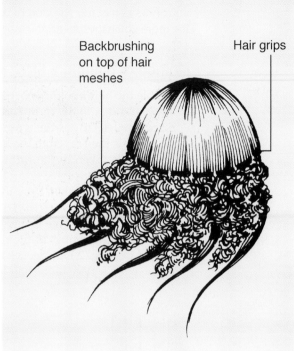

Backbrushing on top of hair meshes

Hair grips

Fig. 2.105

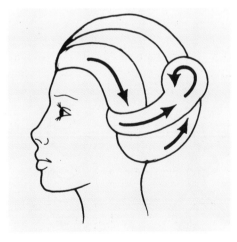

Fig. 2.106

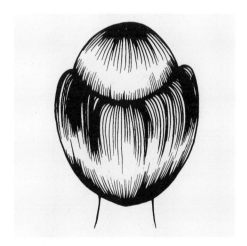

Fig. 2.107

Plaits do not always have to be woven down towards the nape, they can be positioned across the head or plaited from the nape upwards. The way in which the hair is woven, i.e. either under or over the hair strands or a combination of each will also give variety.

When learning to plait, you first need to master how to manipulate your fingers for a three-stem plait. When you are used to weaving the hair strands over each other, experiment by bringing in extra strands, twisting the hair, weaving the hair under instead of over and placing the plait (or any number of plaits) in different positions on the head. Do not worry if your first attempts at plaiting are not very neat and that your fingers feel too wooden to cope; remember that practice makes perfect and that the more you experiment, the more confident and adept you will become.

Method of plaiting a three-stem plait (English plait)

1 Divide the hair into three equal strands (see Fig. 2.108).
2 Take strand A to the right and wrap over strand B. Pull strand B in the opposite direction (left) to aid the wrapping (see Fig. 2.109).
3 Strand C is then taken to the left and wrapped over strand A (see Fig. 2.110).
4 Strand B is taken to the right over strand C in the same direction as strand A (see Fig. 2.111).
5 Strand A is now taken back in the opposite direction and over the centre strand B (see Fig. 2.112).
6 Continue wrapping the strands over each other, always taking the outside strands in towards the centre, in the manner described above until all the hair has been plaited (see Fig. 2.113). Secure the ends of the hair with a covered band or alternatively, wrap a piece of the hair tightly round then tuck in the ends securely.

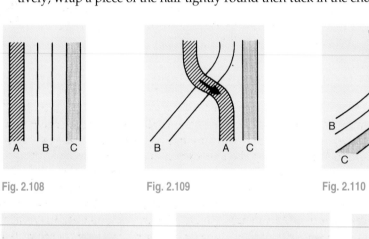

Fig. 2.108   Fig. 2.109   Fig. 2.110

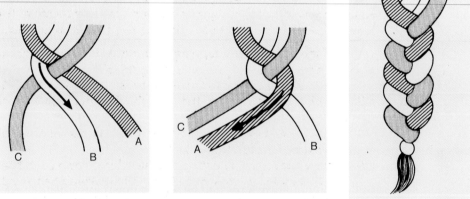

Fig. 2.111   Fig. 2.112   Fig. 2.113

Plaiting the hair to the scalp (French braid)

1 To plait the hair to the scalp, begin by gathering the top hair, from the temples to the crown, into a thin ponytail.

2 Divide this hair into the three equal sections and begin plaiting in the manner described in Figs 2.108 and 2.109. Hold the braid in the right hand keeping the strands separated.

3 With the left hand, take a strand of hair from the front through to the back which is approximately half the width of the originals and draw it back towards the ponytail. Combine this new strand of hair with the left strand and cross over the centre.

4 Hold the plait in the left hand with the strands separated and take a section in the same way as before but on the opposite side of the head, making sure that it is the same width as the previous strand and therefore equal on both sides of the head. Add this newly gathered hair to the right strand and cross over to the centre.

5 Continue taking fine, equal sections of hair from alternate sides of the head until the nape is reached and there is no more hair to section. Plait the remaining hair in an English braid as described previously (see Fig. 2.114).

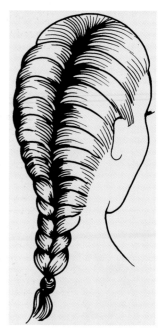

Fig. 2.114 A finished French braid down the centre of the head

Under-plaiting the hair to the scalp

This is carried out in almost the same way as a French braid. The hair is gathered into a fine ponytail from the temples through to the crown and is divided into the three equal sections. Commence plaiting as described previously; however, instead of wrapping the hair **over** it is taken **under**.

Fine strands of hair are then taken alternately from each side of the head and combined with the original strand of hair from that side remembering to cross each strand under the centre instead of over. The finished result is a plait which rests on top of the hair instead of being incorporated into it. Under-plaiting can also be done along the edge of the hair by including sections from only one side of the hair and combining them with the plait strands on that side.

1 Start the plaiting by wrapping strand A *under* strand B. Strand B is taken to the left in the opposite direction (see Fig. 2.115).

2 Strand C is then taken to the left under strand A (see Fig. 2.116).

3 Strand B is taken left, in the opposite direction and then under strand C (see Fig. 2.117).

4 Figure 2.118 shows an under-plait down the centre of the head. Note how the finished plait sits on top of the hair.

5 Under-plaiting can be done along the edge of the hair on both sides of the head. The two plaits are held together with a covered band and the ends are then turned under and secured at the nape with hairgrips (see Fig. 2.119).

Usually referred to as **corn rowing**, the type of plaiting shown in Fig. 2.120 is extremely popular for African Caribbean styling. Many small plaits are used throughout the head and the ends can be secured with cotton thread, or beads to give more decoration. The direction of the plaits creates the style and the variations are almost limitless to the experienced plaiter.

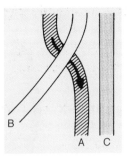

Fig. 2.115

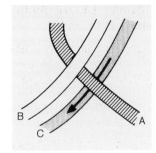

Fig. 2.116

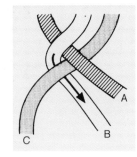

Fig. 2.117

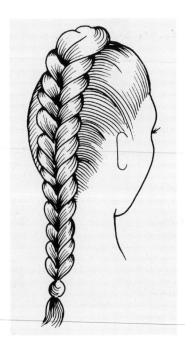

Fig. 2.118

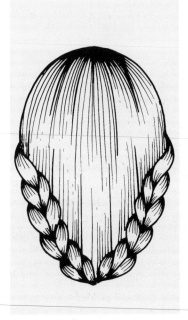

Fig. 2.119

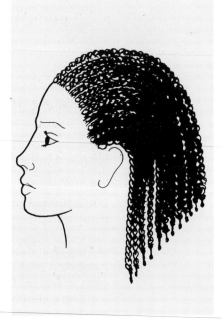

Fig. 2.120

Using ornamentation in the hair

A client with very long hair is not usually able to achieve a change of style by having a new shape cut into the hair. Any new style must therefore be achieved by setting/blowdrying or dressing the hair in different ways. Ornamentation such as ribbons, ornamental grips, decorative combs, beads and embroidery thread, when used imaginatively, can alter the effect of a hairstyle and give the client more variety.

Things to do

Plaiting requires flexible fingers. This assignment has therefore been devised to help you to handle strands of hair more easily and with greater confidence.

You will need:

- A4 size piece of card.
- Large safety pin, scissors and stapler.
- 19 strands of very thick wool about 25 cm (10") long.
- Old cushion.

1 Take three strands of the wool, knot the ends together and attach the safety pin 2.5 cm (1") to the ends of the wool.

2 Attach the safety pin and wool to the cushion and plait the wool into a three-stemmed plait. Secure the ends by twisting one strand of the wool around the others and knot. Remove the safety pin and place the plait to one side.

3 Repeat the procedure using four strands of wool, then five then seven until you have four completed plaits of differing sizes.

4 Draw or collect an illustration of a hairstyle for each type of plait.

5 Attach the plaits to the card with the stapler (or adhesive tape) displaying them to their best advantage together with the relevant illustration. Ornaments or dried flowers, etc., may be used to emphasise the plaiting. Label each plait clearly using block letters.

6 Write a short report on how you carried out the task and any difficulties you encountered.

<table>
<tr><td>**What do you know?**</td><td>Level 2 Unit 11</td><td></td></tr>
<tr><td></td><td>*What holds the polypeptide chains of hair keratin together?*</td><td>☐</td></tr>
<tr><td></td><td>*What is the effect of moisture on a set?*</td><td>☐</td></tr>
<tr><td></td><td>*Give four examples of both dry and wet sets.*</td><td>☐</td></tr>
<tr><td></td><td>*What is meant by 'hair direction'?*</td><td>☐</td></tr>
<tr><td></td><td>*Why should placing rollers in straight, ladder-like rows be avoided?*</td><td>☐</td></tr>
<tr><td></td><td>*What effect does using a hair section too wide for the roller produce?*</td><td>☐</td></tr>
<tr><td></td><td>*List the main types of pincurls.*</td><td>☐</td></tr>
<tr><td></td><td>*How does a setting aid produce a longer lasting set?*</td><td>☐</td></tr>
<tr><td></td><td>*What type of accident is particularly associated with dry setting techniques?*</td><td>☐</td></tr>
<tr><td></td><td>*In wet sets, what causes the cross-linkages to re-form?*</td><td>☐</td></tr>
<tr><td></td><td>*Why should a client not smoke when laquer is being applied?*</td><td>☐</td></tr>
<tr><td></td><td>*Why is it necessary to use dressing creams sparingly?*</td><td>☐</td></tr>
<tr><td></td><td>*Which teeth of the comb are used to smooth out backcombing?*</td><td>☐</td></tr>
<tr><td></td><td>*Where should the hair be backcombed to create lift?*</td><td>☐</td></tr>
<tr><td></td><td>*What is meant by balance in relation to hairstyling?*</td><td>☐</td></tr>
<tr><td></td><td>*Why is dressing cream or oil used when dressing the hair?*</td><td>☐</td></tr>
<tr><td></td><td>*How would you advise the client to look after long hair?*</td><td>☐</td></tr>
<tr><td></td><td>*When dressing the hair into a pleat, why may it be necessary to use some backcombing/brushing?*</td><td>☐</td></tr>
<tr><td></td><td>*What is a plait?*</td><td>☐</td></tr>
<tr><td></td><td>*What is the difference between a French braid and under-plaiting?*</td><td>☐</td></tr>
</table>

BARBERING TECHNIQUES

Trimming beards and moustaches

A beard should suit the client's face shape and size of head. It should also balance the hairstyle giving a 'total' look. Client consultation is very important before commencing the beard trim to determine the client's requirements and overall final length of the beard.

Clippers and attachments are often used for very close beards, for example, 'designer stubble' or when a very short uniform look is required.

The following guidelines usually apply when shaping a beard to suit the face:

- **Round face** – to make the face appear thinner: cut the beard close, or shave the sides and shape the hair to be longer at the chin; shave under the neck.
- **Narrow face with hollow cheeks** – to widen the face and fill out hollows: leave the sides full and create a round shape at the chin; leave the hair a medium length under the chin and just above the collar line.
- **Long chin** – to create the illusion of a shorter chin: cut the beard in a square shape across both the sides and chin area.

Procedure

1 Place the client in a reclined position.
2 Make sure that the client's clothing and eyes are adequately protected. This is done by placing a gown over the client's clothing and covering the eyes with a small cloth.
3 Begin the trim by disentangling the beard, combing the hair in a downward direction.
4 Cut the beard using the scissors or clipper over comb method combing the beard upwards. Take small sections and keep the comb moving as you cut. Remember that the further away from the face that the comb is held then the longer it will leave the hair.

> **SAFETY TIP**
> Small, bristly beard cuttings are sharp, dangerous and can cause infection; therefore it is extremely important to protect the client as much as possible.

5 Take extra care when trimming under the chin and around the lips as it is easy to tickle the client and could result in cutting the skin.

6 Outline any moustache by supporting the scissors with the first finger to prevent cutting the lips, then cut the hair freehand.

7 When enough hair has been removed from the beard, outline the final shape using a razor/shaper or clippers.

8 Remove the beard clippings from the client with a brush and show the client the result in the mirror.

Precautions when trimming a beard and moustache

- *Always* carry out a consultation before starting the beard/moustache trim to ensure client's wishes are taken into consideration.
- Check whether the client requires the finished beard 'blended' into the neck or prefers a definite outline shape.
- Make sure that the client is well protected, particularly the eyes.
- Longer beards are sometimes cut freehand, remember to comb the hair into shape before cutting.
- Beards can be thinned out with the razor, but take care not to make the finished result too wispy.
- Take strong hair growth patterns into consideration when cutting the hair.
- *Always* dispose of sharps safely.

> **TECHNICAL TIP**
> Facial hair can have strong hair growth patterns. If a close-cropped beard is required it is necessary to cut hair **against** the fall of the hair.

Cutting men's hair

Similar skills are needed for cutting both men's and women's hair. However, although there are similarities there are also many differences. Overall, men's hair tends to be shorter and, because of their larger face shape, it is thought to be more masculine if the shape of the finished style is more 'square' (see Figs 2.121 and 2.122).

Similar tools are used, these consist of scissors, clippers, razors and combs. However, clippers and razors are used more extensively in men's, particularly traditional, hairdressing and the scissors tend to be heavier with longer blades. The basic haircutting techniques are the same but they are sometimes applied differently. Below is a brief summary of these techniques, but they can be found in greater detail in Level 2 Unit 4:

- Club cutting.
- Taper cutting.
- Thinning.

Club cutting

Cutting the hair straight across using either the scissors or clippers. Club cutting can be carried out on either wet or dry hair. This technique retains thickness and weight on the ends of the hair, therefore it tends to discourage curl and keeps the hair as thick as possible.

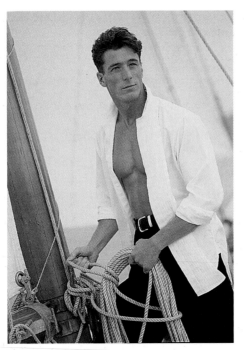

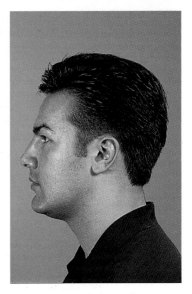

Fig. 2.122 Men's haircut with squared neckline and sideboards

Fig. 2.121 Men's haircut without fringe showing the ears

Taper cutting

This method of cutting is a slicing movement, therefore it also thins the ends of the hair whilst removing the length. It is usually carried out with a razor on wet hair and scissors on dry. It tends to encourage any curl as it has removed some of the weight from the ends of the hair.

Thinning

As its name suggests, this type of cutting thins the hair. It does not necessarily remove length from the hair but because it removes weight it allows the hair to curl more easily.

Methods of cutting

The following methods are used in conjunction with the above techniques to create different 'looks' depending on the wishes of the client, their lifestyle and personality. These methods are also used for some women's haircuts, particularly the very short styles, but not as extensively as in men's styling:

- Scissors over comb.
- Clippers over comb.
- Razor cutting.
- Scissor cutting.

Before cutting the hair

Always carry out a thorough consultation and take note of the factors listed below before deciding on the most suitable style and method of cutting. It is very important to disguise any blemishes or abnormalities and this can sometimes be a difficult task if the required hairstyle is quite short.

- Face shape, including size of ears, thickness of neck, cheekbones, prominence of chin and forehead.
- Head shape and size.
- Hairline, including a front, receding hairline and any difficult hair growth patterns.
- Texture and density of hair.
- Partial baldness.
- Any scarring of the skin.

Cutting a traditional short back and sides

Any barber must master the art of cutting this classic haircut as many of the new styles evolve from it. Take into consideration any balding areas and blend the hair accordingly. Extreme baldness looks better if the hair is cut uniformly short all over the head. Try to dissuade clients from growing side and back sections of the hair long to cover up a bald patch as this emphasises rather than camouflages it.

Procedure

1 Protect the client with gown and towels, disentangle the hair.
2 Place a No. 1 cutter head attachment to the clippers. Use a higher numbered attachment if the hair length needs to be longer.
3 Run the clippers up the neck to below the crown to approximately level with the top of the ear, round the ear and up the sideburns. Just below the required line, ease the clippers away from the head in an outward curving movement to bevel the hair and prevent a hard line.
4 Hold the comb close to the head at the clipper line and, using scissors or clippers over comb (remember to remove attachment!), increase distance from head to blend but produce longer hair length on the crown. Cutting the hair too short in this area will make it stick up and the overall finished shape will be wrongly balanced.
5 Determine the required length on top of the head and, using this as a guide, cut the hair on the top, crown and upper sides to blend in with the short clippered hair.
6 Remove the hair below the haircut shape by shaving clean with razor or clippers.
7 Check in mirror and around head that the style is even and correctly balanced from all angles.
8 Clean client free from hair and advise on after-care of the cut. Dispose of any sharps safely and complete a record of work carried out.

Cutting a crew cut or 'flat top'

These haircuts are derived from the old German 'Boche' cut. Before starting to cut the hair consult with the client to determine whether the hair is to be 'squared' or 'rounded' at the sides. The flat top is very squared whilst the crew cut can be either.

Procedure

1 Assess the hair and scalp, determine whether the finished shape is to be rounded or squared.
2 Cut the back and sides quite short, as with a short back and sides cut. Alternatively, the hair may be left the same length as the top with graduation at the nape only.

3 Make the hair on top of the head stand upright using either brushes or wax. Insert a comb or flat top comb at the front of the head towards the back. Make sure that the comb is level then remove the protruding hair with either scissors or clippers.
4 Repeat this process all over the top of the head to ensure that all the top hair is cut to a uniform length. Use the mirror to check the shape continually.
5 Blend the top hair into the back and sides using scissors or clippers over comb. Clean stray hairs from the nape and sideburn areas with either clippers or razor.
6 Check in the mirror and around the head to ensure that the style is even from all angles. Clean client free from hair. Dispose of sharps safely and complete a record of work carried out.

Dealing with baldness

Men can be extremely sensitive about their loss of hair and it is therefore very important to be very tactful during the consultation process. Always try to style and cut the hair to under-emphasise thinning or hair loss by blending the haircut well with any bald areas and advising the client on a suitable style.

Some men prefer to disguise their loss of hair by the addition of false hair such as a wig or toupee. These must be well cut and of a colour to blend with any existing hair. Unfortunately, because the hair does not 'grow out' it becomes discoloured by sunlight and the atmosphere and may need recolouring from time to time. It is also easy to tear the base of the wig or toupee if it is not treated correctly. Advice and guidance on their care and maintenance is therefore essential.

Measuring the head for a toupee (using a polythene template)

The decision to wear a toupee is usually taken after much thought and deliberation. It is therefore of the utmost importance that the operator allows enough time to be spent making sure that the client has adequate consultation and advice about how the toupee will affect his appearance. It is sometimes a shock to the client to be suddenly confronted with a full head of hair!

It is important to take accurate measurements so that the finished postiche is a perfect fit. Nothing looks more false or attracts the attention more than an ill-fitting toupee, which is just the effect that the client wishes to avoid! As a rule most men wear their hair short which means that there is very little hair with which to blend and disguise the edges of the false hair thus the fit and colour match of the toupee is crucial.

Choosing the colour of the toupee should be done very carefully as the client's existing hair colour could have different shades throughout the head. It will therefore make the finished toupee appear more natural if cuttings of hair are taken from various parts of the head to enable the varying shades to be duplicated. This will also help to blend the toupee more easily into the client's own natural hair.

Procedure
1 Assemble the equipment and protect the client with a gown.
2 Analyse the client's existing hair and allow adequate consultation to determine exact requirements regarding length, density, texture, amount of curl and finished style of the toupee.

3 Place an oblong piece of polythene (approximately 40 cm by 20 cm (16" by 8")) over the bald area of the client's head. For safety reasons the polythene must be kept away from the client's eyes, mouth and nose.

4 Mould the polythene to the head by twisting its ends, then make a firm base by pulling adhesive tape lengthways then across the polythene overlapping the bald area by 2 cm ($\frac{3}{4}$").

5 Mark the bald area by drawing round it carefully with a waterproof marker pen or eyebrow pencil, making sure that it is drawn to the correct size.

6 To outline the front edge, use any stray, wispy hairs that may be visible at the front hairline. If there are none then this will have to be carefully estimated.

7 Indicate with the marker pen the front and back of the template and the direction the hair is to lie on the finished toupee. The length and position of any partings should also be clearly marked on the template.

8 Remove the template from the client's head and wipe the scalp clean of any perspiration caused by the polythene.

9 Cut around the edge of the marked area then check that the completed template fits correctly by replacing it on the client's head.

10 Pad the inside of the template with tissue paper to make sure that it retains its shape, then complete a workroom order in the same manner as a wig. Make sure that all relevant information is included on the order and attach any hair colour samples, indicating their required position on the finished toupee.

11 Dispatch the order to the wigmaker as quickly as possible keeping a record of the transaction for future reference.

Securing a toupee to the head

Before placing the toupee on the client's head the scalp should be clean and free of grease to enable the postiche to stick to the scalp. Draw the toupee over the scalp from the front hairline towards the back making sure that it is in the correct position by checking in the mirror. Attach to the client's scalp with double-sided adhesive tape. Clients with some hair on the top may have the toupee clipped into position and there are now various types of postiche which have been designed with snap-on clips for rigid fastening.

Gently comb the hair into position, blending in the edges of the toupee with the existing hair, taking care not to snag or pull the base of the postiche. Check that there are no hard edges and that the front hairline is styled to make it appear as natural as possible. This part of the toupee is the most noticeable to others, therefore it is always worthwhile paying it special attention to make sure that it is not combed either too far forward or too far back.

On the first, initial fitting the postiche hair may have to be cut into the shape of the existing hairstyle. If it requires restyling then this *must* be carried out by an expert as mistakes at this stage can be extremely costly.

When the toupee has been fitted, make sure that it feels comfortable and that the client is happy with the result. Demonstrate to the client how to attach and remove the hair piece and give advice on its maintenance. Explain how the hair should be combed to prevent tearing the base and that the base must be kept dry (unless specially designed otherwise). Stress that the hair does not grow, therefore the colour may fade due to the effect of natural sunlight and that it may be necessary to professionally refresh the colour (or add extra white hairs) in the future. Make sure that the client is aware of the need for professional maintenance of all the postiche to prolong its 'life'.

Research into the variety and types of added hairpieces available for men.

Present your findings under the following headings:

- Type of added hair
- Uses of each type.
- Maintenance and after-care advice.

Trade journals and trade exhibitions are a good source of information.

Level 2 Unit 12

Why is client consultation necessary before commencing the beard trim? ☐

What is often used to produce a beard with a very short uniform look? ☐

How should the client be positioned for a beard trim? ☐

What happens to the length of the hair when the comb is moved further away from the face? ☐

What technique is used to prevent cutting the lips when outlining the moustache? ☐

What is used to outline the final shape of the beard? ☐

List what needs to be taken into consideration before carrying out a haircut. ☐

Why is it necessary to leave the hair longer on the crown? ☐

How would you remove hair below the hairline shape? ☐

How would you deal with a client requiring a toupee? ☐

MEN'S SHAVING AND FACE MASSAGE

This section covers the key skills needed for men's shaving and face massage. The tools used to provide these services include:

- Razors.
- Vibro machine.

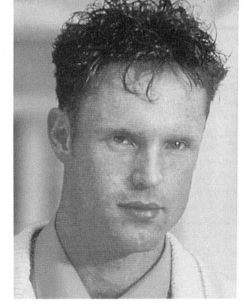

Razors

There are various types of razors that can be used to shave the beard and these can be categorised as either **safety** or **open**.

Traditionally, open razors have been used by barbers to shave beards. However, for safety and hygienic reasons safety razors with disposable blades are now becoming much more popular as each client can have their own new, sterile blade for each shave. The most recently developed safety razor has special blades which can be inserted and removed without the operator having to handle any part of the blade at all.

For those salons that prefer to use open razors, extreme care must be taken to ensure that the razors are kept clean, sharp and sterile and that all possible precautions are taken to prevent cuts to the skin and cross-infection.

Open razors

Open razors are made of steel with a bone, vulcanite or celluloid handle. They can be either **solid** or **hollow-ground**. Hollow-ground razors are finer, more pliable and quicker to set than solid razors which are rigid and kinder to sensitive skin. Solid razors also have the advantage of being suitable for haircutting, thus making

SAFETY TIP
The use of razors in the salon carries a high risk of cutting the client (or hairdresser). It is therefore important to bear in mind the Health and Safety points given earlier in this book.

them more versatile for salon use. However, all razors vary according to steel quality, hardness, grinding and tempering.

The main categories of open razor are: **hollow-ground English, hollow-ground German** and **French** which is smaller in blade length, depth and thickness than the other two types and is known as a solid razor. The most popular open razor for salon use is the 16 mm medium full hollow-ground.

Different razors have different uses and the advantages and disadvantages of each are listed in Table 2.16.

Table 2.16

Type	Advantages	Disadvantages
English/German hollow-ground	Durable, pliable, quicker to set and lighter to handle.	Too hard for sensitive skin types. Will damage cuticle of the hair if used for hair cutting.
French solid	Smooth and soft to the skin therefore good for thin, fine skin. Suitable for haircutting.	Has to be ground and stropped more frequently than hollow-ground as the metal is softer.

Honing and stropping

When magnified, the edge of a razor is like the teeth of a carpenter's saw which becomes worn down as it is used. **Honing** restores the worn edge by creating a new row of teeth while **stropping** is used between honing to help preserve the edge for as long as possible.

The honing process is often called *setting* and is done on a stone known as a **hone**. If it is carried out correctly it will give a perfect cutting edge to the razor's blade. There are various types of hone, each of which has a specific use. Table 2.17 gives a brief summary of the various types.

Table 2.17

Type	Made from	Use	Lubricator
Californian	Fine-grained, natural stone from California set into a slate base.	General purpose.	Usually oil but lather or shampoo may also be used.
Water (slatestone)	Fine quality slate.	Hollow-ground razors.	A sandstone strip dipped in water then rubbed over the hone surface.
Carborundum	Carbon and silicon obtained in various forms.	Very coarse, used to remove any gaps or notches on the blade prior to finer honing.	Usually oil but lather or shampoo may be used.
Pike's	Various compositions.	Hollow-ground and French solid.	Oil lubrication.

Honing (or setting) a hollow-ground razor

1 Place the hone on a tissue. Wipe the surface of the hone to ensure that it is clean and free from hair.
2 Sprinkle the selected lubricant over the surface of the hone and spread evenly with the back of the razor.

3 Stroke the razor blade diagonally across the hone, leading with the cutting edge of the razor. Start with the heel and finish with the toe. The blade should be kept flat on the surface and equal pressure exerted on the razor at all times.

4 Turn the razor on its *back* to commence the second stroke. Using the fingers to roll the razor over and *not* the wrist. As the razor turns over slide it from the bottom to the top of the hone so that the heel is again on the hone.

5 Next draw the razor diagonally across the hone with the cutting edge leading.

6 Repeat this figure of eight movement until the razor is what is known as 'sets', i.e. the cutting edge has been restored. The lubricant will darken during the honing process as the steel is removed from the blade.

7 After setting, wipe the blade on a tissue (along the back to avoid cutting the fingers). Clean the hone and store away carefully with the surface protected so that it does not become chipped.

Honing a French solid razor

The steel of a French solid razor is softer than the hollow-ground and must therefore always be set on a fine grain hone with thin oil or lather as a lubricant.

> **TECHNICAL TIP**
> When honing any type of razor the edge can be blunted and damaged if the razor is turned on its edge instead of its back.

The strokes should be shorter and crisper than those used for the hollow-ground with only the razor edge resting, almost flat, on the hone. The strokes resemble a 'V' with the razor turned on its back at the end of each stroke. As the strokes progress they become steeper and steeper until they are almost perpendicular (see Fig. 2.123).

Testing the razor

This is done by pulling the razor across a moistened thumb nail. The different degrees of sharpness will give a different tactile sensation.

- A perfect or **keen** edge will dig into the nail with a smooth, steady grip.
- A blunt or **dull** edge will pull smoothly across the nail without dragging or cutting.
- A **coarse** edge will feel jerky and dig into the nail.
- An **over-honed** edge will stick to the nail with a harsh, grating sound.
- A **nick** in the razor will feel uneven as it is drawn across the nail.

Stropping

As you have already learned, stropping is done to preserve the cutting edge of the razor between setting. It cleans debris such as soap, skin and hair from the razor's edge and also re-aligns the teeth.

Stropping is carried out on a leather strop which can be of either the hanging or solid (hand) variety. The hanging strop is flexible with leather on one side and canvas on the other, it is used for hollow-ground razors. The solid or hand strop is rigid and is used for solid French razors.

> **TECHNICAL TIP**
> Always store strops away from dust, damp and hair cuttings as any damage to the surface of the strop will ultimately spoil the cutting edge of the razor.

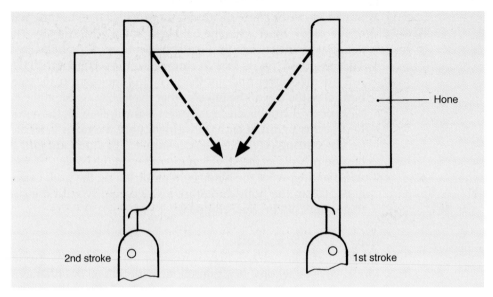

Fig. 2.123 Honing a French solid razor

Before being used for the first time, a new strop must be treated by smearing it with plenty of oil and leaving it to soak overnight. The canvas side of a hanging strop should also be treated by rubbing soap into the canvas. After treating, both surfaces are then rubbed with a round, glass bottle until a glazed surface is obtained.

Stropping a hollow-ground razor

1 Hang the strop on a hook then hold firmly in a horizontal position by gripping the free end with the hand. Hold the razor shaft between the first finger and thumb of the other hand to allow the razor to be revolved easily during stropping.
2 Lie the razor flat and stroke it, with the back leading, away from the operator down the strop. When it has travelled approximately two-thirds of the way down the strop, turn the razor on its back and bring it back up the strop in the opposite direction.
3 Initially, the strokes should be slow and careful as speed only comes with practice. Twelve strokes is usually sufficient (six forward and six back). Over stropping should be avoided as it will spoil the razor edge.

Stropping a solid razor

A solid razor is rigid and therefore does not 'give' when being stropped.

Place the solid strop in a horizontal position. Hold the razor between the thumb and the first finger, but with the back of the razor slightly off the strop with the edge resting flat and even on the strop. Use six strokes backwards and forwards as before but as the steel of the solid razor is softer than the hollow-ground the stropping will have more effect.

Stropping a French solid razor

These razors are also very rigid and the method of stropping is therefore very similar to that of stropping solid razors. French strop paste is mildly abrasive making each stropping of the French razor a mild form of honing. The condition of the edge will determine the number of strokes required. The duller the blade then the more strokes are needed. Six strokes each way is usual for normal stropping rising to twelve strokes each way if the razor has a dull (blunt) edge.

TECHNICAL TIP
It is important to remember that if the razor is turned on its edge during any type of stropping, the strop may cut and split making it useless for further use. Making a mistake of this kind will also damage the razor's edge.

Shaving

Shaving can take place on the whole of the face or partially to leave either a moustache and/or long sideburns. It may also be carried out on nape and sideburn outlines to give a 'clean' finish to the haircut.

A good shave should not be felt by the client and a full facial shave should result in a smooth face. Shaving has three separate phases:

- Preparation of the client.
- Lathering.
- Shaving.

Preparation of the client

For hygienic reasons, ensure that your own hands and nails are clean and that the client's beard is clean and free from grease before commencing the shave. Any grease remaining on the beard will prevent the lather from foaming correctly.

Discuss with the client his requirements then seat him in a reclining chair with a clean paper towel placed over the headrest. Protect the client with a gown then place a towel across his chest and tuck it in firmly at the neck. Position the client's head well back so that the chin and lower face area are easily accessible, then place a paper towel, tissue or shaving square near to the neck.

Examine the face for any abnormalities, broken skin, strong or unusual beard growth patterns and length of sideburns (sideboards). If everything is satisfactory then the client is now ready for the next stage.

Lathering

This process is carried out to soften the beard and help prevent the shave from being painful. The lather is produced by soap and water. Shaving soap can be obtained in foam, powder, cream or liquid form.

SAFETY TIP
Block or tablet soap is not recommended for lathering because it would be unhygienic to use the same block for a large number of clients.

Procedure

1 Steam a sterile towel in a steamer. Place the towel over the beard area. Avoid covering the nose to allow the client to breathe. If an open razor is to be used, this is usually stropped while the face is steaming.
2 Replace the cooled towel with a second steamed towel. Fill a shaving mug or bowl with hot water.
3 Remove the towel and mix the lather by first dipping the brush into the mug of hot water then placing a small amount of the soap to be used into the centre of

the brush bristles. Rotate the brush vigorously (almost like whisking an egg) in the bowl of the shaving mug or a second bowl until a lather is produced.

4 Begin lathering the face by placing the brush under the tip of the chin and rotating it over the chin, cheeks and neck until all the beard is well covered. To lather the upper lip the brush is spread by placing the finger in the centre of the bristles, this prevents the lather from going up the nose or on the lips. Use a thin, watery application at first, increasing the lather later.

5 Keep the brush warm by dipping it into the hot water and remember that the better the lather the easier the beard will be to shave.

Shaving

Any shaving will remove a fine layer of epidermal skin so it is essential that the angle of the razor and the direction of the razor strokes are correct.

When shaving, the blade of the razor must be wiped clean of hair and lather between each razor stroke. It is *very important* to wipe the razor on its back, avoiding the edge otherwise the operator may cut their fingers quite badly and blunt the razor edge.

The temperature of the water should be kept warm. Cold water will cause the razor to drag while hot water swells the face and prevents a close shave.

TECHNICAL TIP
Always stretch the skin taunt when stroking with the razor as this will hold the hair up to the razor and allow it to be cut more closely and will also help to prevent cuts to the skin.

First time over shave

The first time over shave is always done in the same direction as the hair growth, i.e. *with* the grain of the hair. When stretching the skin for this shave, the finger is placed *behind* the razor instead of in front, as it is very difficult to get a firm grip on the skin when the face is slippery with the lather.

TECHNICAL TIP
A right-handed operator should stand and start on the right-hand side while a left-handed one should stand and start on the left.

Procedure

1 Hold the razor loosely with the thumb on the blade. The actual position will vary with the different strokes, and dip the razor into the hot water.

2 Begin the shave on the side nearest to the operator. Always start by holding the dry, unlathered skin at the sideboard area (to prevent the fingers slipping) pulling it taut to commence the shave.

3 Move the razor in a slicing, scythe-like motion following the movements shown in Fig. 2.124.

SAFETY TIP
It is important to start any razor stroke *before* a bony prominence to prevent cutting the client.

4 Each side of the face should be completely shaved before starting the other, with the centre chin section left until last. Try to incorporate each side of the upper lip area when shaving that side of the face, thus leaving just the centre section which is then shaved upwards while pressing the tip of the nose upwards to tighten the skin. Avoid holding the nose as this can be painful to the client and could cause sneezing.

5 When one side of the face has been completed, the client's head is turned towards the operator to make it easier to shave the other side.

6 To shave the point of the chin, pull the skin tight between the finger and thumb then use the middle of the razor blade to shave *across* the chin.

7 Finish by shaving the neck area downwards.

Second time over shave

This shave is necessary to ensure that the hair is cut as closely as possible giving a clean finished result. The hair is cut against the growth in an upward movement.

This is usually the final shave unless the client is very dark haired with a strong beard growth. In this case, it may have to be followed by a sponge shave. This entails soaking a small sponge in hot water then dragging it across the face with the razor following closely.

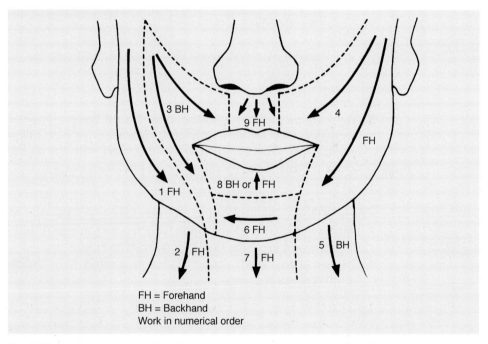

FH = Forehand
BH = Backhand
Work in numerical order

Fig. 2.124 Shaving procedure – first time over

Procedure
1 Re-lather the face in the manner described previously.
2 Begin the shave at the collar area with the fingers again holding the dry, unlathered skin. Move upwards in backhand strokes, completing one side of the face before starting the other as for the first time over shave. See Fig. 2.125 for the order and manner of the strokes.

Men's Shaving and Face Massage 257

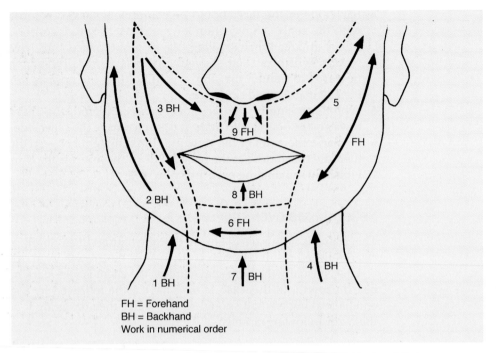

Fig. 2.125 Shaving procedure – second time over

TECHNICAL TIP
Juvenile beards are quite soft and may not therefore require shaving against the growth with upward strokes.

3 Any cuts or punctures to the skin should have a powder or liquid styptic applied to stop the flow of blood. However, for hygienic and health reasons extreme care must be taken to avoid contact with the blood, particularly if the operator has any cuts or punctures to their own skin.

4 Clean the face with a damp, warm towel or sponge then gently pat dry with another clean towel. Apply a small amount of talcum powder to ensure that the skin is thoroughly dry and to prevent chapping of the skin after the shave.

5 Finish with an after-shave lotion, which is an astringent, and will therefore close the pores and leave the skin feeling fresh and clean.

6 Dispose of any sharps (razor blades, etc.) safely in accordance with the salon's health and safety policy.

Men's face massage

The massage is usually carried out after shaving to aid skin elasticity, tone the facial muscles and encourage natural excretion of waste products. However, the main benefit of a face massage is to relax the client and this point should be remembered by the operator while the massage is being carried out.

Before commencing the massage, make sure that the client's clothing and hair are well protected from the massage cream. Check that your hands and nails are clean and assemble equipment.

Procedure

1 Steam the face with two hot towels.

2 Stand behind the client and commence the massage by placing the flat surface of the closed fingers on the forehead at the eyebrows. Stroke the fingers back towards the front hairline then across the forehead in gentle, stroking, effleurage movements until the client is relaxed. (See Level 2 Unit 2 for additional massage information.)

3 Move to the corner of the eyes and rotate the skin in a petrissage movement then continue with the same movements above the nose. Gentle *tapotement* (tapping movements) can be used under the eyes so that the skin is not pulled.

4 Next, stroking effleurage movements are used from the temple down and round the cheekbone to the side of the nostril base. The hands are then turned so that the backs are together with the palms facing outwards. Carry this movement on up the sides of the nose ending between the eyebrows.

5 Placing the third finger of each hand on the side of the nostrils, use small, circular movements up the sides of the nose to help to unblock the pores.

6 With the tips of the fingers held together, gently stroke from the upper lip sliding the fingers sideways and diagonally upwards towards the outer corner of the eye finishing with a circular effleurage movement around the bony part of the eye socket.

7 The lower part of the face is massaged using the flat of the hands in a circular movement from the mouth out towards the ear then from below the mouth to under the ears.

8 The top of the chin and jawline can be massaged by rotatory petrissage movements but tapotement or vibratory movements are more suitable for fleshy or double chins.

9 Finish the massage by rolling the skin upwards between the thumb and the forefinger from the chin to the forehead.

10 Complete the treatment with another hot towel followed by a cool towel and/or an astringent to close the pores and tighten the skin. Finally, a light dusting of powder, cream or lotion may be applied depending on the personal preference of the client.

Vibro massage machine

This is a machine (see Fig. 2.10, page 92) used to provide a mechanical massage. It has three main applicators; spiked applicator fur use on the scalp, flat vulcanite applicator for use on the skin and a sponge applicator for use on the face. The sponge applicator is usually the attachment used when giving a mechanical face massage.

Using vibro massage

The vibro massage gives strong tapotement movements. It can be used in place of a manual hand massage but it is only suitable for the fleshy areas. Great care must be taken when using the vibro on bony areas such as the jawline and forehead as it can be very uncomfortable for the client and it must *never* be used on the nose and around the eyes.

SAFETY TIP

Always be aware of the comfort of the client and use the vibro carefully and gently. If it feels too strong for the client then use the attachments over the hand.

If the vibro is used to replace some of the hand massage movements, it should be used in the same order and direction as the massage movements that it is replacing.

Things to do

Some salons use the traditional 'open' razors which need to be kept both sterile and sharp. The problem with this type of razor is that there is a chance of cross-infection between clients if not properly sterilised and considerable skill is needed to sharpen them (honing and stropping). The best kind to use are 'safety' razors where the blade is changed for a new sterile one between clients, without being touched by the hairdresser. This assignment therefore concentrates on the uses of the 'safety' type of razor.

Shaving the face is a skilled operation which improves with practice. It is, however, the hairdressing operation most likely to cause bleeding and it is important to know what to do if this occurs. This assignment is designed to help you to develop your practical skills and hygiene operations.

1   Using an inflated balloon of about head size, lather, and shave as you would a face. You know instantly if you have cut into it! You can use a peach instead of a balloon but this lacks the realistic size.

2   If you cut a client while shaving (or at any other time):

   • use styptic to stop the bleeding; put the styptic onto a tissue and give this to the client for them to hold on the cut
   • if any blood has fallen onto surfaces, wipe with neat bleach and wash off with plenty of water and detergent

   Explain each of these steps.

What do you know?

Level 2 Unit 13

Give the advantages and disadvantages of hollow-ground and solid razors. ☐

What does honing do to the edge of the razor? ☐

List four types of hone and give their uses. ☐

What will happen if the razor is turned on its edge instead of its back during honing? ☐

How is the razor edge tested for sharpness? ☐

What is the purpose of stropping? ☐

What are the three phases of shaving? ☐

What should you look for when examining the face prior to shaving? ☐

Why is the face lathered before shaving? ☐

Why is the skin stretched taut when stroking with the razor? ☐

How often is the razor wiped clean when shaving? ☐

How is the razor wiped and what could happen if it was wiped along its edge? ☐

What is the main benefit of a face massage? ☐

Which type of massage movement is used first to relax the client? ☐

What type of movements are more suitable for fleshy or double chins? ☐

What is the purpose of an astringent? ☐

What is the vibro massager suitable for? ☐

Where must the vibro massager never be used? ☐

What can be done to aid client comfort if the vibro feels too strong for the client? ☐

Level 3

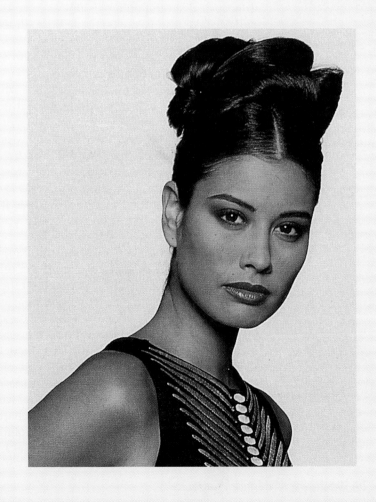

MAINTAINING AND DEVELOPING CLIENT CARE

Always remember that clients are indispensable to your business and your behaviour towards them should show that you value them and their custom. Talking to the client prior to their treatment will not only determine their specific needs but will also help to develop a positive relationship between the stylist and the client. Listen carefully to find out *exactly* what the client requires and check your understanding by repeating their request. Talk to them in a language they understand – using specialist terminology is fine as long as everyone understands what is being said! Mistakes can easily be made through the differing perceptions of both client and stylist.

In addition to determining the client's wishes, any consultation should include an examination of the head and face shape, and also the texture, length and condition of the hair to ensure that what the client actually wants is compatible with their hair type and facial features. When diagnosing the hair before carrying out a chemical treatment, it is very important to determine which, if any, chemicals have been used previously on the hair. This can be done through feeling and looking at the hair and also by questioning the client. Sometimes a client may be less than truthful in their response due to embarrassment or not realising how long a product will remain on/in the hair. If in doubt, *always* carry out a suitable test – not only does it prevent harmful mistakes, it also shows professionalism and saves any argument as to the suitability of the required service.

Clients are not always aware of the range of products and services that the salon has to offer, so a discussion of the relevance and benefits of these to the client, and their related cost, can highlight the expertise of the stylist and make the client feel that they are receiving individual attention.

Client consultation is an ongoing process and, although the major part of the diagnosis will be carried out prior to the service, there should be continuing dialogue between the stylist and the client both during and at the end of the service. All staff should be familiar with the range of products used and sold in the salon to enable them to offer advice and guidance regarding improvements to the client's hair and which after-care products would be suitable for home use. Up-to-date records should be kept of all client services and products used or recommended, to help with future consultations.

These areas are covered in detail in Level 1 Unit 3 and Level 2 Unit 1.

Supervising client consultation

There are two main areas involved when supervising junior staff members, trainees or students carrying out a client consultation:

- Training.
- Monitoring progress.

Training

Carrying out a consultation with a client requires good interpersonal skills on behalf of the trainee and these skills usually have to be taught if they are to form the basis of a good relationship between the client and the salon staff. All salons have their own image and will expect a certain standard of conduct from their personnel. However, it is unrealistic to expect staff to know exactly what is required of them without their being fully briefed so it is essential that they are all given training on how the organisation expects them to behave in a client–staff relationship. The actual training plan will usually be devised by the manager or employer but it is often the role of the supervisor to oversee the actual training and ensure that employees reach the required standard. A clear induction of new staff is very helpful, outlining the salon 'ground rules' with regard to customer care, together with regular practice sessions (for junior staff) which encourage the use of role-play to rehearse their interpersonal skills.

Consultation also includes giving advice and guidance to the client. This is impossible without a thorough knowledge of the products and services used in the salon. The more a product is used then the greater understanding the staff acquire of its possible uses and effects. Encouraging staff to use the products as frequently as possible, insisting that the manufacturers' instructions are read and carried out correctly, and asking the manufacturers to demonstrate their products in the salon are all means of increasing product knowledge and understanding.

Points to include in training for client care

Good client care begins with personal attitude. All trainees need to be made aware of the importance of the client, and their attitude towards the client should reflect this. Without clients the salon cannot function and it is therefore vital to provide an environment in which the client can relax and enjoy their visit. A client may book an appointment for a technical service but in reality they are also booking a salon 'experience' in which the relationship between the stylist and the client is of paramount importance. Indeed, most clients continue to return to the salon not only because of the skill and expertise of the stylist but also because of the way they are treated and valued as a person.

Building up a relationship of trust is not easy and requires a combination of good interpersonal skills, sound product knowledge and a genuine empathy with the client's requirements. Offering the client help and advice is all part of the hairdressing service and as has been mentioned in previous units, the advice given *must* be based on a sound understanding of the client needs combined with expertise gained through experience and thorough product knowledge. Remember that what you recommend for the client should do what it is supposed to do – if it does not then the client has every right to mistrust your judgement and will probably seek future advice elsewhere!

Client care should be an integral part of any training programme and should be constantly reinforced by the example set by senior stylists in the way they themselves treat their clients. However, it is well worth regularly reminding trainees, and possibly all staff, of the following ten points which will help to focus client care at the forefront of their work.

1 Remember that the client is essential to the business.
2 Develop a trusting relationship with the client.
3 Find out **exactly** what the client requires and make sure that you are able to give it.
4 Always **listen** to clients and try to understand their points of view.
5 Make sure that your behaviour tells clients that you value them and their business.
6 Try not to keep clients waiting and **never** ignore them.
7 Check that clients are happy with the outcome of their visit.
8 Treat all complaints seriously – deal with them courteously and **immediately**.
9 Always record and analyse any complaints to enable you to improve future services.
10 All staff members should apply 'client care' to each other within the salon as well as to those outside.

Monitoring progress

Whilst they are acquiring the skills necessary for client consultation, it is important to encourage the trainees to practise these skills as frequently as possible. The more the trainee is exposed to different hair types, face shapes and abnormalities, etc., then the more adept the trainee will become in identifying them. Allowing them to practise under supervision and monitoring their progress will ensure that staff learn as quickly as possible to the standards expected by the organisation.

Supportive help and guidance should be given – it is a good idea to apply customer care to 'customers' *within* the organisation as well as outside! Judgements are inevitable when supervising the trainee's performance but any criticism should be constructive and carried out in private in a debriefing session. Emphasis should be placed on the confidentiality of any consultation, the importance of good interpersonal skills, accurate record keeping, and the health and safety requirements of manufacturers, the salon and current legislation.

POINTS TO REMEMBER

- Listen to what the client is saying, not just the words but the implications and body language.
- Carry out a thorough diagnosis of the hair, face, scalp and total image of the client.
- When in doubt *always* test the hair.
- Keep clear, precise and up-to-date records.
- Treat any client consultation with confidentiality.

Promotion of after-care procedures and future salon services

This topic is covered in Level 2 Unit 1, page 73. The key points to summarise are that after-care is important.

- To the **client** – in terms of knowing what to do/what not to do with their hair following a salon service.
- For the **salon** – due to the importance of after-care advice in the professional image and operation of a salon.

This is an important factor in client satisfaction and helps develop return custom and positive personal recommendation – both of which are **very** important to the salon business.

Promoting and developing effective working relationships with clients

A salon cannot exist for long without clients! Hairdressing is a highly competitive service industry and success depends on developing and keeping a good client base. What makes a client return to a salon? What makes a client recommend the salon to someone else?

The key to success is *communicating a positive attitude*. Is the salon a welcoming, friendly place? Will a client feel valued? Will they feel they have experienced a thoroughly professional service?

Difficult situations in communicating with clients

'Difficult' situations are bound to arise with some clients. There are two areas in particular.

1 The need to refer a client to hairdressing or non-hairdressing services because of some diagnosed problems.
2 Dealing with client complaints.

Referring clients to other services

The need to refer clients to other services, hairdressing or non-hairdressing (such as medical) will arise from time to time. This may well be as a result of client consultation and assessment of the condition of a client's hair and scalp (see Level 2 Unit 1). The outcome of the hair and scalp assessment may be relatively unimportant (such as using a different type of mousse) or be more sensitive (such as the presence of head lice). Sometimes a client will have a hair or scalp condition which is beyond the salon's ability to help. In this case, the person may be referred to professional medical treatment. Scalp ringworm is an example of such a condition. On other occasions referral to other professionals such as trichologists may be appropriate (psoriasis is an example). For full details of scalp and hair conditions and what action to take see Level 2 Unit 1.

On any occasion requiring referral of a client, the key word is tact. The information is confidential; treat it so. Talk quietly, be positive, listen to the client, reassure them. Explain that they will:

● Need expert opinion to confirm the diagnosis.
● Be welcome to return to the salon if the condition turns out to be non-infectious.
● Understand the need to suspend hairdressing operations (should this be necessary) in order to prevent infecting others.

Dealing with a client complaint

Most people, if dealt with pleasantly and correctly, are easy to please, but there will always be one client who has some grievance, whether real or imagined. Tactful dealing with the client is essential to keep their goodwill and create a good impression of the salon. It is very tempting to feel that the salon would be better off without this type of client but remember that when a client is lost, the salon also loses many more potential clients because the unsatisfied client will almost certainly give a bad impression of the salon's service to others. The best practice is to **anticipate** problems. Most people will 'leak' their dissatisfaction in a non-verbal way. Look out for:

- Body movements.
- Body posture.
- Facial expressions.

which indicate that the client is not very happy.

If a complaint does occur it must be dealt with immediately, whatever the cause. If it is a complaint against the service, it should be dealt with to their complete satisfaction. For example, in the case of an unsatisfactory perm – it is no use trying to persuade the client that it is satisfactory. Instead, you should deal with the incident without fuss and re-perm where necessary, giving a quiet explanation as to the failure. This is a far more professional attitude and more acceptable than an argument, which does not solve anything.

If a client is loud in their protests and embarrassing to yourself and other clients, you should take them quietly to a private part of the salon to rectify the complaint. If it concerns another member of staff it must be rectified with that member of staff present.

Even in the best-run salons, mistakes sometimes happen. A colour does not come up to expectations or a perm may be limp. If this occurs it is often the best policy to tell the client, before they complain, that you are not satisfied with the result and will rectify it immediately. This promotes goodwill and the client will have more trust, feeling that the stylist cares about their hair and will not be satisfied with second-best results. Their recommendations to others could win many new clients and is an extremely effective way of advertising.

Looking after clients is good business. The wages of the staff depend upon clients returning regularly to the salon. If a client has enjoyed their visit and feels that they have had a first-class service, they will almost certainly return.

Obtaining feedback from clients

Obtaining feedback from clients is very important in evaluating the quality of a person's experience of the salon and its services. At the end of their treatment the client is asked something along the lines of 'Are you happy with that?' If a client is very dissatisfied they will let the salon staff know. Many people, however, if only slightly unhappy say 'fine' or something neutral and then leave. Very few salons obtain 'formal' structured feedback by using a questionnaire. This is well worth considering. Questionnaires can be short (even 'tick the box' types) and are anonymous and confidential. The idea is to pick up lower levels of dissatisfaction and people's general impressions of the way they have been treated. By being quick to complete and anonymous it is hoped that clients will be more honest than if they are asked by the stylist outright.

Other forms of feedback which are more often used are the client:

- Returning to the salon.
- Recommending the salon to other people.

Both of these are good indicators of the client's perception of the salon's service.

1 Every professional product used in the salon is accompanied by a detailed set of instructions. The information contained in the instructions covers the company in case there are any problems with the product, e.g. reaction to the client's skin.

   Read and collect as many different manufacturers' instruction leaflets as you can, covering the following services:

   - perming
   - colouring
   - relaxing
   - retail products
   - cutting tools
   - hair pieces/extensions

   Make notes on any important points which need to be brought to the attention of the other trainees and staff members. Hold a briefing session or meeting to share the information.

2 Take an example of a client complaint. This could be simulated but a 'real' example is better. Make out a report, including a **portfolio** of information about the incident.

Level 3 Unit 1

List what should be included in a client consultation. ☐

Give a brief account of how and when you would explain the benefits and uses of the range of products and services the salon has to offer. ☐

*Give **three** ideas for ensuring that junior staff reach the required standard for customer care.* ☐

Which areas need to be emphasised to the trainee regarding consultation procedures? ☐

Explain how you would supervise a trainee carrying out a client consultation. ☐

Why does a salon need clients? ☐

*Give **two** reasons why it is important for clients to have a positive impression of the salon and its services.* ☐

How can 'feedback' be obtained from clients? ☐

Explain why non-verbal communication is so important in the salon. ☐

*List **two** strategies that will make a client feel 'valued'.* ☐

How should a client referral to other services be handled? ☐

List the key points in dealing with a client complaint. ☐

How may client satisfaction with the salon and its services be measured? ☐

Explain the importance of client consultation. ☐

*List **three** non-verbal signs of client satisfaction.* ☐

SPECIALISED CUTTING TECHNIQUES

Specialist haircutting techniques are innovative ways of solving problems – the problem being how to achieve a certain visual effect with the hair. Several techniques may actually give the same effect showing that the 'problem' has been approached from different angles. Before attempting to employ or create new techniques, it is essential that the stylist has an understanding of the basic methods of cutting hair and the principles of shape, texture and balance. Once these precepts have been learnt, it is then possible to increase this knowledge through practice and experimentation. The expertise of being able to create different shapes and textures in the hair comes from having a thorough knowledge of the effects that can be created by the basic cutting methods then having the courage to 'mix' these methods together to create new shapes and styles.

Review of basic cutting shapes

There are five main basic shapes which can be cut into the hair:

1 **Solid form** (e.g. bob) – this is a squared shape with all the hair cut to one length at a single base line.
2 **Uniform layering** – the hair is cut so that the inner length is the same as the outer length. Thus, it is cut to the shape of the head and a rounded shape is produced.
3 **Low layering** (e.g. wedge) – the low graduation of this cut creates a triangular shape. The hair is cut so that the inner hair length is longer than the outer hair length.
4 **Reverse graduation** – this hair is also cut so that the inner hair length is longer than the outer hair length but in this case, the inner hair length is also longer than the actual base line. Used for pageboy styles.
5 **Increased layering** – when the inner hair length is shorter than the outer hair length. This creates a shape which is shorter on the crown. Can be used when cutting longer hair to give height on top of the head.

Cutting methods

The basic methods include **tapering** which removes length as well as bulk and therefore increases the hair's tendency to curl; **club** or **blunt** cutting which reduces length only, keeping the weight on the ends of the hair thereby reducing the hair's tendency to curl; **thinning** and **texturising** which both reduce bulk from the hair; and scissors or **clippers over comb**, both of which reduce the length only and enable the hair to be cut much shorter than the other methods; **freehand** cutting of the hair without holding it in place. These cutting methods are dealt with in detail in Level 2 Unit 4.

> **Preventing RSI**
> Keep your wrist in a straight line from middle finger to elbow. This is one of the best ways to pre-vent pain in the wrist. Don't let your wrists arch, dip or angle to either side.

Specialised techniques

Once the basic principles have been acquired and practical confidence gained, more complex techniques can be used to create a variety of effects. These techniques will vary considerably depending upon individual preference. Two separate hairdressers could cut a head of hair into the same style using different techniques and finish with exactly the same style.

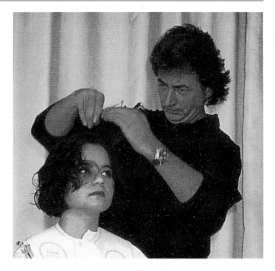

Hair fashions are continually changing and to be able to create current styles the stylist must be able to adapt a variety of techniques to keep up-to-date. It is possible to produce high fashion work by utilising a variety of basic techniques and working imaginatively. If the technique used produces a good result and the client is satisfied then that technique is right in that particular case. However, it is always useful (and more interesting for the stylist) to be able to use additional skills as and when necessary. The range and variety of techniques is only limited by the imagination of the stylist and it is therefore impossible to list each one. A selection of the more popular methods are:

- Bevel cutting.
- Slide or slither cutting.
- Specialised texturising.

Bevel cutting

This technique consists of cutting the hair on a curve. The section of hair is held between the fingers and then bent up and towards the scalp, thus curving the hair round. The hair is then cut straight across, creating graduation on the ends of the hair. This is a useful technique to use in conjunction with low layering to soften and prevent a definite line or step on the edges of the bobbed or wedged hair.

Slide or slither cutting

This is a method of cutting used to blend extremes of hair lengths, e.g. very long outer perimeter line and short interior hair. A fine section of hair is taken which includes the short and long hair lengths, and the scissor or razor blades then slide down the section without cutting the length of the longer hair blending the two lengths together.

Specialised texturising

Texturising, as the name suggests, makes the hair appear visually more textured. This is a means of removing bulk without reducing length and by cutting selected areas shorter, the cut hair acts as a support for the longer hair giving lift and volume to the style. The removal of weight from the hair encourages any natural movement in addition to the non-uniform effect which can also be achieved. There are many ways of texturising the hair and the choice of technique/s will depend on the type of hair the stylist is working with and the required final result. A selection of techniques are as follows:

- Chipping in.
- Channel cutting (scaffolding).
- Weave cutting.
- Under cutting.
- Twisting.

Chipping in

This technique will 'break up' a solid outline and take away bulk from the very ends of the hair. A section of hair is held out of the head at right angles. The points of the scissors are inserted into the section, towards the scalp, but at an angle, and about 5 mm ($\frac{1}{4}$″) of the hair is snipped away to form a 'V' shape along the length of the section. This technique can also be employed around the front hairline and fringe to soften, or even, spike the front hair onto the face by combing the hair forward onto the face then snipping away the hair as it lies flat on the skin (see Fig. 3.1).

SAFETY TIP
Remember to be very careful when using the points of the scissors near the eyes and ears.

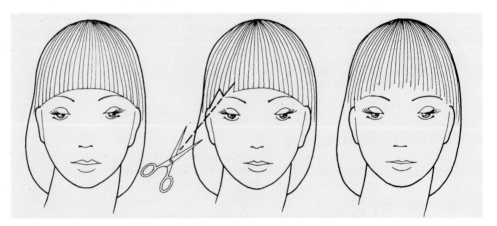

Fig. 3.1 Chipping in on front hair line

Channel cutting (scaffolding)

This is the drastic removal of hair to produce a 'spiky' effect. A 'grid' of shorter hair is cut to support the longer hair lengths. The hair is cut first one way and then across the other to create the grid effect.

Weave cutting

The hair to be left long is woven out using either a tail comb or the closed scissors. This hair is then held out of the way while the remaining hair in the section is cut. It can be drastic or subtle depending on how much of the hair is woven out and the effect required (see Fig. 3.2).

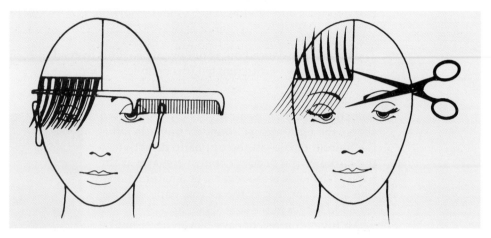

Fig. 3.2 Weave cutting

Under cutting

The underneath sections of the mesh of hair are cut shorter to support the longer lengths. This technique can be done using either the scissors or a razor. If a razor is used, hold the blade at a slight angle to the section and make light, slicing movements underneath the section of the hair from the roots up towards the points.

Twisting

This technique will thin the hair out generally and is a very useful method of 'wisping' and softening the hair around the face. A section of hair approximately 2 cm (1") square is taken and combed out from the head at right angles. The section is then twisted until the whole length of the hair is twisted from points to root. With one hand firmly holding the twisted hair, the scissors snip into and down the length of twists at an angle. Care must be taken not to inadvertently cut the hair straight across.

Perimeter lines and shapes

The perimeter line is the outside line or shape of the haircut. When designing the finished style, it is important to ensure that the shape is complementary to the facial features, body size and head shape of the client. Some common terms used are:

- Base line.
- Symmetrical.

- Asymmetrical.
- Concave.
- Convex.

Base line

This is the perimeter edge or the line to which the hair is cut. A haircut can have more than one base line and interesting effects can be achieved by incorporating several base lines and a variety of techniques on one head.

Symmetrical

This is when a haircut is evenly balanced and each part is in the same proportion. A basic bob is an example of a symmetrical hairstyle with each side being similar.

Asymmetrical

The haircut is balanced but is not evenly so, thus instead of each side being similar they are usually of different lengths or style.

Concave

Sometimes known as an inversion or inverted shape, the term means 'rounded inwards', thus the haircut curves in the opposite direction to the curve of the head. A concave shape at the nape of the neck is the reverse of a natural nape-line and is shorter in the centre nape curving round to longer at the side. (See Fig. 3.3)

An inversion or concave shape need not be limited to the hairline alone, it can be cut into the bulk of the hairstyle to produce unlimited effects on both short and long hair. If a concave shape is cut into the top hair, the centre will be the shortest point. Hair will always fall away from its shortest point, therefore width will be created just above the temple area, giving a 'squared-off' shape to the final dressing.

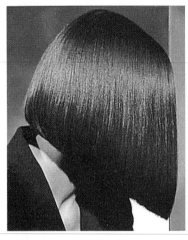

Fig. 3.3 Concave shape

Convex

This shape is the opposite of a concave shape. Therefore, when cut into the nape, it will follow the hair's natural hairline and will be longer in the centre curving round to shorter at the sides. A convex perimeter line gives a 'rounded' shape which can sometimes be more flattering for mature clients than the more angular shapes.

Restyle cutting the hair

Restyle cutting is about designing an individualised haircut for the client which is suited to their lifestyle, in keeping with current trends and uses the full potential of the hair.

Client consultation

A restyle is intended to give a completely new image. This means that the client should be made aware of how the finished style may alter the way they look, and they will also require advice and guidance on how to maintain this new look.

A thorough discussion with the client *before* commencing the treatment is absolutely essential to prevent any misunderstanding of the client's wishes and gives the stylist the opportunity to offer any help and advice that may be necessary. Remember that the finished style must complement the client's personality, appearance and lifestyle but, above all, they should be pleased with the finished result! A disappointed client will not return for another appointment and will also give the salon negative, adverse publicity.

Influencing factors

There are many things to look for before advising the client, these are known as influencing factors. Very often one of these factors prevents the hair being suitable for the client's chosen style, in which case it may be necessary to devise a compromise.

Factors that will influence the finished style include:

- Cutting techniques, equipment and suitable tools.
- Type of finishing technique.
- Appropriate use of products.
- Texture, density, length, condition and amount of curl in the hair – often one of these factors prevents the hair being suitable for the client's chosen style.
- The 'look' that is to be achieved.

Hairstyles can be broadly divided into three main 'looks':

- Classic.
- Fashion.
- Avant garde.

Classic

This look withstands the test of time! A good example of this type of timeless style is the 'bob'. The bob of the 1960s looks just as good in the 1990s. Mature or business clients often prefer smart, classical styles which flatter their image.

Fashion

Fashion styles are the look of the moment and therefore often change quite quickly. Interestingly, classsic haircuts can frequently be adapted to meet new fashion trends.

Avant garde

Unusual, different, striking and often fun are descriptions of the avant garde style. Not usually suitable for the quiet, shy type of client! However, these styles are often adapted to become the fashion styles of the future.

Preventing RSI

Make sure you keep up to date with the most recent innovations in design. There may be a better design for scissors that will allow for improved hand position and less strain. When such a design surfaces, you want to know about it. The same applies to your other tools, appliances, supplies and equipment.

Sectioning for restyle cutting

There are no hard and fast rules for sectioning the hair and it should be sectioned as and where required. Often the hair is sectioned down the centre of the head from the front through to the nape but any partings, fringes, etc., should be taken into consideration and sectioned off separately.

Procedure for restyle cutting

This will depend on the result required. However, if the style is to be clean and precise it is often easier to cut the hair in a straight line, either horizontally or vertically. By considering carefully the shape of the finished style, then taking into account where the hair needs to be short and where the length needs to be kept, it is often possible to use the shape of the head to create the angles needed for the amount of graduation required. Hair usually needs to be kept thoroughly wet during cutting to ensure that cutting sections are smooth and straight from root to point.

A skilled haircutter can often cut the hair freehand, by identifying where and how much hair needs to be removed. This is not a precise method of cutting but can produce interesting results.

During the haircutting procedure care should always be taken to ensure that health and safety regulations are adhered to and that adequate hygiene precautions are taken. When dealing with sharp objects which could puncture the skin, it is important that all tools and equipment are correctly sterilised and that reasonable care is taken to guarantee customer comfort and safety. Sharps such as used razor blades should be disposed of safely in accordance with salon procedures and any local by-laws. All records should be clear and up to date with adequate information including any after-care advice given to the client.

> **SAFETY TIP**
>
> Working with sharp tools and equipment can be dangerous and therefore has implications for the health and safety of both clients and staff. There is legislation regarding Health and Safety in the workplace and also liability to the client. In addition, the salon will usually have their own policy which must be adhered to. Because of the additional implication of transmission of disease to both staff and clients, the sterilisation, storage and disposal of sharp equipment and tools used in the salon is very important.

Considerations when cutting long hair

1 The longer the hair, the heavier it becomes. Therefore, if the client requires height on the top it will be necessary to cut this area shorter to prevent it from flopping.
2 Hair does not grow evenly, thus, long hair will require cutting every 8–10 weeks. However, it is important not to remove too much of the length as hair only grows at approximately 1.25 cm ($\frac{1}{2}$") per month; therefore if the stylist removes more than 2.5 cm (1") each time the hair is cut then it will never appear to grow any longer!
3 Before layering long hair which is all the same length (e.g. bobbed) make sure that the client has been adequately informed of the likely effect and implications as it can take several years to grow out layers if the hair is very long and the client is unhappy with the style.
4 Increased layering can often make the hair *appear* longer because it takes away the width at the sides and gives more height on top.
5 Any split ends (*fragilitis crinium*) should be removed by cutting them off. If they are left they will become worse and make the hair appear dull and lifeless.

6 If the hair is very long, then the client may have to stand while it is being cut. If this is the case then always make sure that the client's head is held at the correct angle while cutting the hair.

7 To ensure that the guideline at the nape/back is absolutely level and precise it may be necessary to remove or alter the position of the gown and towel around the client. However, it is still important to keep the client's clothing protected.

Cutting African Caribbean hair

African Caribbean hair requires specialist cutting techniques. The amount of curl present in this hair type and the diversity of hair growth patterns throughout the head combine to make many of the previously mentioned cutting methods unsuitable.

When cutting African Caribbean hair the hair is usually combed out from the head using a wide-toothed African Caribbean comb and then shaped freehand using either scissors or clippers depending upon how short the hair is to be cut. Very short styles are better cut using the clippers and dramatic effects can be created using this method.

Straightened African Caribbean hair can often be cut in the same manner as other hair types. If the cut is to be carried out at the same time as the straightening process, then it is easier to cut the hair after it has been straightened. However, care should be taken to avoid the use of excessive tension on the hair when cutting as it will be in a sensitised, weakened state after the straightening process.

Things to do

To ensure that you fully understand the requirements of current legislation and the policy of your organisation, complete the task below. You can use the information you collect to keep in your portfolio as evidence of your knowledge in this area.

● Collect information regarding health and safety at work. (This can usually be obtained from your local environmental health officer.)

● Research into the methods of sterilisation for metal and electrical tools.

● List the requirements and procedures of sterilisation, storage and the disposal of sharp tools and equipment and also electrical tools.

● Place all your evidence in your portfolio.

What do you know?

Level 3 Unit 2

Name the five main basic shapes which can be cut into the hair. ☐

*Give a definition of **bevel** cutting.* ☐

*Explain, in detail, **three** specialised texturising techniques.* ☐

Name the perimeter lines and shapes. ☐

Give a definition of a base line. ☐

Explain the difference between a symmetrical and an asymmetrical shape. ☐

Explain the difference between a concave and a convex napeline. ☐

Why do some stylists prefer to see the hair wet before cutting? ☐

What would you include in a client consultation prior to carrying out a haircut? ☐

What health, hygiene and safety procedures would be necessary when cutting hair? ☐

SPECIALISED PERMING AND COLOURING TECHNIQUES

Fashion permanent waves

There are many types of fashion permanent waves and many techniques are employed to achieve the desired effect. However, the main objective of each is to give curl and/or body to the style wherever it is required.

It is often more desirable when fashion perming to wind the hair with water and then post damp with the perm lotion when the wind is completed. This enables winding to be commenced anywhere on the head as the lotion is only in contact with the hair when the whole head has been wound. It also ensures a more even curl throughout the head as the processing time is the same for each strand of hair. However, the resistance of certain areas of the head, e.g. the nape, must be taken into consideration and the size of the perm rods in these areas must be adjusted accordingly, otherwise the finished curl will be too loose in comparison with the rest of the head.

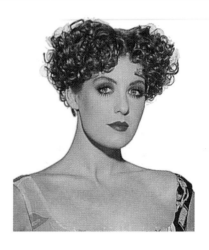

The cutting of the hair for fashion perming is of the utmost importance. Tapering before a basic permanent wave gives the best results, but to achieve a particular fashion style or shape the hair very often requires club cutting. Winding hair that has been club cut is more difficult than winding tapered hair because of the thickness or bulk left on the points. Very often it is preferable, and gives a better result, to perm the hair first and then cut the style into the curl.

Sectioning for a fashion permanent wave depends largely on the direction of the wind and the finished hairstyle. Any sectioning of the hair is used to help not hinder the operator by keeping the hair out of the way and under control while winding. However, when perm winding directionally, i.e. in the direction of the finished style, any sections should be placed where they are required, to make the actual winding easier. It is impossible to give any hard and fast rules as to how and where to section the hair for fashion perming and it is up to the individual to decide exactly where the sections are necessary for each particular head according to the technique used and the direction of the finished style.

Particular care must be taken when the hair is permed and left to dry naturally, without setting or blowdrying. Mistakes in this case cannot be hidden so they must not be made! Avoid some of the perming pitfalls by taking the following precautions:

1 Communicate fully with the client to ensure that their ideas and requirements are fully understood.
2 Decide on the finished effect before starting on the perming process so that there is a very clear picture in the mind as to what is required and the best method to achieve it.
3 Before perming porous or impoverished hair always treat it with a pre-perming treatment or a restructurant to give it strength. Remember to take a pre-perm test if in doubt.
4 Choose the correct strength of lotion for the hair type: if it is too strong the hair will frizz or break; if it is too weak the curl will not be strong enough.
5 Choose the technique and size of perm rods carefully to give the correct amount of curl where it is needed.
6 Watch processing carefully. Over-processing will make the hair frizzy; under-processing will leave it 'floppy'.
7 Depending upon the desired result, it is often more successful to cut the hair after perming. This has the following advantages:
   • if the finished curl is slightly tighter on the ends, this can be easily rectified when it is cut
   • if the hair is very short it prevents a frizzy effect by having to use too small a rod
   • if the perm is softer or curlier than required, the style can be made to suit the amount of curl present
8 When leaving the perm to 'natural dry', do not brush or comb the hair while it is drying. Comb into place when wet then leave until dry or mould or scrunch dry with the fingers to give more lift. Use an Afro comb with wide teeth or use the fingers when the hair is dry.
9 Always advise the client on after-care. Explain that permed hair goes curlier when wet, therefore, if it should go flat during the week, redamp with water to reintroduce the curl. Advise that a conditioner be used regularly to counteract the drying properties of most permanent waves.

> **TECHNICAL TIP**
> It is often better to apply the reagent after winding to prevent over-processing and to give a more even curl.

Perm winding techniques

There are a number of ways of winding hair for a fashion permanent wave. It would be impossible to list and describe all of these but a brief summary of the most popular types of fashion wind are listed below. However, it must be stressed that a competent stylist can develop their own techniques by thinking carefully about what effect is to be achieved. New techniques are born by using the basic skills and experimenting with differing sizes of rods at various angles and positions.

Spiral winding

This is used on longer hair to create an even curl along its length. The hair is wound *down* the rod, usually from the roots to the points, unlike other perming techniques such as croquignole which is wound from the points to the roots.

Any short layers in the hair make it unsuitable for this type of wind as the hair must have enough length to be wound down the rod. If very long hair has been given short layers on top then it may be necessary to wind the shorter hair in a croquignole manner and only the long hair spirally.

Sectioning the hair for spiral winding

Divide the hair off into the first major section which must be the required width usually 1.25–2.50 cm ($\frac{1}{2}$–1″) wide. Curve the section to run parallel with the nape hairline and pin the remaining hair firmly out of the way (see Fig. 3.4).

Divide the major section into squares for the actual wind. When all the first major section has been wound, continue up the head dividing the hair into major sections before winding the square sections (see Fig. 3.5).

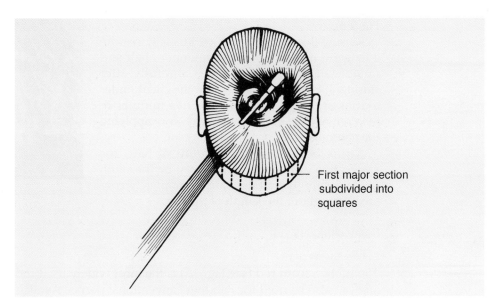

First major section subdivided into squares

Fig. 3.4

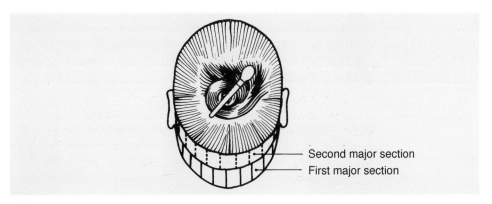

Second major section
First major section

Fig. 3.5

Winding

The winding of a spiral perm should always start on the underneath layers of hair, usually at the nape, as the wound rods hang down and would therefore get in the way of any unwound, underneath hair.

The sections should be square, with the size depending on the size of rod and the amount of curl required. Remember that the smaller the diameter of the rod, then the tighter the curl. Never take too large a section or the finished curl will be too loose.

Processing and neutralising

Checking a spiral wind for development can be quite difficult as it does not always form the same type of 'S' shape as a conventional wind. Using a self-timing perm or placing a few *croquignole* wound rods, to use as test curls, in a position that is not obvious are ways that can resolve this problem.

Make sure that any heat used to cut down the development time is evenly applied, as the head when fully spirally wound is quite a size and difficult to place under a conventional drier (see Fig. 3.6).

Rinsing this type of wind will usually require a longer time because of the amount of hair and number of rods. Blot the rods carefully after rinsing; it is also useful to place the client under a drier or use a hand drier for five minutes to help remove the excess moisture before applying the neutraliser.

Again, because of the amount of hair, the application of the neutraliser must be thorough to make sure that all the hair is completely covered throughout the length of the rod.

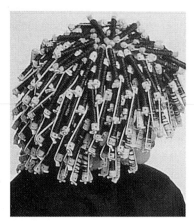

Fig. 3.6 Completed spiral wind

Rod techniques

Rubber/foam rods

The rubber/foam rod (see Fig. 3.7) is the most widely used rod for spiral winding and can also be used for winding conventional perms. Available in four sizes, the rod is made of either rubber or foam and usually has a wire running through its centre which allows it to bend wherever needed. Twisting the hair during winding will give added volume.

Take a square section of hair. Cover hair points with an end paper then start winding down the length of the rod (see Fig. 3.8). Secure the hair by bending the rod (see Fig. 3.9). Adjust the amount of curl by winding close together or further apart (see Figs 3.10 (a) and (b)).

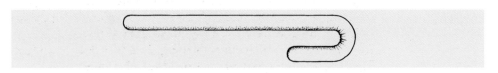

Fig. 3.7 Rubber/foam rod

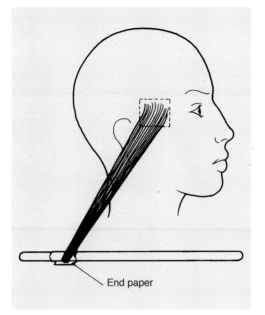

Fig. 3.8

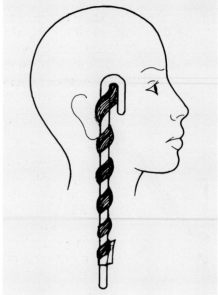

Fig. 3.9

End paper

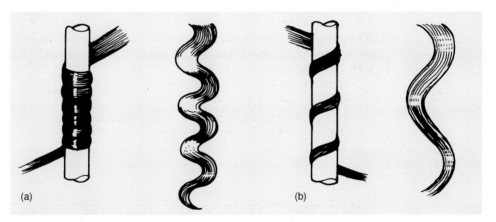

(a)

(b)

Fig. 3.10 (a) Tighter curl (b) Looser curl

Spiral rods

Spiral rods are made of plastic and are available in five sizes with left and right sloping spirals and an end securer (see Figs 3.11 (a) and (b)). Because of the uniform ridges along the length of the rod they produce a uniform curl down the hair shaft.

Take a square section of hair approximately 1.25 cm long ($\frac{1}{2}''$) (see Fig. 3.12 (a)). Hook the section of hair onto the rod. Wind spirally down the rod then fasten with the end securer (see Fig. 3.12 (b)). See Fig. 3.13 for the types of curl produced by small and large rods.

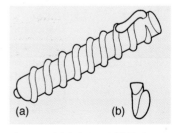

(a)   (b)

Fig. 3.11 (a) Spiral rod (b) End securer

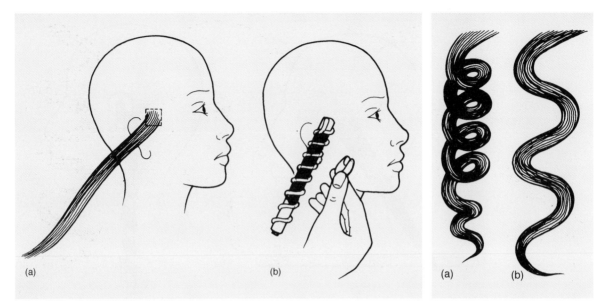

(a)   (b)   (a)   (b)

Fig. 3.12

Fig. 3.13 (a) Expected curl using a small rod (b) Expected curl using a large rod

Chop sticks

Made of plastic, these are available in only one size. Because of their angular shape, chop sticks produce considerable volume with uniform, angular curl along the length of the hair (see Fig. 3.14).

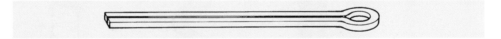

Fig. 3.14 Chop sticks

Take a small section of hair, wrap two end papers around the points of the hair. Place the section of hair through the loop of the chop stick and hold securely (see Fig. 3.15). Wind hair down chop sticks in a figure of eight holding them apart. Secure with a rubber band over the end paper, *not* the hair (see Fig. 3.16). (See Fig. 3.17 for the type of curl produced.)

U-stick rod

These are made of plastic and are available in three sizes. U-sticks are wound in a similar way to chop sticks but because the ends of the roots come together when wound they produce a looser curl at the roots rather than at the points of the hair (see Fig. 3.18).

Take a small section of hair and pull through the middle of the U-stick. Wind the hair in a figure of eight over A, then between the sticks, over B and repeat down the length of the stick (see Fig. 3.19). Place two end papers over the points of the hair and secure with a rubber band over the end papers not the hair (see Fig. 3.20). Figure 3.21 illustrates the results of this method.

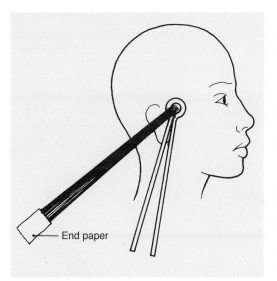

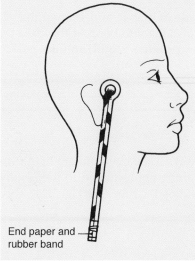

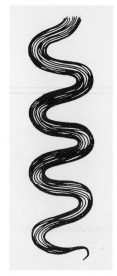

End paper

Fig. 3.15

End paper and
rubber band

Fig. 3.16

Fig. 3.17 Expected curl

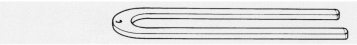

Fig. 3.18 U-Stick rod

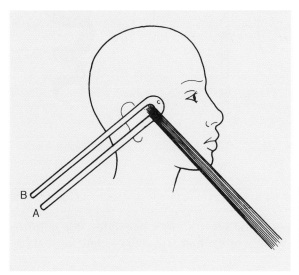

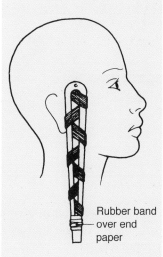

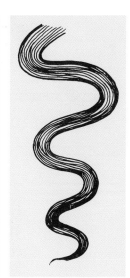

B
A

Fig. 3.19

Rubber band
over end
paper

Fig. 3.20

Fig. 3.21 Expected curl

Pen rods

Made of plastic, these are available in only one size. The degree of curl will be determined by the way the hair is wound down the rod. The closer together the hair is wound, the tighter the curl will be. The expected curl would be the same as for rubber/foam rods (see Fig. 3.10).

Crystal rods

Available in two sizes, these produce an angular uniform curl because of the way in which the hair is wound behind the bars.

Tube rods

Made of plastic and shaped like straws, tubes have a corrugated section which allows them to bend in this area (see Fig. 3.22). Because of their small diameters they produce a tight, uniform curl throughout the length of the hair.

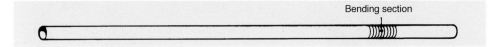

Fig. 3.22 Tube rods

. Take a square section of hair. Cover the points with an end paper. Start winding A at the opposite end to the bending section B (see Fig. 3.23). Secure the hair by bending the tube (see Fig. 3.24). Figure 3.25 shows the resulting curl.

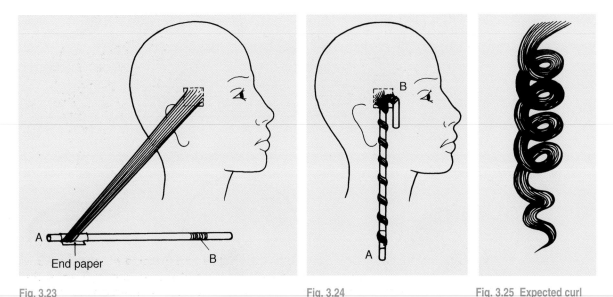

Fig. 3.23   Fig. 3.24   Fig. 3.25 Expected curl

Root perming

This technique is used to give support and lift to shorter hairstyles. It is not usually suitable for longer hair as the weight of the hair will pull out any lift that has been obtained.

Lift at the root area only can be achieved by various methods, for example, winding the hair with water and coating the mid-lengths and ends of the hair with hair gel or oil, then wrapping this part of the hair in tin foil to prevent penetration of the perm into these areas. The hair should then be post damped with the perm lotion, thus allowing the root area only to be affected.

Manufacturers have now produced a gel perming lotion which is applied after winding is complete. Because of its viscous nature, this type of perm lotion does not penetrate through the hair mesh and is therefore active on the root area only.

However it must be remembered that the intended effect of a root perm is to give support and *not* curl to the hair. It is therefore suitable only for certain types of hairstyles and is not advisable for clients who require a substantial amount of curl or body in their hair.

SAFETY TIP

Permanent wave reagents are potentially hazardous chemicals and due care and attention must be paid at all times to health, hygiene and safety procedures to satisfy current legislation, manufacturers', and salon guidelines.

Edge or perimeter winding

This puts curl on the ends of shorter or longer hair. The wind is usually used on hair that does not require height or lift on top. The hair is dragged at the root and wound sideways giving curl at the ends of the hair. This is a useful type of wind to use in conjunction with other methods, e.g. edge wind on the fringe area to keep the fringe low onto the face while the remaining hair is wound as required.

Figure 3.26 shows the whole of the crown area edge wound which will result in no lift on top of the head but volume and curl around the edges.

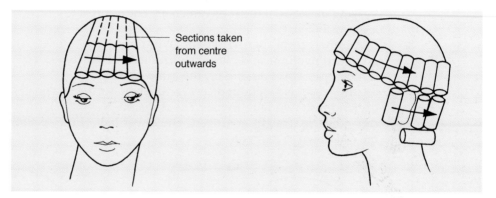

Sections taken from centre outwards

Fig. 3.26

Partial winding

As the name suggests, only some areas of the head are permed to create volume and texture where required. This may be to a small area of the style or to the majority leaving only a small area unpermed. There are unlimited variations to this type of wind and it is a method that can be used on long or short hair.

Figure 3.27(a) shows a partial wind at the front of the head to create volume at this area. The rods can be placed in any direction that may be required by the style.

Figure 3.27(b) shows the top and fringe area left straight with the back and side areas permed. Again, the rods may be placed in any direction or, indeed, wound by any method depending upon the required finished effect.

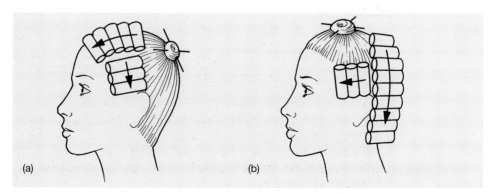

(a)   (b)

Fig 3.27

Piggyback winding

This is used on long hair (usually over 15–20 cm (6–8″)) to give an even curl movement along the length of the hair. It also allows a more even penetration of both the perm lotion and the neutraliser, which is always a problem when perming very long hair.

Taking normal partings, the hair is wound from mid-way down the length of the hair section to the root, leaving the end unwound (Fig. 3.28). The ends are then wound down to the centre of the section using another rod of the same size (Fig. 3.29), which is secured with a plastic pin inserted between the bands of the rods to hold them securely (Fig. 3.30). Varying the sizes of the rods can create endless possibilities.

Another form of piggyback winding gives extra volume and curl to shorter hair. In this case, a section of hair, the same size as the rod, is sectioned off and then divided into two lengthwise. The division

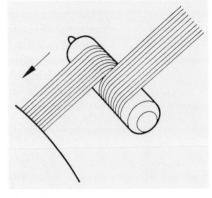

Fig. 3.28

can either be straight or woven. The lower half of the section is wound around the rod down to the root.

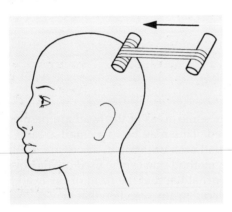

Fig. 3.29

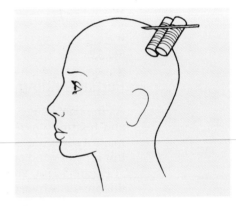

Fig. 3.30

The remaining hair from the top half of the section is then wound down using another rod of the same size (see Fig. 3.31).

This second rod is forced to lie on top of the first one as the size of the section will only accommodate one of the rods. By varying the sizes of the rods different effects can be achieved, e.g. a large rod at the root, small rod on top will create a looser movement at the root with varying degrees of curl throughout the ends.

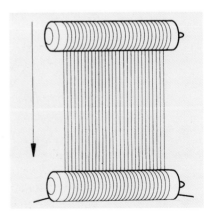

Fig. 3.31

Weave winding

Weave winding creates a natural, undisciplined textured effect on shorter or mid-length hair and is particularly good for fine hair and thick coarse hair.

TECHNICAL TIP
To ensure the correct result, take small sections. For less root support and more curl, reverse the curler sizes.

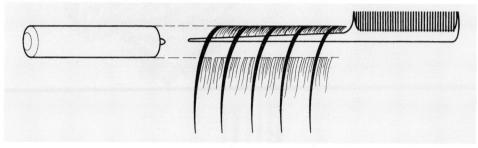

Fig. 3.32

A section of hair, the same size as the rod is taken and fine strands of hair are woven out of the section and clipped out of the way (shown in Fig. 3.32). The remaining hair is then wound as normal (see Fig. 3.33).

This technique is used on each section throughout the head with the result that the bulk of the hair is permed but fine strands are left straight. Alternatively, the strands may be wound on a larger sized rod; both techniques create a natural, unruly effect.

Weave winding can be done on individual areas of the head, e.g. when partial winding the top area of the head, weave winding the last few rods before the straight nape area will help to blend the permed area into the straight area without too strong a division.

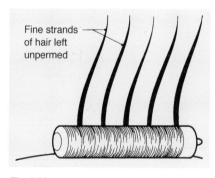

Fine strands of hair left unpermed

Fig. 3.33

Weave sectioning the hair instead of straight sectioning when using the basic perm method helps to prevent rod divisions on certain hair types although this does not necessarily mean that all hair types should be treated in this manner. (See Fig. 3.34 for the completed wind.)

Candlestick wind

This technique produces a soft, natural spiral curl with strong root movement. A triangular section corresponding to the diameter of the roller is taken and the hair is wound vertically in a spiral fashion. At the roots, the roller is turned vertically so that it stands on its own base. The hair should be secured with pins through the base of the roller (see Fig. 3.35).

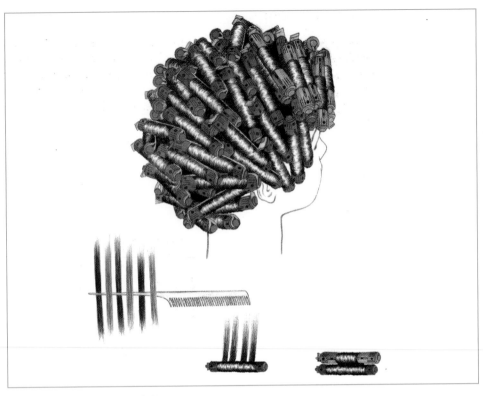

Fig. 3.34 Completed weave wind

TECHNICAL TIP
The candlestick technique is most commonly used on the crown area only.

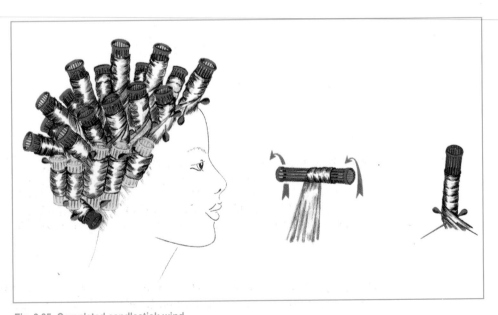

Fig. 3.35 Completed candlestick wind

Hopscotch wind

This wind produces irregular volume and movement with natural looking curls. A section of hair is taken in the normal way, and thickly woven (see Fig. 3.36). The rod is placed in the back half of the woven section, and this winding technique is continued until there are four or five rods in a row with the unwound pieces sitting between. These pieces are then wound so that the rods are sitting vertically on the previously wound section.

> **TECHNICAL TIP**
> The hopscotch wind can be used on the whole head or on areas which require irregular curl formation.

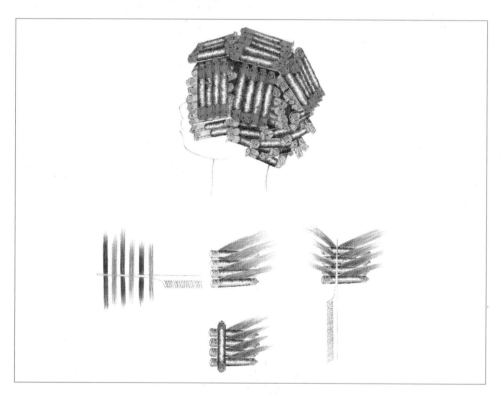

Fig. 3.36 Completed hopscotch wind

Double winding

The section of hair is wound down from the points to approximately the middle of the hair length. Another rod is then placed underneath the wound hair and both rods are used together, as one large rod, to wind the remaining hair down to the root. Because of the greater circumference of the combined rods, the final result is a looser movement at the root with greater curl on the ends of the hair.

Pin curl perm

This type of perm is used on short hair which requires a soft wave movement without root lift. The hair is wound with lotion following the direction of the style.

Triangular sections are taken and an end paper is placed around the hair and curls are clipped carefully according to the desired finished result. For example, an open middle will provide soft movement whereas a tighter middle will produce a stronger movement. A flat curl will result in no root movement and a barrel curl will produce slight root lift. A net is placed over the pin curls to ensure that they are not disturbed during neutralising (see Fig. 3.37).

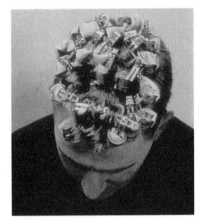

Fig. 3.37 Pin curl perm

Combination techniques

When perming any head of hair, always remember to put the curl or volume *where it is needed*, even though this may mean that a variety of techniques will have to be used on the same head to create the desired effect. Bearing this in mind, the variations and effects that can be achieved when perming the hair are limitless. By experimenting with various techniques it is possible to meet any new needs of the client as hair fashions change and also to invent new techniques by adapting the basic methods (see Fig. 3.38).

TECHNICAL TIP
Ensure that an end paper is always used, and that the centre of the curl is open – this will avoid the hair becoming frizzy.

POINTS TO REMEMBER

Always keep precise records of each treatment. Fashion perming offers an individualised service, to suit the individual needs of the client, and it will therefore be extremely difficult to remember exactly the techniques and procedures used if the client requires a repeat treatment in the future.

Perming and colouring

This technique is ideal for clients with short natural hair who wish to enhance their hairstyle with a hint of colour and for those people who don't have the time to have both services done separately.

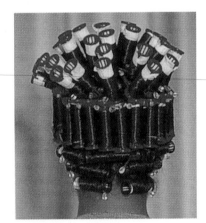

Fig. 3.38 Candlestick, directional and brickwind

Winding (without lotion) is commenced at the front of the hair where the lights (colour) are to be featured. One or two rods are wound, then a section is taken and woven for lights. The colour product is then applied using easi-meche. This pattern is continued and then, according to hair type, post-damping should take place ten to fifteen minutes before completion of colour development. Ensuring that the packets are secured, the lotion is then rinsed out and the hair is neutralised. Packets are then removed before rinsing (see Fig. 3.39).

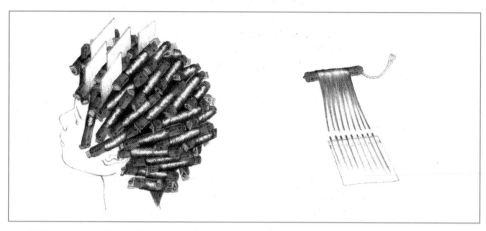

Fig. 3.39 Perming and colouring

Considerations when chemically processing long hair

1 Always remember that the ends of the hair have been there for a long time and have been subjected to much physical (e.g. brushing, heated appliances, etc.) and atmospheric (e.g. sun, wind, rain, etc.) influences. Therefore, the ends of the hair will be far more porous than the remaining hair and will process more quickly when perming, tinting and bleaching.

2 The client must be made fully aware of the long-term implications of using potentially damaging chemicals such as perm lotion, tint and bleach on the hair. If these chemicals should damage the hair then it is extremely difficult to rectify and often the only real remedy is to remove the damaged hair by cutting. It is extremely upsetting for a client who has grown their hair over a number of years to have to have it cut off because a chemical process has damaged it.

3 Always protect the hair with restructurants, pre-chemical or post-chemical treatments.

4 Use only good quality products which will do the least damage to the hair. Do not use excessively high hydrogen peroxide strengths or harsh lotions.

5 Do *not* over-process the hair. However, when perming long hair also make sure that it is not under-processed as it is not usually advisable to re-perm on this length of hair.

6 Always advise the client on how to look after their hair by protecting it from the sun, regular conditioning, using a suitable shampoo, using oils and waxes and on the effects of over-using heated appliances such as curling tongs, hot brushes, heated rollers, etc.

Fashion colouring techniques

Fashion colouring techniques are usually used to improve the look of a hairstyle or haircut. Colour can emphasise a shape, give the illusion of increasing weight or of lightening heaviness, depending upon how and where it is applied. Most important of all, fashion colouring techniques can be fun. The more outrageous or different the equipment and methods used, the more interest is stimulated. Clients are often unaware of the many effects that can be achieved using colour, so it is the responsibility of the stylist to suggest various techniques that can be used to improve the hairstyle of the client. Most clients want to improve their image and once made aware of the subtle effects that can be achieved on their hair are prompted to do something positive.

Fashion colouring techniques are a natural progression from the basic colouring techniques. Once the stylist has become skilled in the art of hair colouring, with a little imagination and the confidence to try out new ideas, the opportunities and variations of colour are endless.

> **TECHNICAL TIP**
> When using two colours, mix together in a bowl before adding hydrogen peroxide or applying to the hair.

Recent trends in hair colouring are to use more than one colour or partial colouring in one form or another, on one head. Most colour shades are intermixable and when used in conjunction with bleach or lightening agents allow complete freedom to achieve anything from the subtlest form of coloration to the most outrageous. With confidence and experience it is possible for the stylist to create personal techniques to achieve the effect desired.

A few of the popular techniques are indicated below.

Block colouring

This is a good technique to emphasise the shape of short hairstyles. Two, three or even four colours can be used, but there should be at least two shades difference between the colours. The darkest shade is usually used at the nape, graduating to the lighter shade at the front. Zig-zag the partings or divisions to prevent a hard line between the shades. Cotton wool/foil strips can be used to block out each section as it is completed to prevent the colours from touching each other, although a more subtle effect is created if the tint is carefully combed together up from the nape to the crown when application is complete.

Subtle effects are created by using similar colour tones to the client's own hair. Dramatic effects can be created by using contrasting colours, e.g. dark brown at the nape graduating to bright red-orange at the front.

POINTS TO REMEMBER

1 When tinting lighter, allow for the effect of body heat at the scalp; the mid-lengths and ends must be tinted before the roots. When tinting darker, the tint can be applied from the roots through to the ends. It may, therefore, be necessary to use both techniques on one head when block tinting.
2 The hair is naturally lighter at the front and crown area because of the effect of sunlight, etc.; by using lighter shades in these areas a more natural effect is achieved. To give a very dramatic effect, reverse the colours, i.e. darker shades at the front and lighter shades at the nape.

3 Darker shades make the hair appear more dense and, therefore, heavier. Lighter shades give the illusion of less weight. This is a useful fact to bear in mind when emphasising a hairstyle with colour.

Painted lights (flying colours)

This technique adds colour and depth to a particular hairstyle. The hair is combed into shape and a decision is made as to where the style needs accentuating. This may be at the nape, sides or crown. A semi-permanent colour or permanent tint is then painted on to the hair using a vent brush, a wide-toothed comb or a fine artist's paint brush. Apply the tint in the direction of the style (bleach can also be applied in this manner) but try not to work in straight lines as this can give a heavy effect (see Fig. 3.40).

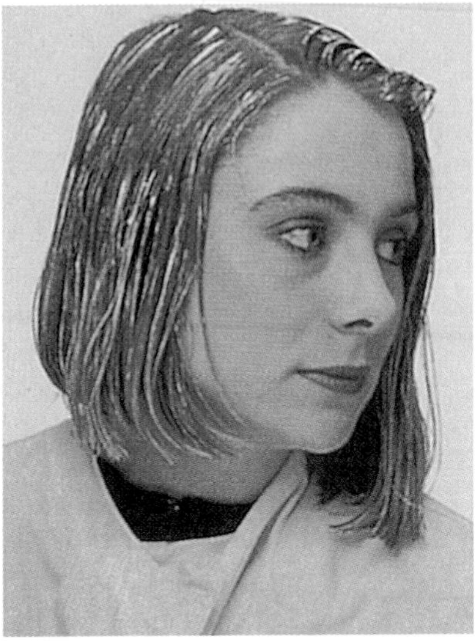

Fig. 3.40 Application of painted lights

POINTS TO REMEMBER

1 A number of shades can be used throughout the head. Lighter shades at the front and darker shades at the sides and nape will give a shimmering effect.
2 This is a good method to add interest to dark hair. Paint the hair with strong red or burgundy shades of tint.
3 A tinting gun can be used instead of a vent brush, etc.; this creates interest in the salon but it requires plenty of practice so handle it with caution.
4 Painted lights are a very quick method of adding colour and are an invaluable way of using up odd quarter tubes of tint, etc., but remember not to get too enthusiastic. Applying too much tint (particularly tint lightener) in too great an area can defeat the object of the method and give a patchy result.

Shimmer lights

This has the same effect as painted lights. Shampoo and towel dry the hair thoroughly then comb into the desired style with gel, using a wide-toothed comb. This will create 'tram-lines' in the direction of the hairstyle. Using a tint at least two shades lighter and of a brighter tone than the natural colour, apply carefully along the raised lines with a fine artist's brush or a tinting gun.

This method can be used all over the head or just on certain areas, depending upon the effect desired.

Colour flashes

This technique can be used on its own or in conjunction with other techniques. It is equally effective on long, short, curly or straight hair.

A fine or thick band around the front hairline is lightened with a tint lightener. If a bright colour is required the band is pre-bleached to the degree of lightness required and then a permanent tint is applied to this area. Similarly, after banding, a semi-permanent colour can be applied all over the whole head to brighten all of the hair and create a lighter tone of the same colour at the front.

1 Use zig-zag partings to soften the demarcation line.
2 Colour flashes can be used in conjunction with fine highlights of the same colour through the back of the head to give added interest or to emphasise and soften the front hairline.
3 Another use of colour flashing is to lighten the weight of a heavy forward fringe. Take out a section at the front hairline of the fringe (zig-zag parting) about 10–20 mm ($\frac{3}{8}$ – $\frac{3}{4}$″) wide, and use a tint lightener in this area. When all of the fringe is combed forward, the darker back section of the fringe will blend with the front section, creating a wispier, lighter effect.

Scrunching

This gives a good effect on either long or short curly hairstyles but is not suitable for long straight styles. This quick and easy technique adds colour and depth to the ends of the hair, thus emphasising the outline of the hairstyle.

The hair is shampooed then rough-dried into shape. Mix the desired shade of tint (usually tint lightener). The operator must wear rubber gloves. The tint is then spread evenly onto the palms of the rubber gloves and the ends of the hair are squeezed or 'scrunched' between the fingers; this deposits the tint on the ends of the hair only. Apply throughout the head, or wherever required.

POINTS TO REMEMBER

1 If the hair is longer and tends to flop, backcomb the hair thoroughly at the roots in the areas that require scrunching, then carefully lacquer the roots with a fine hairspray. This will prevent the tint from running or flopping onto the root area.
2 More than one shade of tint can be used, depending upon the result required.
3 Bleach may be used in preference to tint, but care must be taken only to lighten a few shades. When bleach is developed and removed, a semi-permanent tint can be applied over the whole head to give lighter and darker tones of the same colour.
4 This method is excellent for the client who enjoys changing their hair colour frequently or for brightening dull hair during the winter months. Because only the ends of the hair are tinted or bleached lighter, they are soon removed by cutting.

Combination tint and bleach highlighting

Highlighting gives a very natural effect, particularly on lighter hair. Fine streaks are pulled through a streaking cap and bleach is applied. When the hair has been lifted sufficiently, the bleach is removed and a full-head permanent or semi-permanent tint is applied. An alternative method after removing the bleach is to weave out more fine strands of hair over both the previously bleached and the natural, virgin hair. A tint lightener is applied to these strands which are then wrapped in tin foil or plastic. This method produces a much lighter overall result.

Tortoiseshell lowlights

This technique gives a richer effect than the usual lowlights and is suitable for any length of hair.

Three to four different colours are used, ranging from one shade darker to two to three shades lighter than the natural base shade. The different colours are applied separately and alternately to fine woven streaks of hair that have either been pulled through a streaking cap or woven with easi-meche (see Fig. 3.41). A variation on this method, although it does not give the same effect, is to use the shades in bands of colour from the nape up towards the front. The lightest shade is usually used on the front and the darkest shade at the nape. Figure 3.42 shows the finished result.

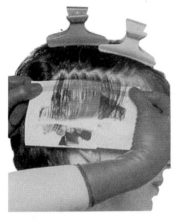

Fig. 3.41 Application of tortoise-shell lowlights

Glimmering (polishing)

This is a very quick technique for any length of hair, but particularly good on very short nape hair where it is difficult to use other techniques.
 Comb the hair into style. Take a piece of tin foil or cellophane and paint the surface with the chosen shade of tint. Hold the tin foil or cellophane in both hands and allow it to touch the ends of the hair, then gently stroke backwards and forwards in a polishing motion in the direction of the style. Pull away and repeat over the whole head or just the areas that will emphasise the style.

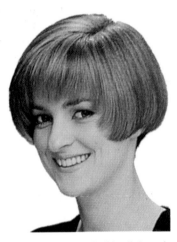

POINTS TO REMEMBER

1 Do not be afraid to use bold colours as this technique gives a subtle effect.
2 Do not become too enthusiastic and cover all of the hair – it is usually just the ends of the hair that are tinted.
3 Polish the hair gently otherwise the tint may be inadvertently placed where it is not required.

Fig. 3.42 Tortoiseshell lowlights – finished results

Slicing or tramming

A very dramatic effect can be produced with this technique and it is a very bold method of coloration.

Comb the hair into style and decide which area of the head requires emphasising (slicing usually looks more effective on the front section of the head). Section the remaining hair away from this area. Take a section of hair about the size of a perm rod from the area to be coloured and apply the tint to this section. Wrap in tin foil, easi-meche or cling film then leave out a fine 6 mm ($\frac{1}{4}$″) section and take the next section in the same manner as before. Continue across the area to be covered, tinting a section and leaving a section until completed. Leave to develop.

TECHNICAL TIP
Always ensure there is no seepage of the tint from the easi-meche, foil or cling film, otherwise the results could be disastrous.

1 More than one colour may be used depending upon the desired result.
2 Because the hair is not woven the colour is far more dense in certain areas and therefore more dramatic. Do not use this technique on clients who wish to have subtle coloration only.
3 The brighter and more vibrant the colour shade used, the more dramatic the effect will be, particularly if it is in total contrast with the client's own hair.
4 Work methodically from one side of the area to the other. The fine sections that do not require tinting can be kept out of the way by winding on a perm rod.

Precautions for fashion colouring techniques

1 Introduce the client to colour with subtle coloration. Once they have gained confidence they will become more aware of what the salon has to offer and be willing to be more adventurous.
2 Use colour as an extension of the client's personality, but do not use too bright or very dark colours on older clients, it can be ageing.
3 When a subtle effect is required always look at the natural base shade carefully, there are usually golden or reddish glints to be seen that can be emphasised and highlighted. When using two or more colours on the hair try to keep within the same colour tones, and use different depths of these tones, e.g. red tones, gold tones, beige tones, etc. This will produce a more natural effect.
4 Do not be afraid to experiment with more than one technique on one head. With confidence, the operator will develop his/her own personal techniques.
5 When using tin foil to add lights to the hair, ensure that there is no seepage at the roots by wrapping a doubled strip of tin foil round the packet at the root.
6 Always discard rubber streaking caps when holes become too large. The bleach or tint can seep through these holes onto the scalp and hair with disastrous results.
7 Some of the fashion tinting techniques are so quick that it is a great temptation to tint more of the hair than necessary. Remember that it is better to apply to too few areas than too many. More highlights, slices, etc., can be added but they could prove time consuming to remove.
8 The main mistake when highlighting hair is to weave or pull the meshes of hair too thickly. This can give an unsightly striped effect and make the hair so light overall that a regrowth can soon be seen.
9 Always advise the client on the after-care of their coloration. The condition of the hair is of prime importance, as tinted hair only looks good when it is healthy. The client will also need advice on the upkeep of their colour and on how often salon visits will be necessary.
10 Be aware of the health and safety of the client and yourself at all times.

Scrunch bleaching

This is a very quick and commercial method of adding lighter glints to the hair and is suitable for thicker hair, usually with some movement to the style.

Scrunch bleaching does not give the same effect as highlighting, since the hair is only lightened at the points and not throughout the length, but it can look very effective on darker as well as lighter hair, especially if used in conjunction with semi-permanent colours. No retouching is necessary – the bleached area has usually been cut from the hair after a couple of months when retouching would normally become necessary.

Method of application

There are two main methods of application, one using two tinting brushes, the other using the hands only.

Method 1 (two tinting brushes)

1 Assemble materials and equipment.
2 Comb the hair into style. On short hair it is usually the crown and front areas that require scrunching. On longer hair the entire head is usually scrunched, although this depends on the client's personal preference.
3 Backcomb thoroughly the areas to be scrunched, pushing the hair well down to the roots to prevent the hair falling back on itself when the bleach is applied. Backcombing the hair also makes the final result less dense as some of the hair points will be omitted from the bleach.
4 Using a fine hairspray, lacquer the roots of the backcombed hair.
5 Mix the hydrogen peroxide with the bleach to form a stiff paste.
6 Using two tinting brushes, apply the bleach to the points of the hair, making sure that both sides of the meshes are completely covered
7 Allow the bleach to develop naturally, without heat. Do not allow the bleach to go too light, otherwise the contrast between the darker and the bleached hair will be too great.
8 When the hair has lightened sufficiently, gently comb out the backcombing and rinse the hair thoroughly. Apply an acid balance shampoo, rinse and condition with a mild acid balance conditioner.
9 If a semi-permanent colour is required, this should now be applied to the whole head in the normal manner. The final effect of this gives lighter tones of the same colour to the ends of the hair.
10 Complete a record of the work carried out.

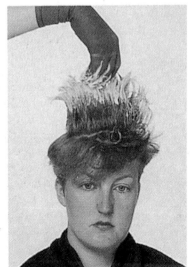

Fig. 3.43 Scrunch bleaching

Method 2 (without brushes)

Proceed as for Method 1 but instead of applying the bleach with two tinting brushes, evenly spread the bleach onto the palms of the operator's gloves. Then scrunch the points of the hair where required with the fingers, imparting the bleach from the gloves onto the points of the hair (see Fig. 3.43). It is important to ensure that the points of the hair are kept lifted out from the scalp away from the root area.

Await bleach development and then proceed as for Method 1.

Bleach toners

These are used to neutralise any unwanted golden tones produced by the bleaching process.

It is important to remember that even careful bleaching will damage the cuticle scales and in some cases creates a highly porous state. The biggest problem is that after bleaching the hair may have an *uneven* porosity, either along the hair, or throughout the entire head. Toners must therefore be applied with extra care, following the manufacturer's instructions, to avoid a patchy and uneven result.

Types of toners

There are three main types:

- Temporary toners.
- Semi-permanent toners.
- Permanent toners.

Temporary toners

These are rinses that are applied to the hair after shampooing. They usually last from one shampoo to the next. However, because of the highly porous nature of bleached hair there is often a colour build-up if these rinses are used continuously over a period of time. To correct this fault, apply the rinse to the root area only until the colour fades from the ends of the hair. It is preferable to apply the rinse with a tinting brush to ensure an even coverage.

Semi-permanent toners

These toners last from one bleach retouch to the next, although when applied to bleached hair they can fade more quickly than when applied to untreated hair. Application should be made with a brush to the roots of the hair first as they are not as porous as the points of the hair. The manufacturer's instructions should be carefully followed (some manufacturers produce semi-permanent tints specifically designed for bleached hair).

Check the development of the application carefully. Because of the damage to the cuticle scales by the bleach, the toner is absorbed quickly but is also easily removed; therefore development may appear complete, but on rinsing the colour may almost disappear! Alternatively, the development may be rapid and if the toner is left in contact with the hair too long the finished result will be too dark.

> **SAFETY TIP**
> Protect the skin with barrier cream – this also prevents staining.

A semi-permanent toner used regularly after each bleach retouch may create a colour build-up on the ends of the hair after a period of time. To rectify this, apply the toner to the root area only, then comb through to the ends of the hair, if and when necessary.

Permanent toners

No toner used on bleached hair can be truly permanent. The degree of porosity of bleached hair causes any toner to fade quite quickly.

A permanent toner is usually a 'para' dye, which is mixed with 10 vol. (3%) hydrogen peroxide. If this type of toner is used, a skin test is necessary because of the possibility of a reaction to the 'para' compound. Care must be taken not to damage the hair still further by the use of too high a volume strength of hydrogen peroxide with the tint.

Toning the hair after highlighting with a cap

When toning the hair after highlighting with a toner that is mixed with hydrogen peroxide, remember that the hydrogen peroxide could alter the natural base shade of the client. To prevent this, apply the toner to the highlights before the highlighting cap is removed, thus colouring only the highlights.

If using a semi-permanent toner without hydrogen peroxide, apply in same manner as above or remove the highlighting cap and apply the toner to the whole head.

Returning bleached hair to a natural colour (prepigmentation)

This is not as simple nor as straightforward as returning tinted hair to its natural colour.

During the bleaching process, the chemical action of the oxygen liberated from the hydrogen peroxide causes the hair to progress through several colour changes, from the base shade of the hair to pale yellow or white. However, the red shade of pigment (produced by pheomelanin) is the most difficult colour to convert and there is usually a lot of this colour pigment present in the hair shaft. If brown pigment, which is a mixture of red + blue + yellow is added to the bleached hair, the hair absorbs the red from the brown pigment, leaving a green (blue + yellow) discoloration of the hair.

To avoid this discoloration, **prepigmentation** of the hair is necessary, using red colour particles. The red colour particles can be obtained in a temporary, semi-permanent or permanent tint, the choice of which depends on the porosity of the hair and the needs of the client.

Method of prepigmentation

1 Take a test cutting of the hair.
2 Ensure that the client has had a skin test if using a 'para' dye.
3 Assemble materials and equipment. Protect client's and operator's clothing.
4 Disentangle the hair and check for cuts and abrasions on the scalp.
5 Section hair into six major sections as for permanent tinting.
6 Apply a red semi-permanent tint using a brush, sponge or nozzle, to the bleached areas only (see Fig. 3.44). It is preferable to use a semi-permanent that does not require the addition of hydrogen peroxide so that the hair is damaged as little as possible.
7 When the application is complete, check that the semi-permanent is evenly and thoroughly applied to all the bleached areas (see Fig. 3.45).

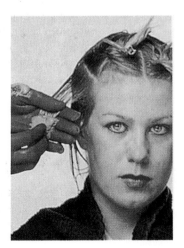

Fig. 3.44 Applying red colour to the bleached hair

Specialised Perming and Colouring Techniques 301

8 Leave to develop according to the manufacturer's instructions but check the development frequently with a swab of damp cotton wool.

9 When the development is complete, rinse the semi-permanent from the hair with warm water until the water runs clear.

10 Dry the hair and re-section into six as before.

11 Proceed then as for a normal full-head tint, using the shade of tint required but applying to the prepigmented areas only.

12 Complete a record of work carried out.

13 Advise the client on the after-care of the hair. Although the hair may appear to be the client's natural colour it must be emphasised that the hair will now probably be in a highly porous state due to all the chemicals that it has been subjected to. It will be necessary to treat the hair with conditioning and/or restructurant preparations until the treated hair has been removed by cutting. This could take 6–12 months depending on how short the client wears their hair. If the client requires other chemical processes on the hair, e.g. perming,

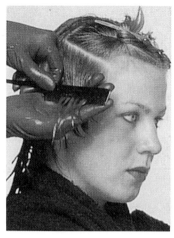

Fig. 3.45 Ensuring even coverage

the porosity of the hair must be given due consideration when selecting the strength of reagent to use; always test the hair before embarking on perming this type of hair.

The porosity of the hair may also cause fading of the new colour after a few weeks. In this case, the tint should be re-applied but without prepigmentation.

Hair discoloration and unwanted colour tones

An unwanted discoloration of the hair can often be masked by the addition of another colour. This is because brown hair colour is made up of three primary colours (blue, yellow and red).

By mixing the primary colours it is possible to produce the secondary colours. These three secondary colours are produced as follows:

Primary		Secondary
Blue + Yellow	=	*Green*
Yellow + Red	=	*Orange*
Red + Blue	=	*Purple*

If all the three primary colours are mixed together, they produce brown, which is a neutral or *tertiary* colour.

Blue + Yellow + Red = Brown

Using this fact, any peculiar discoloration of the hair can be masked and brought to a neutral brown colour by the addition of the missing colour. For example, a green discoloration can be brought to brown by the addition of red:

Green = Yellow + Blue
but *Yellow + Blue + **Red** = Brown*

By drawing two triangles, one with the primary colours and the other with the secondary colours, then superimposing the two triangles to form a star, it is possible to see quite easily which colour can be masked by the addition of another colour (see Fig. 3.46).

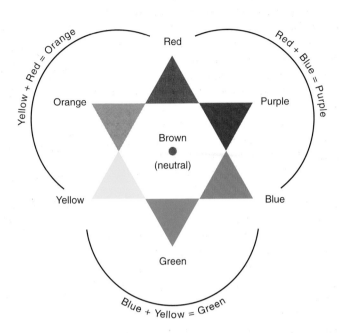

Fig. 3.46 Colour mixing triangles

TECHNICAL TIP
When masking unwanted colour tones by adding a contrasting colour, remember that the depth of both colours must be the same, e.g. pale yellow can be masked by pale purple (mauve) to produce pale brown (beige).

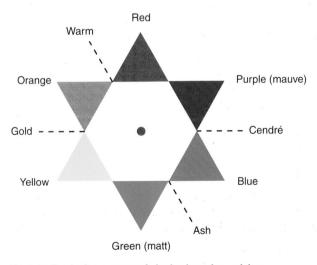

Fig. 3.47 Producing a range of shades by colour mixing

Manufacturers take the characters from around the colour star and add them to various depths to create a range of shades (see Fig. 3.47).

From Fig. 3.47, it is possible to see that any discoloration can be masked by the opposite contrasting colour. Thus:

- Orange discoloration is masked by **blue**.
- Yellow discoloration is masked by **purple** (mauve).
- Red discoloration is masked by **green** (matt).
- Gold discoloration is masked by **cendré**.
- Warm tones are masked by **ash**.

Colour reducing

People often like to change their hair colour, even if it is already tinted, but sometimes the tinting results are not successful. Some of the worst cases of unwanted colour tones are caused by home hairdressing and, in such cases, partial or complete removal of the original tint followed by recolouring may be necessary. Sometimes, the colour can be improved with only a slight correction but when more drastic treatment is needed it can be a long, slow, painstaking process that may also cause considerable hair damage.

Colour removal should always be carried out methodically and with extreme care. Every head is particular to each individual and so creates different problems; therefore, test cuttings *must* be taken to ensure that the colour can be successfully removed. The results of the tests should be shown to the client so that they will know in advance what to expect.

Thorough consultation is very important in order to find out what products have been previously used on the hair and what the client expects from the treatment. Using shade charts and pictures helps to identify the exact requirements and whether they may be attainable. If the client has practised 'home tinting', an incompatibility test is necessary to ensure that the product they have used does not contain any metallic salts. If the client has had it tinted by another hairdresser, try to find out the manufacturer of the previous tint as most colouring manufacturers have an advisory service and can give valuable assistance to the hairdresser.

Do not take details of a previous treatment at face value. Clients are often reluctant to admit what they have actually used on their hair, particularly when the results have been unsatisfactory. They also do not realise that a permanent product applied to the hair several months previously could still be present on the ends of the hair; therefore, it is extremely important to check all the facts thoroughly before deciding upon the best method of colour correction to use.

Before commencing any form of colour removal the following information must be assimilated and assessed.

- Condition of the hair and the scalp.
- Porosity of the hair.
- History of any skin troubles.
- Make and type of the previous treatment(s).
- Shade of the previous tint(s).
- General colour state – patchy, dull, multicoloured, etc.
- Final colour shade required.

If the condition of the hair and skin is satisfactory, a skin test, incompatibility test and test cutting should be taken. When all these tests have been completed and it is shown that the hair colour can be removed satisfactorily, with no adverse effects to the hair or the client, it is safe to proceed with the colour removal.

Reduction

This is an acid removal which involves the chemical process known as **reduction**. The oxygen is removed from the converted colour molecules which are then converted into colourless **leuco-compounds**. This means that only the artificial colour pigment is removed and that the natural colour pigment is left unlightened, it also means that the lightening power of the reducers is limited. Colour reducers, or reducters as they are sometimes known, are usually in liquid or powder form and may be mixed with either water or peroxide. They must be used in strict accordance with the manufacturer's instructions. For simple cases the reducer is mixed with water and this will take the hair colour down by approximately one shade. If the hair is dark through colour build-up and requires more lightening, the reducer is mixed with 10 or 20 vol. (3% or 6%) hydrogen peroxide. Occasionally, for very dark shades and dramatic removal, 30 vol. (9%) hydrogen peroxide may be used, but never stronger than this.

It is not possible to obtain cold or flat shades when reducing as some of the red pigment will stay in the hair. A toning shade of matt will therefore be necessary to mask any unwanted warm shades.

Colour reducers make the hair more porous; therefore a tint applied after reducing is likely to process more quickly or produce a deeper shade than required. To counteract this it is advisable to use a tint a shade lighter than the one required to achieve the best results.

The condition of the hair is also affected by colour reducers. Thus, it is important to condition the hair thoroughly after the treatment and extra care should be taken when perming decoloured hair.

> **TECHNICAL TIP**
> Take test cuttings from various parts of the head, particularly if the unwanted colour is patchy.

Method of removal by reduction
1 Check all tests to ensure that they are satisfactory.
2 Protect the client's clothing with dark gown, towels, etc.
3 Check the scalp for cuts and abrasions.
4 Divide the hair into four major sections (forehead to nape and ear to ear across the top of the head).
5 Mix the reducer in a non-metallic bowl (do not allow the mixture to come into contact with metal comb or clips).
6 Commence application with a sponge or tinting brush, taking intersecting partings across the crown.
7 Application must be done speedily and thoroughly. Apply the mixture to the tinted hair *only*, and avoid the root section if there is a natural colour regrowth. The natural regrowth can be blocked out with cotton wool strips if necessary.
8 When the application is complete, comb through thoroughly to ensure complete penetration of the hair, but do not allow the reducer to come into contact with the root area. Pay particular attention to the front hairline and the ends of the hair as this usually has the highest concentration of tint.

9 Leave to develop, usually up to 50 minutes, but check with the manufacturer's instructions.

10 When development time is complete, check that the hair has sufficiently lightened, then rinse thoroughly and shampoo.

11 Rinse hair with a stabilising solution of 10 vol. (3%) hydrogen peroxide and comb through gently. This will show whether all the colour pigment has been removed from the hair.

12 If the hair redarkens after combing through, it means that the pigment has not been successfully removed and it will be necessary to repeat the application.

13 Dry the hair to check the colour. If patchy, re-apply the reducer to the patches. If the colour is even but the shade is too orange, red or brassy, tone out with a semi-permanent or permanent tint in the usual manner.

14 Condition the hair well.

15 Complete a record of work carried out.

16 Advise on after-care conditioning treatments.

> **TECHNICAL TIP**
> *Never* apply the reducer to the untreated (virgin) parts of the hair.

Contra-indications for colour removal

Do not proceed with colour removal in any of the following cases:

- Contagious/infectious disease of the hair and/or scalp.
- Excessively weak and porous hair.
- Incompatible chemicals present on the hair shaft.
- Adverse reaction to the test cuttings.
- Adverse reaction to the skin test (if using para after the decolouring) in which case it may be necessary to mask any unwanted colour tones with a semi-permanent colour that does not contain para.
- Highly sensitive scalp.
- Build-up of very dark products that are impossible to remove.

Precautions and considerations for colour removal

1 Always check the client's final requirements thoroughly. It may not be possible to achieve the exact desired colour due to the previous treatments, and the client should be made aware of this fact.

2 Always test the hair before commencing a decolouring process.

3 Ensure that the hair is in reasonable condition before strong colour stripping.

4 Be aware of the health and safety of yourself and the client at all times.

Oxidation colour removal

This is an alkaline method of removal done with bleaching preparations. It will lighten both the artificial and natural colour pigments. The bleach mixture is applied to the tinted area of the hair only, in the same manner as a reducer. It may, however, be necessary to bleach the hair a shade or two lighter than the required colour to allow for corrective tinting afterwards. When an even, bleached base has been achieved a permanent tint can then be applied to obtain the colour that is required.

It is very important when carrying out colour removal to test the hair for breakage and tensile strength during the processing (this is done by pulling the hair between the fingers). Remember that the hair is probably in a very porous state before colour removal and the addition of still more chemicals to the hair can be very damaging. The importance of test cutting prior to the application cannot be stressed too strongly nor too often. The client will also require advice on after-care conditioning treatments to counteract the damaging effect of the chemicals.

Things to do

1 Mistakes sometimes happen with even the most experienced stylist but this does not make the result less upsetting for the client! It is therefore extremely important that any mistakes are identified as soon as possible and remedial action taken immediately.

The following table has been devised to enable you to identify some common faults which occur if due care and attention has not been paid during the perming process.

Fill in the blank spaces on the chart below. If you are unsure, you can check your knowledge by reading the relevant section on perming in Level 2.

You may also wish to keep the completed chart to use as evidence of your knowledge for your portfolio.

Perming Faults and Corrections

Fault	Possible cause	Correction
Perm slow to process		
Hairline and scalp irritation		
Pull-burn		
Straight finished result (no curl)		
Hair not curly enough		
Frizz (hair looks curly when wet and straight when dry)		
Hair too curly		

2 The following case study is a means of testing your understanding of colour correction principles by asking you to apply those principles to solve a problem which could occur in the salon.

A member of staff asks you to look discretely at a client's hair after having woven highlights. The product has swollen over the packet and has left lines of colour on the roots.

Describe how you would handle this situation with reference to:
- the interpersonal skills necessary to prevent losing the client
- the interpersonal skills needed and the discussion you would have with the staff member
- correction of the colouring mistake
- any advice needed for the client and staff member

Level 3 Unit 3

What curl effect does a spiral wind give to long hair? ☐

Where on the head is winding commenced for a spiral perm? ☐

Why and when is a pre-perm treatment used on the hair? ☐

How is the hair tested for development when spirally wound? ☐

What type of curl movement is obtained from a double wind perm? ☐

Where on the head is winding usually commenced for a brick wind? ☐

Give **two** methods/products used for 'blocking out' the ends of certain types of root perms. ☐

Why is it important to pay due care and attention to health, hygiene and safety procedures? ☐

List the legislation which needs to be considered when perming the hair. ☐

List the information required before commencing a colour reduction. ☐

What tests should be carried out prior to a colour reduction? ☐

What is the difference between removing colour by bleach and removing colour by a reducer? ☐

What is meant by the term 'highlighting' the hair? ☐

List the three types of bleach toners and give the possible uses of each. ☐

What is meant by the term 'prepigmentation'? ☐

How would you mask an orange discoloration? ☐

List the primary colours. ☐

Explain how you would carry out **four** fashion colouring techniques. ☐

Why is it important to be constantly aware of the health and safety of both yourself and the client? ☐

EFFECTIVE TEAMWORK

Teams do not just 'happen'. Indeed, to encourage a group of people to work efficiently and creatively together as a team requires planning, organisation and sheer hard work on behalf of the supervisor/manager. Part of the role a supervisor/manager plays within the team is that of a 'role model'. This includes setting a good example to other staff members by acting professionally at all times and maintaining standards by supporting the salon's procedures and activities. Other areas requiring consideration include:

- Managing and developing own work role.
- Working and supporting others in the team.
- Allocating and supervising work.

Managing and developing own work role

A particular work 'role' consists of the duties and responsibilities defined in the 'job description'. An important starting point therefore is, does a *detailed* job description exist for a particular role in the salon? If not, then one should be developed and if a job description does exist what are the arrangements for reviewing and updating this? A job description is necessary to define the limits of a person's authority and autonomy – that is, which areas they are/are not responsible for. Given that a relevant, up-to-date and detailed description of the work role exists, then the next step is to ask these questions:

1 Where am I up to in terms of the competencies I need in order to fulfil this role effectively?
2 In what areas do I need training and development?
3 What are the best development activities to meet these identified needs?

All the above three are best carried out with other people to ensure the analysis is reasonable and planning is realistic. The people involved could be one or more of:

- Immediate manager.
- Personnel or training specialist.
- Other team members.

Some further questions are:

4. How is my achievement to be assessed?
5. When will this review happen and who will be involved?
6. What will be the outcome?

This is the progress review stage. It should be organised as a basis for future development and may be part of a general appraisal system. This feedback from other people is vital in assessing a person's own performance and to decide future development objectives. The people involved can be the same as those who helped the training needs analysis stage as mentioned above.

How to structure self-development within a job role

This process revolves around the 'How am I doing?' question which is at the heart of any self-evaluation. This self-evaluation needs to be *structured*. To do this it is helpful to think of the categories of objectives which could be involved in a review of how effectively a work role is being carried out. These could be listed as:

- Short-term objectives.
- Long-term objectives.
- Salon business objectives.
- Personal objectives.
- Team objectives.
- What specific achievement should be made in a specified time before a progress review?

Some notes made under whichever of these headings is appropriate are a useful starting point for discussion with others.

Having identified and refined some general objectives the next step is to make these as **specific** as possible. The more precise these objectives the better. It can be very useful to use already existing lists of criteria. These criteria are available from a number of sources, including:

- National Vocational Qualification – both in hairdressing and in other areas such as team leadership, management, accountancy procedures, etc. All NVQ programmes are organised as **competence statements** and these provide a useful checklist to use as a basis for a skills/competencies audit.
- Personal identification of the competencies needed for the job role.
- Detailed job description, outlining the work role and team requirements.
- Appraisal/review criteria used in the organisation which may include additional performance criteria.
- Informal comments by people whose opinion you would particularly value.

Once specific competence-based objectives have been identified the next step is to develop an individual development action plan.

How to write an individual development action plan

The easiest way to do this is to refer to Level 3 Unit 11, page 380, and use the **SMART** action plan system. Relate it to your own needs.

The specific training and development activities can be selected from a variety of exercises, which include:

- Work activities – to develop skills.
- Training courses and seminars.
- Open learning activities – which are flexible and can be accomplished at an individual's own speed.
- Assignments and projects – which can be part of external programmes or developed by individuals or teams in the salon.
- Job rotation – on a planned basis to fill in gaps in work experience.
- Mentoring and coaching activities to develop competencies in supervisory and management skills.
- Job shadowing – to develop an appreciation of the qualities, skills and competencies required for a particular role. Conversely, an individual can agree to be 'shadowed' so that their performance can be evaluated as a means of identifying points for personal development.

Working and supporting others in the team

There is coverage of the practical aspects of operating and enhancing the salon team in Level 2 Unit 8, page 204. However, the following is of particular importance to those in the salon who are operating in a supervisory or managerial role.

Organisational structure

Each member of staff has his or her own role and responsibilities within the salon organisation. To enable the salon to function as efficiently as possible, these roles and responsibilities must be clearly defined, as previously discussed, through a **job description** (**specification**), so that each member of staff understands fully what is expected of them.

The organisation of the salon will depend largely on its size. A large company with a chain of salons will obviously require more managers, supervisors and other specialist staff to organise and oversee their large workforce than a smaller salon which may have to combine a number of roles to create just one manager/supervisor. However, regardless of the salon size, someone within the organisation must have overall responsibility for managing the workforce and ensuring that the salon's policies and procedures are carried out. This can be a supervisor or manager who is specifically employed to carry out this task or it can be the salon owner.

Lines of communication

To prevent friction, staff should be aware of the organisational hierarchy and in particular their immediate **line manager**. This is the person to whom they should talk regarding any problems or grievances. Often the 'line of command' will be stated in the **Contract of Employment** which must be issued to all staff members giving their rights and working conditions (**conditions of service**) within the organisation. The conditions of service will vary depending upon the company's policy although there is also **statutory** legislation which the salon organisation must adhere to.

Role and qualities of a manager

The manager's role is to seek to achieve the objectives of an organisation by controlling and organising its resources, including human resources, in the most efficient way possible. The manager acts as a link between the employer and the workforce and so must be a good communicator and well aware of current legislation in addition to the salon's rules, procedures and policies and how they affect the workforce.

Managers are not always expected to carry out manual work as their role is to delegate tasks to other people, leaving themselves free to oversee the running of the salon, solve problems and make decisions as and when necessary. In order to delegate effectively, the manager must be fully aware of the abilities of each staff member including their strengths and their weaknesses. Knowing their strengths enables them to select the most suitable person for each task while knowing their weaknesses allows extra training to be given where it is needed (often called 'staff development').

A manager must also have good administration skills and be able to write reports, keep or check records of staff attendance and try to ensure that all the salon paperwork is in order. In addition, it is usually the manager's responsibility to listen to the views and problems of both staff and clients which are often relayed through the supervisor. A good manager should identify and solve each problem as it arises, *before* it has a chance to affect the efficiency and goodwill of the salon.

Role and qualities of a supervisor

According to the Hairdressing Training Board, a supervisor is a 'person responsible for others but also having operative duties with limited formal authority and with responsibility to management'. The supervisor is expected to keep the manager informed of what is happening within the salon and to contribute ideas for improvement. However, he or she must be very much a 'people' person with a key role in ensuring that the salon runs efficiently with a well-motivated team producing work of a high standard. The main duties and qualities of a supervisor include:

- Set a good example to the other salon staff and know where the limits of their authority lie.
- Know when to operate on their own and when to involve management.
- Work with the rotas and schedules as the other staff are expected to.
- Provide a lead in working to organisational standards.
- Show a high awareness of health and safety.
- Prioritise work efficiently and carry it out effectively and within a recognised time limit.
- Encourage co-operation between staff and set a good example of this through liaising constructively with the salon management.
- Participate in an appraisal system which identifies problem areas and seek help and advice on these areas from salon management.
- Be prepared for unforeseen events and emergencies where changes to the planned work schedule become necessary.
- Show a lead in client care, taking client requirements into account in their operations.

Work, team and individual requirements

Team needs

It cannot be stressed too often that to create the right atmosphere within the salon and to work efficiently and effectively, the staff **must** work as an integrated team.

Building a team requires special skills of the supervisor as it is never easy to bring together a group of people with different personalities and backgrounds to work together in harmony. However, the following points can be helpful to satisfy the needs of the team and aid cohesion:

- Make use of individual talents.
- Speak up for the team and put their views to management.
- Consult the team and involve them in the organisation and decision-making process.
- Establish standards and maintain them with the help of the team.
- Encourage group identity and help the team to give other members mutual support.
- Book a regular meeting slot and keep the team fully informed of what is happening.

Individual needs

Various studies have shown that work plays an important role in most people's lives. People do not always work for financial rewards alone although this is obviously an important incentive. Often people work for other reasons such as personal satisfaction, challenge, status, etc. People do **not** work well if there are bad working conditions, fear of redundancy or change, personal worries, lack of incentives or information, lack of importance, boredom or poor relationships with colleagues. The supervisor must therefore take into consideration the needs of the individual and try to provide the right atmosphere and opportunity for personal growth and satisfaction. This can be done in the following ways:

- Ensure that the working environment is as pleasant as possible.
- Understand the organisation's policies and keep staff fully informed of any decisions and changes by holding regular meetings.
- Be approachable, so that staff feel that they can discuss any problems freely and with confidentiality.
- Ensure that there is a structured training programme with a system for progression within the organisation.
- Encourage staff to use and broaden their individual talents and skills.
- Delegate responsibility and encourage staff to take pride in their work and the salon.
- Offer incentives to increase productivity and standards.

Giving information and advice

An important role of the supervisor is to help staff with any queries or problems, offering help and guidance as and when necessary. Good interpersonal skills are essential to be able to communicate with other staff members at a variety of levels.

Communication is defined as the transfer of information from one person to others. It sounds easy but poor communication is the cause of more interpersonal problems than almost anything else in the salon. Communication goes wrong due to a combination of the speaker not being clear about their message and/or the listener picking out (perceiving) things in the message that are not there or taking the wrong emphasis.

The important thing is to be clear as to the key points of the message and relate this carefully to the listener. Good communicators do not have to speak loudly, fast or often. They put the message clearly, simply and make sure the listener understands. This is as true of written as it is of oral information. Information and advice can be transmitted via:

- Meetings.
- One-to-one discussion.
- Telephone conversation.
- Written communication.

Meetings

Meetings are an excellent means of passing on information and receiving staff opinions, ideas and suggestions – if they are conducted properly.

They should be held on a regular basis at a regular time slot to ensure that all staff are available. If possible, they should be well planned in advance and staff should be informed of the topics that are to be discussed. To be successful, the meeting should be kept strictly to time and within the limits of the agreed topics on the agenda. If other issues are raised these should be included at the end under 'Any other business' or retained for a future meeting. Make sure that any decisions made are implemented as soon as possible and any tasks allocated to staff are followed up soon after the meeting to ensure that they have been done or are in hand.

One-to-one discussion

During a busy working day this is not always as simple as it seems. However, finding time to talk to staff very often pays dividends as problems are more easily solved and good ideas can be implemented. Being available to staff also enables the supervisor to be aware of the opinions and feelings of their team and therefore puts them in a better position to put their point of view across to higher management when required.

Telephone conversation

A business telephone is not for social 'chatting' and any conversation or instructions need to be kept **clear** and **short**. It is important to identify the **essential** information and concentrate on this. Question the listener to ensure that they have taken in the message and that it has no ambiguity.

Written communication

Written communication can be in the form of a business letter or a report. In giving a report or set of instructions to salon personnel (at a staff meeting for example), write down and try out (rehearse) what you want to say. A 'memo' is the most usual form of written communication used in the salon. It is a condensed message and the key points to remember are to keep it clear and short, as with a telephone conversation. Use note form and include lists as often as possible.

Record keeping

Good record keeping is essential to the smooth operation of the salon and enables senior management to acquire any relevant information which it may require as quickly as possible. The supervisor usually has responsibility for keeping the following records accessible and up to date:

- Recording of work done by each stylist and other staff members to enable any training needs to be quickly identified.
- Staff attendance and sickness.
- Staff appraisal, training and assessment so that the progress of each member of staff is monitored.
- Any disputes, grievances and discipline procedures.

- Updating of personnel records of employees to ensure that any change in address, circumstances, staff development, etc., is duly recorded for future reference.
- Results of any marketing exercises.
- Resource allocation including stock control and maintenance of equipment.

Allocating and supervising work

To ensure that the salon runs smoothly and that all staff are treated fairly, the supervisor should draw up, then supervise, staff rotas and schedules.

How to devise staff rotas/schedules

A rota is essentially a plan of when staff are in. It will include breaks and lunch times, holidays and time out of the salon for training or other reasons. It will also indicate when people are working overtime and in larger salons may well include a 'floating' person who can assist and fill in where required during usual salon operations and is available if someone is missing due to sickness or holidays.

The schedule of staffing will reflect the usual cycles of activity in the salon. Typically these cycles are *weekly* (see Fig. 3.48) and *seasonal*.

Training and updating activities also need to be incorporated into the rota. Many trade shows and seminars are on Mondays as this is usually the quietest day. Trainees' attendance at off-the-job sessions at college or training centres may be later in the week and these will need to be staggered in the staffing schedule to avoid too many people being out of the salon at once.

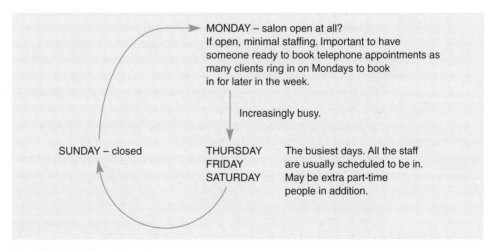

Fig. 3.48 A typical weekly cycle

The seasonal cycle follows the major holiday times. The time before Christmas, Easter and the summer holidays is particularly busy, with January and February being fairly slack times. The dates of the school holidays are good clues as to the busy times.

Both the weekly and seasonal cycle are fairly predictable and can be planned for. There are, of course, other situations which occur from time to time and for which **contingency plans** must be made.

> **Preventing RSI**
>
> Pressures of time may force the stylist to do things the fastest way instead of the safest way. Try to use any waiting time as a rest period. Whenever possible, vary tasks so that you do not do three cuts, for example, in a row. By providing variety, muscles get a chance to rest and recover.

Contingency plans

These are needed to cover abnormal staffing situations which can arise due to:

- Staff absence through sickness – an extreme example would be all the staff away through illness!
- Unexpected increase in clients – a nearby salon closing could cause this.

Contingency plans have to deal with the probable – a large salon is more likely to have someone off sick and the larger the salon the greater the chance of this. Most contingencies will require additional people to work in the salon and these can be:

- Trainees from a college or training organisation – although this usually means relative lack of experience and unfamiliarity with the salon's modes of operation. It does provide the trainees with experience.
- Part-timers – who may work regularly to cover anticipated busy times or staff absence. The problem here is that it is often difficult for part-time staff to be available at short notice and be able to work flexible hours.

Good relationships with college/training organisations and part-time staff make contingency planning a lot easier.

Staff absence

Staff absence can be part of a planned programme of training and development, or anticipated in terms of going into hospital or having some sort of domestic commitment. These have been agreed and authorised. Unauthorised absence is when a person fails to turn up for work for some reason – usually through illness.

All staff need to inform the salon as early as possible as to the cause of their absence and likely duration. This needs to be done first thing or even better, before the salon opens by contacting the supervisor at home. Repeated and unauthorised absence may require disciplinary action if necessary. See page 320 for details of this.

How to allocate work to individual members of staff

Who does what in the salon is a very important area. Decisions on this may be made in conjunction with management and will take into account an individual's competencies and personal qualities. This needs to be based on an objective and fair assessment which involves individual appraisals. How to operate appraisal/ review systems is introduced in Level 1 Unit 4 and covered in detail in Level 3 Unit 11.

In summary, a good appraisal system is about identifying current competencies, reviewing how tasks have been carried out and recognising problems, if any. A common reason for problems developing is a lack of understanding of what is required. It is very important to give information in a way that suits the individual and that people are encouraged to ask questions and seek clarification if anything is not clear. A supervisor needs to be receptive and encouraging in this as it is very easy to put people off asking questions. It is also important that people appreciate when to ask for help and where the limits of their authority and autonomy lie.

For routine salon operations, it is well worth considering writing down a set of instructions which clearly identify the nature of the operation. People can read and reread instructions and have time to think through areas of uncertainty. Listening to verbal instructions does not allow this, although more information can be transferred more quickly and flexibly. Where possible, use written instructions. Other tasks, such as being asked to manage the salon for a short period, need careful verbal instructions if there is not enough time to communicate in writing.

What to do if things go wrong

The allocation of work to an individual may not be appropriate for a variety of reasons. Usually this occurs when there has been a lack of accurate assessment by the person concerned, the supervisor, or both, as to a person's level of competence and willingness to undertake the task. An unrealistic allocation needs to be discussed with management.

Where reallocation of work is necessary this needs to be planned so as to **minimise** the disruption to staff in the salon. There can be a significant 'ripple' effect of such changes and this needs to be carefully considered and reduced as much as possible. Changes in workloads can cause resentment and reduce motivation if not properly explained.

> **Preventing RSI**
> Appointments should be scheduled with strain in mind whenever possible. A *variety* of tasks and physical demands, together with good practice, will help to avoid repetitive strain injury.

The supervision and support of individuals as they perform allocated tasks

How much help and support a person needs involves a delicate balance between too much and not enough. When the requirements of work activities have been identified and written down it facilitates the mutual process of deciding how much support an individual feels they need and in which areas. It is well worth keeping a record for each individual and the task carried out (see Fig. 3.49).

Involving both the individual and the supervisor means that:

- Problem areas can be precisely and objectively defined.
- Agreement is reached on what action to take, the nature of the action and the time span. This action may involve other members of staff who can help the individual develop their competence. There needs to be agreement on when and how this assistance is to be provided and the person involved informed.
- Feedback to individuals is objective and positive. The objectivity is provided if a person's performance is rated against specific criteria rather than just on a subjective 'it seems to me' basis. Objectivity keeps feelings out of the process as far as possible.

Working with management

Establishing a good working relationship between supervisor and manager is very important for, although the manager has overall responsibility, the supervisor is

SUPERVISION RECORD				
Time and Date	Place	Services performed and by whom	Comments	Signed

Fig. 3.49 Sample supervision record card

the person who acts as a 'go between' by liaising between higher management and the work group. A supervisor **must** be able to communicate effectively between the two parties as lack of communication can result in conflict and a shortage of co-operation.

Two of the areas where the supervisor and manager will need to work closely together are:

- Providing information and advice.
- Making proposals for action.

Providing information and advice

This is very much a two-way process. The supervisor should feel free to seek advice and guidance regarding salon rules and procedures, codes of practice, current legislation, and issues relating to quality assurance within the salon. Likewise, the manager will expect the supervisor to provide accurate information on the current activities within the organisation and any problem areas. The information supplied, either informally/formally, verbally or in writing should be clearly stated to ensure that it is not misinterpreted. Always check that the other person has **fully** understood the meaning of the exchange.

The supervisor *must* be fully aware of their specific areas of responsibility and that of their immediate line manager. Otherwise, they could be accused of not fulfilling their role obligations or they could offend the manager by making decisions or taking a course of action that is beyond their remit.

Making proposals for action

If there is a good working relationship and mutual respect between the supervisor and the manager then both parties will feel more confident in offering ideas and suggestions for improving the systems and services of the salon. If there is friction between the two, a supervisor could feel too insecure to offer suggestions or, alternatively, the manager may dismiss good ideas out of hand, without considering them fully, because of personal animosity.

When putting forward any proposals, always make sure that they have been thought through thoroughly. It is a good idea to write down any ideas on paper, then try to imagine any difficulties and how they can be overcome. By preparing in advance, proposals are more likely to be considered and accepted.

Handling conflict

Conflict can arise for any number of reasons – a difference of opinion, a personality clash, someone breaking the rules or behaving inappropriately, sexist or racist issues or it could merely be caused by a misunderstanding. How the conflict is handled depends on the gravity of the situation and the issues involved. The important thing to note is that any potential disagreement is identified as soon as possible and dealt with in an appropriate manner **immediately** to prevent the situation getting out of control. If small problems are not resolved quickly they can snowball with the next small problem until eventually the supervisor has a crisis on their hands!

The supervisor *must* be aware of the legal rights of the staff as ignorance of the law is no excuse for wrong decisions and, certainly, issues involving equal opportunities, racism, sexism and working conditions are all covered by legislation in addition to any salon policy. However, trying to resolve disputes informally through good communication skills is usually preferable to more formal disciplinary action or eventual legal proceedings.

Because of their liaising role, the supervisor will have to learn to deal not only with different **forms** of conflict but also contention between staff on the one hand and management on the other.

Dealing with staff conflict

Misunderstandings can be minimised if all staff know the standards they are expected to adhere to. This includes not only their practical skills but their behaviour towards the clients and each other. If they are disruptive or behaving inappropriately, the supervisor will need to find out the reason why. There must therefore be opportunities available for staff members to talk over their problems or difficulties in a quiet place away from interruptions. It is advisable to keep confidential records of both informal and formal interactions and also to ensure that management is aware of any difficulties and how, if at all, they are being resolved.

The main point in this situation is listening to, as opposed to solving, problems. There is always a natural inclination to try and find solutions for other people's problems but this is not what the listening role is about. If the solutions offered are unsuccessful then the situation will be made far worse as the 'blame' will be automatically transferred to the person giving the advice! You need to be a sympathetic ear and, if necessary, a shoulder to cry on. Any 'solutions' need to come from within the person and not from the outside.

It is important to bear in mind the confidential nature of the conversations. The staff should feel they can talk to you and be absolutely sure you will not divulge any of what they tell you. Even if you feel that the manager ought to know about the conversation, you must first obtain the permission of the staff member.

Although this rarely happens, it is possible that someone who has told you of various troubles will then use your knowledge of this to attempt to manipulate you over such matters as pace and standard of work. If you feel this is the case, tell the individual concerned that this is not really fair and that at the end of the day, however sympathetic you are, there is a limit to the amount of consideration a person can have in a salon operating as a business in a competitive environment.

It is essential to be very careful in any form of counselling role and refer the person to professional counselling help if appropriate.

Handling conflict with management

Any disagreements with the line manager should be sorted out as amicably as possible – at the end of the day, both parties usually still have to work together! It is also demotivating to the staff and detrimental to the organisation if senior staff members are continually at loggerheads with each other.

It is often difficult to give criticism and even harder to accept, particularly if you feel it is unjustified or at too personal a level. Conflict is almost always disturbing to deal with and it is therefore important to keep calm, stick to the facts and act in an adult fashion. Do not revert to 'child' mode and have a tantrum if things do not go exactly as you would wish!

Very often people only listen selectively to what they hear and therefore misinterpret what is being said, particularly if one or both of the two parties lack interpersonal skills. The golden rule is to **listen** to the comments, **weigh up** what is being said and then make a reasoned **judgement** before deciding on the course of action.

Assisting with disciplinary and grievance procedures

Maintaining discipline in the salon does not necessarily mean 'domination'. If staff are treated fairly and with respect they are more likely to be loyal and hard working in return. Even so, it is inevitable that on occasions the supervisor will have to assist with the discipline of someone with poor or unacceptable performance. It is unfortunate that even when a supervisor has identified a problem, and dealt with it immediately in an efficient manner, there will still be instances when the informal procedures have just not worked and more formal action has to be taken.

Disciplining staff

The manager should **always** be aware of any disciplinary matters and it is their responsibility to decide whether the situation is best dealt with by the supervisor, manager or the employer. Situations which may need disciplinary action include:

- Persistent lateness or excessive time off work.
- Attitude problems shown by being offhand or rude to colleagues and clients.
- Slovenly or low standards of practical skills.

The disciplinary process should be carried out quietly, objectively and privately – away from the other members of staff. Prepare carefully for the disciplinary interview by collecting together all the facts and making sure that they are correct, with dates and times if applicable. Most salons have a book in which to record when staff are off work (it is usual to let the salon know before 9.00 am when a member of staff needs time off for sickness or other reasons).

During the interview, if appropriate, the **positive** aspects of the individual's performance should be stressed. Such phrases as: 'I'm surprised at this lateness because your general attitude is so good. Is there a problem?' should be used. Always record the matter and what action was taken in accordance with the salon's disciplinary procedure. These procedures are usually contained in the contract of employment and a common system is:

1 Two verbal warnings.
2 Two written warnings (the final one of which is usually the dismissal notice).
3 Dismissal.

POINTS TO REMEMBER

It is important to ensure that all individuals are aware of disciplinary procedures and that it is the responsibility of the manager or employer to instigate disciplinary strategies and to deal with any serious misdemeanours.

Grievance procedures

The employee has the right to complain if they believe that they have been treated unfairly. It is usual, in the first instance, to talk to their line manager and the procedure should be clearly stated in the employee's Contract of Employment. In addition to the organisational policy, all staff members should be aware of their statutory rights. The Offices, Shops and Railway Premises Act and the Health and Safety at Work Act are designed to give protection and reasonable working conditions to everyone in the workplace and it is also against the law to discriminate against individuals because of their gender, race or beliefs. The laws pertaining to these issues are; Sex Discrimination Act 1975, 1986; Race Relations Act 1976; Equal Opportunities Act.

If there is a Trade Union operating within the organisation then any dispute with the management regarding company policy or infringement of the law should be referred to the **union representative** whose role it is to support and advise their members.

Any disciplinary or grievance procedure must be treated in the utmost confidence and an accurate record kept of both the procedure followed and the ultimate outcome. This record, although confidential, should be made available to the relevant parties if and when required.

Things to do

1 You have been asked to help organise the training of a trainee in fashion colouring techniques. What method (or methods) of training would you use? Explain your choice.

   How would feedback on the person's performance be provided?

2 List:
   ● Those areas of the salon's activities which are fully under your control.
   ● Those areas decided jointly by yourself and salon management.
   ● Those areas decided by management.

3 Collect relevant literature, e.g. pamphlets, instructional material, etc., on current national and local legislation on the following areas:

- Health and Safety at Work Act 1974.
- Offices, Shops and Railway Premises Act.
- COSHH 1988 Regulations.
- Sex Discrimination Acts 1975, 1986.
- Race Relations Act 1976.
- Equal Opportunities Act.

Highlight the sections which are relevant to the hairdressing industry and your salon.

Create a file containing the relevant sections of the information collected above which can be kept in the staff-room as a source of reference for the employees.

You may also use this file as evidence towards your underpinning knowledge of working relationships and Health and Safety in the salon.

4 Using the following case study, organise a rota for seven staff members who wish to take two weeks holiday each during the summer months and a further week at some other time. Two of the trainees have requested leave to go on holiday together and one of the senior stylists must be given the last week of July as part of their two weeks as he is getting married at that time.

You are the supervisor of an extremely busy hairdressing salon in a small seaside town. The staff consist of two senior stylists, two junior stylists and three trainees in addition to yourself and the manager.

When you have completed your provisional rota answer the questions below:

- What were the major considerations when trying to work out the rota?
- What difficulties for the salon do you foresee if two of the trainees take their annual holiday together?
- Explain how you would deal with the situation and any difficulties as outlined in the previous question.
- How far in advance do you think that the rota should be organised?

What do you know?

Level 3 Unit 4

*What is meant by the **induction** of new staff?*

*List **six** areas that an Induction Programme may cover.*

List the most important rules/guidelines which exist in your salon.

What is a Contract of Employment?

What is usually included in a Contract of Employment?

Give your ideas of how staff within your organisation could be made more aware of Health and Safety within the salon.

State the staff members of your organisation and list their specific responsibilities.

What is the main aim of any Appraisal System?

What are the key areas of Product Knowledge?

What is meant by 'Client Care'?

List the four major 'resources' in the salon.

Define the main role of a supervisor in the use of the salon's resources.

Outline the requirements of the 'rota system' both weekly and seasonal.

What is meant by 'contingency'? Identify **two** likely contingencies in the salon. ☐

Explain for each how responses to these could be planned for. ☐

Outline the procedures involved in staff absences. ☐

List the main things to consider when allocating work to members of staff. ☐

List **four** features of good communication in the salon. Explain how each of these can be incorporated into the allocation of work in the salon. ☐

List **three** reasons why salon staff may require some support from the supervisor. ☐

Outline the actions that should be taken if the allocation of work to an individual appears to be inappropriate. ☐

Explain why the evaluation of a person's performance should involve both the individual and the supervisor. ☐

List the main features of an effective performance-evaluation system in the salon. ☐

What is a job description? ☐

What statutory legislation is concerned with the working conditions of staff? ☐

List **five** qualities of a manager. ☐

Give a definition of a supervisor. ☐

What records is a supervisor usually responsible for? ☐

Give **four** means of transmitting information and advice. ☐

Why is it important that a supervisor is fully aware of their specific areas of responsibility? ☐

Explain how you would deal with staff conflict. ☐

Give **three** situations where disciplinary action may be necessary. ☐

SALON FINANCE

There are a large number of places in this book where the 'salon as a business' is emphasised. This really means the salon as a successful business; that is, one that cares about its staff and clients and makes a profit. Profit is what keeps a salon in business and it is easy to define:

Total income – Total cost to operate business = Profit

From this is follows that there are two key areas in the profitability of a business:

- Maximising income.
- Minimising costs.

Both of these activities revolve around:

- Resources.
- Salon productivity.

Resources

A 'resource' is something that can be used and has a value. A list of resources for a hairdressing salon includes:

- People, human resources – the staff and clients.
- Financial – the income generated by salon sales and services.
- Information systems – these may be paper-based or more usually computerised.
- Utilities – electricity, gas, water, telephone, fax.
- Tools and equipment.
- Time – there is the old saying 'time is money'.
- Space – making best use of this to provide effective displays, secure storage, etc.

The use of these resources is governed by legal and internal organisational factors which are covered elsewhere in this book. For example:

- **Legal factors** – see Level 3 Unit 6 for information on health and safety and Level 2 Unit 9, for further details on stock control.
- **Internal, organisational factors** – see Level 2 Unit 9, for information on waste/spillage and Level 2 Unit 9, for further details on reception displays.

It is important that resource use is carefully monitored and controlled as the potential consequences of missing resources can

- Be dangerous.
- Indirectly affect staff wages through reduction in commission.
- Result in disciplinary action.

Human resources

The development and maintenance of effective team operation in the salon is covered in Level 3 Unit 4. The major problems in 'misuse' of human resources is overloading someone with too much work, or responsibility, or both.

It is very important that people are clear about:

- Levels of responsibility and limits to authority of themselves and other salon staff. This needs to be made clear in all job descriptions.
- The 'steps' in the ladder of salon communications.
- Effective/communication by means of memos, staff meetings, training sessions and notices.

Another possible reason for a person being overloaded is of their own making, due to mobile or working-at-home hairdressing. This is work which is over and above that of the salon where they work and too much of this work is to be discouraged. Some salons as a policy do not allow their staff to be involved in any other hairdressing.

Financial resources

This is a common area for problems in the salon. Examples include the accidental giving of wrong change or mishandling of non-cash payments and the deliberate theft of money or stock. Non-cash payments are covered in Level 2 Unit 9. With cash payments it is good practice to

- Put notes on the till until change has been given.
- Say 'you've given me a £10/£20 note'.

Another aspect of the control of financial resources is commission. Some salons work on a commission-only basis. Others use a basic wage with commission earned on top. The commission is an incentive and may be calculated on the actual income generated or a fixed payment for particular services.

Whenever commission is involved it is in everyone's interests to ensure it is accurately worked out. Most salons use a 'validation' system which checks services against the appointments made (some more details on this is included in the next section on page 326). Stock control is important as commission is often paid on retail goods as well as on salon services.

Information

Information is a resource. It is very important that this is kept **confidential**. There are:

- **Commercial confidentiality** on such areas of pay, pay structure and pricing of goods and services.
- **Client details** which may be of a sensitive nature or more usually this information is important to give the client a feeling of being valued when the time and effort is made to record details which are referred to on later appointments.

People like to be remembered and made to feel important. Salons have strict rules about confidentiality of client details and, in many salons, failure to keep to the rules results in dismissal. The Data Protection Act means that a breach of confidence in computer records can be prosecuted.

Utilities

Salons use a lot of water and electricity, and may also use gas. The main factor is misuse by wasting energy or water – particularly hot water. The procedures to reduce waste of these commodities should be automatic and routine and are covered in Level 2 Unit 9, page 209.

Misuse of the salon phone can be included in this section. The phone should only be used for salon business, not just because of the cost but due to creating difficulties for clients and potential clients when phoning in.

Tools and equipment

The main thing is to ensure that tools and equipment are:

- Properly looked after and maintained.
- Used for their intended purpose – that is, hairdressing in the salon and not for something else!

Time

People's time is an important resource and should not be wasted. This has a lot to do with self-motivation of staff. Staff sitting about gives a very poor impression. The 'final something to do' rule is important here. There are always things that need doing in the salon.

Effective use of space

The careful use of space is important in the salon. Space is often at a premium and things can go wrong:

- At **reception** – to much clutter on chairs, surfaces, untidy displays which get in the way.
- In the **salon** – with staff bags, coats and personal possessions.

The salon layout needs to be planned to give people room to work, clients room to wait, display areas, reception and storage areas. Badly planned space can be a constant problem and good communication systems, such as staff meetings, can help develop better practice and suggestions for better space utilisation.

Salon productivity

Salon productivity is the amount of work carried out (and so the amount of turnover) in a given length of time. Many salons use incentives, particularly commission payment to staff, in order to enhance productivity. As mentioned in the section on resources, some salons operate a 'commission only' payment system to staff, whilst others operate a basic payment with commission added on. In some salons the commission is based on the numbers of operations, whilst in others it is on the income generated by the services provided. In any event it is important for all salon staff to be aware that their own work and how they do it (their work performance) are important to the success of the salon business. This can be encouraged by:

- Providing opportunities to review salon services in terms of improving productivity. This gets people to think about what they are doing.
- Promotion of self and salon by workshops, training sessions, marketing, retailing and shows. This helps staff to identify commercial opportunities and new products as well as encouraging team building.

Setting productivity levels

Setting realistic targets for performance is a key aspect of salon management. This can be through one-to-one discussions (including formal appraisal in larger salons), staff meetings or setting general expected levels of activity. This helps to prevent the abuse sometimes encountered in salons where too few clients are deliberately booked in (or even non-existent bogus clients are put down!) to give an easy time to a stylist. Another problem (mostly by accident) is the failure to pass on in the client's bill the proper cost of the resources used, e.g. payment for a cheaper alkaline perm when in fact a more expensive acid perm has been used.

Setting targets also helps to clarify how long a service or process should take and then identify if problems in working speeds are present.

In many salons staff keep a work log as an independent method of recording (in addition to the appointment record) what they have done over a period of time. This is often used in calculations for commission or bonus payments for exceeding targets.

It is important to maintain the motivation and enthusiasm of staff and key aspects of this are:

- Clear and realistic target setting.
- Good, effective, two-way communication.
- Staff seeing action taken where necessary to ensure implementation of salon and legal requirements of operations, e.g. dismissal for breach of confidentiality, misappropriation of stock, etc.

1   Complete the diagram for an actual salon.

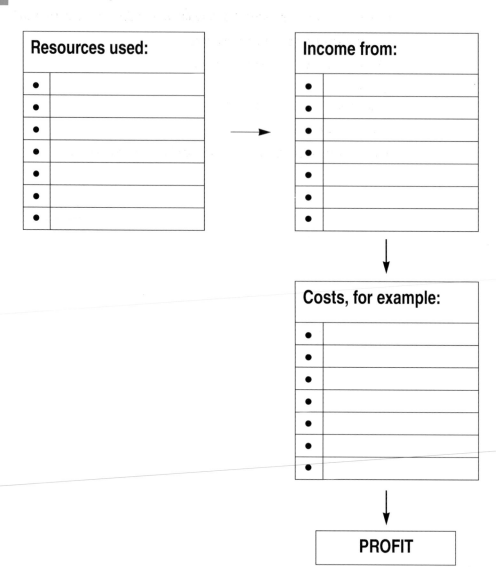

2   Carry out a study of the use of resources in a salon. Suggest **improvements** that could realistically be made.

3   What is meant by **salon productivity**?

- make a list of factors which influence productivity for an actual salon
- from your list select some areas where improvements could be made and explain how this could be realistically achieved.

Level 3 Unit 5

*Can you list **seven** types of resources used in salons?*   ☐

*Explain the **legal** and **organisational** factors which influence resource use.*   ☐

What are the potential consequences of misusing resources?   ☐

How does waste affect profit? ☐

Can you identify who is responsible for resource allocation and use in the salon? ☐

List some effective types of communication. ☐

Why is effective communication important? ☐

- *cash*
- *non-cash payments in the salon* ☐

What is 'productivity'? ☐

How can contributions to improving salon productivity be encouraged? ☐

SALON HEALTH, SAFETY AND SECURITY

Background information

A large hairdressing salon on a busy day may have over one hundred clients using the premises. Most of those people will be concerned only with the finished style and few, if any, will give any thought to the possible hazards in the salon. The hairdresser needs to be much more aware of these Health and Safety issues so that possible accidents or infections can be prevented. To some extent both the hairdresser and the client can be put at risk from a number of possible sources. These can be grouped into:

1 **Physical hazards** – which include:
   - physical injury (e.g. cuts and knocks)
   - fire and heat burns
   - electricity (e.g. electric shock)
2 **Chemical hazards** – which involve:
   - chemical burns (including chemicals on the skin and the eyes)
   - storage and disposal of chemicals (e.g. hydrogen peroxide and aerosol containers)
   - dermatitis or eczema (e.g. from hair dyes)
3 **Biological hazards** – which can be:
   - infections – caused by micro-organisms (germs), e.g. impetigo
   - infestations – caused by animal parasites, e.g. head lice

Hairdressers have a responsibility to protect themselves and their clients both in a moral sense, in that it is wrong to cause pain or discomfort, and in a practical way, due to:

- The **legal responsibilities** placed on the salon owner and worker.
- The **bad publicity** which results from accidents or infections taking place in the salon.

This unit develops further the areas covered in Levels 1 and 2 and the relevant health and safety legislation required for Level 3.

The legal requirements for health and safety in the salon

The legislation, regulations and guidance advice in this area are under constant review and change. What follows is a brief outline of the legislation and regulations of particular importance to hairdressing. These are correct at the time of writing but it is strongly advised that current information be sought if significant time has passed.

Where to get information on health and safety

There are a variety of sources:

- Trade publications.
- Manufacturers, wholesalers.
- Local environmental health officer.
- Community health organisations.
- Health and Safety Executive.

The Health and Safety Executive (HSE) have regional offices (in the phone book) and are an extremely good source of up-to-date information. They produce a range of leaflets and pamphlets on the legislation/regulations and practical guides to implementation. The HSE produce, for example:

- How to use hair preparations safely in the salon.
- Guidelines on Aids and Hepatitis B for hairdressers.
- Five steps for completing a COSHH assessment.

The HSE has information and publication centres, information on which can be obtained through regional offices.

An outline of important health and safety legislation/regulations

These include:

- Management of Health and Safety at Work Regulations 1992.
- Health and Safety at Work Act 1974.
- Workplace (Health, Safety and Welfare) Regulations 1992.
- Manual Handling Operations Regulations 1992.
- Personal Protective Equipment at Work Regulations 1992.
- Control of Substances Hazardous to Health Regulations 1988 – 'COSHH' for short.
- Health and Safety (Training for Employment) Regulations 1988.
- Reporting of Injuries, Diseases and Dangerous Occurrences Regulations 1985.
- Health and Safety Information to Employees Regulations 1989.
- Health and Safety (First Aid) Regulations 1981.
- Electricity at Work Regulations 1989.

Management of Health and Safety at Work Regulations 1992 involves setting up codes of practice to carry out aspects of both the Health and Safety at Work Act and COSHH. Examples would be:

- Risk assessment.
- Keeping records.
- Preventive measures.
- Training.

The Health and Safety Information to Employees Regulations 1989 place a duty on employers to inform employees on exposure and risk as well as policies and procedures on health and safety.

- **Electricity at Work Regulations 1989** state that electrical equipment must be used safely and be checked every year by a 'competent person'.
- **Provision and Use of Work Equipment Regulations 1992** have a very wide scope and will eventually cover both new and old equipment. They regulate areas such as the use, repair, maintenance, and cleaning of equipment and place

a duty on the employer to protect the employee. The regulations cover equipment used in hairdressing and extend to lighting.

- **Workplace (Health, Safety and Welfare) Regulations 1992** replace large parts of the older Factories Act 1961 and the Offices, Shops and Railway Premises Act 1963. They contain large numbers of areas relevant to hairdressing.

The regulations cover areas such as:

- Equipment maintenance – 'good working order and in good repair'.
- Ventilation – 'sufficient' fresh air/purified air.
- Workplace, temperature – at least 16°C.
- Lighting – 'suitable and sufficient'.
- Cleanliness – covering the workplace, furniture and fittings.

The regulations cover floors and indoor traffic routes which should be cleaned 'at least once a week' and should be 'non-slip' and not cause a person to drop anything.

Work stations and seating need to be 'suitable' for the stylist and client, and there should be places to put a person's own clothing and overalls, and facilities for changing. There should also be facilities for rest and meals, including protecting non-smokers from the discomfort caused by smokers. Toilets and wash facilities must also be provided.

Health and Safety at Work Act 1974 and associated regulations

This extends to all working situations and sets out the responsibilities of both the employer and the employee in terms of:

- General health and safety.
- First aid arrangements and reporting of accidents.
- Enforcement of the Act.

General health and safety

The duties of the *employer* include:

- Care and maintenance of equipment.
- Prevention of risk in the storage and use of materials.
- Instruction and training employees in safe practices.
- Maintaining the place of work so that it is safe.
- With five or more employees, the employer needs to produce a written policy statement in terms of the general policy operated concerning health and safety.

For the *employee* the duties are:

- To take reasonable care for the health and safety of themselves and others who may be affected by their actions.
- To co-operate with the employer and others to ensure health and safety at work.

The Act also lists 'dangerous occurrences' and recommends that these must be reported and a record kept – this is taken further in the Notification of Accidents and Dangerous Occurrences Regulations 1980 which stipulate that 'dangerous occurrences' must be noted whether a person is injured or not.

Enforcement of the Act

Enforcement is carried out by Area Offices of the Health and Safety Executive by means of Health and Safety Inspectors. These have the right of entry to premises and the power to:

- Order improvements to be made.
- Prohibit the use of apparatus or premises.
- Seize, render harmless or destroy dangerous equipment.

The Health and Safety (Training for Employment) Regulations 1988 extended health and safety legislation to cover trainees and those on work experience.

Control of Substances Hazardous to Health (COSHH – 'cosh')

This regulation is concerned with chemical hazards. The main principles of these regulations (which took effect on 1 January 1990) are:

- Assessment of risk from substances – much of this depends on information supplied by manufacturer.
- Provision, use and upkeep of adequate control measure for chemicals – the main point is to prevent exposure if practicable or have adequate control.
- Monitoring exposure of employees to potential hazards.
- Health surveillance of employees – this means monitoring the health of people exposed to potential hazards.
- Education and training of employees – in terms of:
  - purpose of personal protective clothing
  - how to avoid endangering themselves and others
  - storage and disposal
  - emergency procedures

Maintaining a healthy and safe working environment

The 'working environment' includes the:

- Salon.
- Access to and from the salon.
- Stockroom.
- Toilets, wash areas, rest rooms.
- Offices.

Having covered the underpinning legislation/regulations on salon health and safety, what follows is an outline of practical health, safety and hygiene theory and practice. Other information is given in Level 1 Unit 6 and Level 2 Unit 10.

Checking and maintaining equipment and tools

Properly maintained equipment can give long and good service.

- Every client should have a clean brush and comb used on their hair. Combs should be kept in antiseptic and brushes in a sterilising cabinet.
- Chairs should be kept clean and free from hair. A vinyl covering makes cleaning easier. They should be wiped down every day, including the backs of the chairs and the legs as these tend to get splashed with lotions. Any splitting or tearing of the material must be attended to immediately to avoid it getting worse.

- Light fittings should be kept clean. It is important that the salon is well lit from all angles.
- Driers do long duty hours. If kept clean and dust free, the wear and tear on them is kept to a minimum. Regularly unscrew the top and remove dust and fluff from the fan, otherwise there is a real risk of fire. Arrange a yearly contract for servicing – there are firms that specialise in this service.
- Steamers and infra-red lamps should be cleaned after use. Always ensure that the water bottle on the steamer has enough water in it before use (distilled water should be used) and the steamer should be cleaned out regularly. Infra-red bulbs should be checked before use and any faulty bulbs replaced. Servicing once a year will prolong the life of this equipment and maintain its safety of use.
- Vapour and ultraviolet cabinets. Make sure that the vapour steriliser cabinet is checked each day and refilled with sterilising solution. Keep cabinets clean inside and out.

POINTS TO REMEMBER

Routine hygiene practices and procedures should ALWAYS be followed by all staff.

Electricity

People can be at risk for two different reasons: either overheating of electrical appliances or electrical shock.

The amount of electricity and hence the severity of the electric shock depends on:

- The **voltage** and **current** of the electrical supply involved.
- The **electrical resistance** between the person and the item from which they receive the shock.

The electricity supplied to and used in most salons has a voltage of 240 volts and a current of 13 amps. This is sufficient to produce a severe shock, especially if the electrical resistance between the person's body and the item causing the shock is low. A good example of this is when wet hands are used to plug in, switch on, or handle electrical apparatus. Water is a conductor of electricity and this lowers the resistance between a person and whatever they are touching. The water could also get inside plugs, sockets, switches and equipment and conduct (carry) the electricity into a person. Therefore, always use dry hands to plug in, switch on or handle electrical equipment.

A further factor in the amount of electricity received by the body is the **earthing** of equipment. In outline, the function of the earth (E) cable is to carry electricity from metal parts of electrical equipment into the earth (or ground). This provides an easy route for electricity to flow and it will take this path rather than pass through the person's body and produce an electric shock.

Regular and expert checking is important to detect faults likely to cause electric shocks and to ensure that the earthing circuit is functioning properly.

Using electricity safely

In the UK electricity is supplied to consumers, including hairdressing salons, in quantities which can be very dangerous, either directly by electric shock or indirectly by fire. Fuses (or circuit breakers) are deliberately placed in circuits for reasons of safety. Basically, the fuses help prevent fires and earthing, already referred to above, prevents electric shock.

Many of the accidents that occur when using electricity are simply due to thoughtlessness, carelessness or downright bad practice.

Ventilation

Routine activities in the hairdressing salon produce damp, warm, contaminated (stale) air, which tends to rise to the ceiling as warm air is lighter than cooler air. The aim of a good ventilation system is to provide fresh air (i.e. less humid, cooler and with fewer micro-organisms) but without producing any draughts or low temperatures in the salon and therefore making conditions uncomfortable.

> **Preventing RSI**
> Arrange your station and your client so that you are not looking into the light, at a white wall or at a mirror reflecting either. The glare can be very tiring and irritating to your eyes.

Effects of bad ventilation in the salon

On client and staff comfort

The body cooling system depends on the evaporation of sweat from the skin. In conditions of high humidity (i.e. moist air) the evaporation process is reduced so the body tends to overheat very slightly. This produces feelings of drowsiness in clients and staff, or even feelings of being uncomfortably hot, if combined with warmth.

On hygiene

One type of micro-organism (germ) is a virus, some of which attack humans and are described as **pathogenic**, e.g. cold and influenza ('flu'). These are mostly spread in tiny droplets of moisture which shoot out of a person's mouth and nose when they cough or sneeze. The more humid the air, the slower these droplets evaporate and the longer the viruses survive, thus increasing the chance of them being breathed in by other clients and staff.

Another type of micro-organism, bacteria, also thrives in damp conditions.

On hair

The major influence is due to the hair's ability to absorb water from the atmosphere, that is, its tendency to be **hygroscopic**.

The more humid the air the more quickly this happens, so it is more difficult to carry out both wet and dry setting and blowdrying in conditions where the hair is continually reabsorbing water from humid air.

Chemical hazards

Hairdressing operations very often involve the use of chemicals on the hair and some of these are sprayed on to the hair using pressurised containers, e.g. hair lacquers. The chemical hazards in the salon come from three main sources:

- Chemicals getting onto the skin or into the eyes.
- Storage and disposal.
- Dermatitis (eczema).

Chemicals getting onto the skin or into the eyes

The main prevention here is to be aware of the risk involved in carrying out any hairdressing operation (even shampooing) that involves chemicals and to handle chemicals with care. Chemicals can be swallowed, especially by children, so care should be taken to put these out of reach.

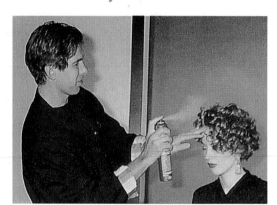

Accidental spills can be avoided by replacing caps and stoppers on containers immediately after use.

Do not use **caustic soda** (sodium hydroxide) to clear blocked drains, get a plumber instead to clear the blockage. Caustic soda can cause severe skin burns.

Storage and disposal

All salon reagents should be stored in well-labelled containers and not put onto high shelves where there is always a risk of dropping when taking them down. Particular care needs to be taken with stored hydrogen peroxide and pressurised aerosol sprays. Both can explode if heated so they should never be stored near heaters or in direct sunlight.

If a container has lost its label or the contents cannot be identified with certainty for any other reason, then dispose of it. Careful disposal of empty pressurised cans is important. These should not be punctured or burned (incinerated) as the pressure left inside could cause an explosion. Warnings about this are printed on the container.

Dermatitis (eczema)

Basically, this involves the body 'over-reacting' to a substance to which it has been exposed. Many of the chemicals used in hairdressing may cause dermatitis, but **paraphenylenediamine** used in some tints is strongly linked to people developing dermatitis. Both the hairdresser and the client are at risk, with the hairdresser at greatest risk due to their repeated and long-term exposure to hairdressing chemicals. The client can be protected against 'para' dye dermatitis by carrying out a skin test before going ahead with the tint. The hairdresser can be protected by using rubber gloves for any hairdressing operation that involves chemicals, including shampooing.

Biological hazards

These consist of infections and infestations both caused by living organisms.

They are either **infectious** or **contagious**; that is they can be passed between people or transmitted in the salon.

Infections

These are caused by harmful germs or, more properly, **pathogenic micro-organisms**. Examples commonly encountered in the salon include:

- Impetigo.
- Boils.
- Eye infections, e.g. conjunctivitis.
- Ringworm.
- Cold sores (herpes).
- Some types of wart.

It is important to be able to recognise these conditions and distinguish between the infectious or contagious complaints and the non-infectious or non-contagious conditions. Also you should know which of these prohibit hairdressing operations. Of the examples listed above impetigo, eye infections and ringworm *definitely* mean that hairdressing operations should not start (or should stop if already started). For more information see Level 2 Unit 1.

Aids and Hepatitis B

These are both very serious infections which can be transmitted by small amounts of blood or serum (clear liquid in blisters) from one person to another. The risk to hairdressers is slight.

There is a useful pamphlet produced by the government's Health Department with notes for guidance. Transmission of both diseases can be avoided by using simple and routine hygiene practices, sterilisation of tools and equipment and prevention of infection or infestation.

Infestations

These refer to larger animal parasites living on the body and include:

- Head and body lice.
- Fleas.
- Itchmites (which cause scabies).

With head lice particularly, the hairdresser can be the first person to definitely detect the presence of these parasites. In all the examples above, hairdressing operations should not start (or should stop if already begun). For more information see Level 2 Unit 1.

Prevention of infection or infestation

To prevent any infection or infestation developing you must:

1 Be able to recognise which scalp conditions are infectious/contagious and know what to do if they are.

2 Carry out routine hygienic procedures in the salon, coupled with design considerations, like the choice of wall and floor coverings, upholstery, ventilation and temperature control.

Routine hygienic procedures include such practices as:

- **Between clients** washing your hands; sterilising personal tools and equipment; cleaning shampoo basins.
- **For each client** preparing a clean towel (or towels) and neck strip; sterilising any tools accidentally dropped onto the floor; not keeping tools and equipment in pockets.
- **Regular** washing down of walls, floors, work surfaces with an alcohol-based disinfectant; sweeping up hair clippings and putting waste into a closed container.
- **Personal routine** not putting hair pins and clips in the mouth; wearing closed-in shoes with low heels.
- **General** not allowing animals in the salon; ensuring an adequate ventilation and heating system.

First aid

First aid can be defined as 'the skilled application of accepted principles of treatment on the occurrence of any injury or sudden illness, using facilities available at the time. It is the approved method of treating a casualty until placed, if necessary, in the care of a doctor or removed to hospital' (authorised manual of St John Ambulance, St Andrews Ambulance Association, British Red Cross Society).

The best thing to do with accidents is to prevent them. However, even in the best run salons, accidents will sometimes happen. There are also cases where events occur which are not under the control of anyone in the salon, a client suffering a heart attack for example. It is important to know what to do and the best method of learning this is to complete a first aid course. There are a number of these organised by the St John Ambulance, Red Cross, or at your local College of Further Education. It is an extremely good idea to have at least one trained first aider in the salon. See Table 3.1 for suggested contents of a **first aid** kit.

A brief outline of some first aid procedures

There is no real substitute for completing a proper first aid course. Here, for guidance, is an outline of what to do if someone suffers:

Cuts
- For **minor wounds** – cover the wound as soon as possible with a sterile dressing.
- For **major wounds** – send for expert help immediately. Try to control the bleeding by pulling the sides of the wound together and hold firmly until the bleeding stops. Apply a pad of sterile dressings and hold in place (use disposable plastic gloves if possible). If these become soaked with blood add more dressings.
- For **blood spills** – pour neat bleach onto the blood. Leave for a few minutes. Put on disposable plastic gloves. Wash off with a large amount of hot water with some washing up liquid or shampoo added.

Table 3.1

Item	Number of employees		
	1–5	6–10	11–50
Card giving general first aid guidance	1	1	1
Individually wrapped sterile, adhesive dressings	10	20	40
Sterile eye pads, with attachment	1	2	4
Triangular bandage	1	2	4
Sterile dressing for serious wounds*	1	2	4
Safety pins	6	6	12
Sterile, unmedicated wound dressings:			
medium size	3	6	8
large	1	2	4
extra large	1	2	4

*These should be provided if the triangular bandages are not sterile

Burns

- **Heat burns** – cool immediately under cold water. If the person is seriously burnt, send for expert medical help. If the burn is widespread, cover it with loose dressings. Do not attempt to remove clothing sticking to the burnt area.
- **Chemical burns** – wash off with plenty of cold water. Remove any clothing which may have chemical on it. Apply a sterile dressing. Refer the person to expert medical help if necessary.

Eye injuries

These include:

- Object in the eye.
- Chemical in the eye.

Attempt to remove the object with the moistened corner of a sterile dressing. If it cannot be removed or the eye is still painful after the object has been removed, cover with an eye patch and quickly send the person to a hospital or a doctor.

If a chemical has run into the eye, wash out with a large amount of cold water. Force the eye open if necessary. Cover with an eye pad and either send the person to a hospital or a doctor or summon expert help depending on the injury.

Collapse

If a person collapses it could be due to a number of reasons, which include:

- Electric shock.
- Heart attack.
- Epileptic fit.
- Fainting.

The person may be partly conscious or completely unconscious. In either case, talk reassuringly to them. They may also have knocked or cut themselves while falling.

ELECTRIC SHOCK

- Switch off the supply. If this is not possible then use an insulator (rug, clothing, paper or plastic) to pull the person away from the source of the shock.

- If they are partly conscious keep talking and reassuring them. Keep them warm and if they do not recover within a few minutes send for expert medical help.
- If they are unconscious then:
  - send immediately for expert help
  - check their heartbeat by trying to find the pulse in the neck
  - check breathing by either watching for breathing movements or by holding a mirror, e.g. compact lid mirror or watchglass, over their mouth and looking for 'misting'
  - if the heart has stopped, start external cardiac massage and/or if breathing has stopped, start mouth-to-mouth resuscitation (the 'kiss of life')
  - continue cardiac massage and/or mouth-to-mouth resuscitation until help arrives
  - keep talking in a reassuring manner, even if they are unconscious.

HEART ATTACK

- If the person is partly conscious they will most likely complain of chest pains (often severe). They may have some medication with them. Loosen clothes; talk reassuringly to them. Send for expert medical help.
- If the person is unconscious treat them as for electric shock above.

EPILEPTIC FIT

These can vary from a mild attack with only a brief loss of consciousness (much like fainting) to severe attacks involving the person becoming unconscious, going stiff and having convulsions, e.g. arms and legs twitching violently.

Try to prevent them hurting themselves by protecting the head. The attack will pass. Again, keep talking reassuringly.

> **SAFETY TIP**
> To learn how to find the pulse and how to carry out cardiac massage and mouth-to-mouth resuscitation complete a first aid course!

FAINTING

It can be partial or complete. If partial, the person will feel faint but will not be unconscious. Put their head between their knees or lie them down with their feet raised above their head. Loosen tight clothing. Keep them warm and supply fresh air.

If they have fainted fully and are unconscious, lie them down with their feet raised above their head. Loosen clothing and keep warm. They should recover rapidly, but if they do not, summon expert medical help.

Security in the salon

This topic has been covered in Level 1 Unit 5, page 38. The key is **prevention** of theft of money, stock and people's belongings. Salons will have their own security arrangements and policies on, for example, what to do if a member of staff is caught pilfering. Crime Prevention Officers can give valuable help on both the physical security and the management of security of both people and premises.

Security audits

These are regular reviews of the security of the salon – both while open and when closed. Team involvement is important as team members:

- Can see security being taken seriously, which reassures the honest and may deter the dishonest.
- Can contribute a variety of views and ideas.

A good approach is to consider how the premises could be broken into, and how stock and money could be stolen. When can someone steal unobserved? Put yourself in the place of someone intending to steal.

Stock control procedures

See Level 1 Unit 5, page 35 and Level 2 Unit 9, page 209. Stock control procedures are very important in the prevention of security problems. They are needed to cross-check what has been used and how much money has been taken and by whom.

Things to do

Good hygiene and safety practices are essential in any working environment and great care must always be taken when dealing with any potentially hazardous tools, chemicals or equipment.

The following tasks have been devised to help you to be aware of any potential dangers and the precautions that can be taken to ensure that your salon is a safe place for both yourself and the clients.

1.
   - Use your workplace or training salon to identify any items/situations which could be a safety hazard.
   - Make a chart listing the potentially hazardous items/situations together with any precautions which could minimise the risk to health and safety.

   Use the following layout for your chart:

Item/situation	Precautions
e.g. Frayed electrical wires	Check all wires before using any electrical equipment. Rewire if necessary.

2. Find out from your salon employment or work placement the procedure in case of fire on the premises.

   Design a bright, noticeable poster for display in the salon staff-room which illustrates the risks of fire and your own salon's procedure should a fire occur.

   The poster should be on A5 size paper of any colour using whatever medium or combination of mediums that you consider suitable, e.g. paint, pastels, ink, collage, etc.

3. Carry out a **case study** on the security arrangements of a salon. Include in your review:

   - stock
   - money
   - people's possessions
   - prevention of break-ins when the salon is closed

   Suggest where improvements could be made.

Level 3 Unit 6

List the **three** major groups of hazards to which a client or hairdresser may be exposed. ☐

Give **two** reasons for regularly cleaning the salon. ☐

List the regulations of particular importance to the salon. ☐

Why is it necessary to unplug electrical apparatus before cleaning? ☐

What **two** types of accident are particularly linked to using electrical apparatus? ☐

What is the first action if a chemical has run onto the skin or into the eyes? ☐

What precautions need to be taken in the use, storage and disposal of aerosol spray cans? ☐

What is the difference between infection and infestation? ☐

How in particular can a hairdresser avoid dermatitis? ☐

Name **three** dangers linked to trailing electrical flexes. ☐

CREATING IMAGES

One of the most exciting aspects of hairdressing is being able to express yourself creatively. Unfortunately, unless you work in an avant garde salon, a lot of the day-to-day styling carried out in the average salon is of a more mundane, commercial nature and it is only the occasional client who will allow experimentation of alternative styling on their hair.

However, creativity is the life blood of the hairdressing industry and without it fashions would never change and new techniques would never be born. Keeping your own creativity alive and actively encouraging all staff members to also work imaginatively promotes an enthusiastic team spirit within the salon and is also good for business!

There are various strategies that can be used to allow stylists and junior staff members the opportunity to practise and use their creative skills, these include:

- Competition work.
- Hairstyling for photographic work.
- Staging a hair or fashion show.
- Styling hair for special occasions.
- Using added hair.

Competition work

This type of work stretches practical ability giving more confidence to try out new techniques and ideas. Local colleges and the National Hairdressing Federation (NHF) usually hold local hairdressing competitions which have different events for all levels of experience. Encouraging junior staff members to enter these competitions helps to foster a culture of creativity within the salon right from the beginning.

Competition styling is often quite different from commercial styling, particularly at a more experienced level. It is the opportunity to show off artistic ability and therefore may have little to do with commercial wearability!

Planning competition work

Planning, preparation and practice, then even more practice, is the secret of successful competition work. The following suggestions are by no means complete but could be helpful to the novice competition worker:

1 Attend some competitions before actually entering them. This will give an insight into what is expected. Look carefully at the 'winning' heads, and take photographs to give you ideas on the types of hairstyles and how they differ from commercial work.

2 Choose a suitable model. Ideally they should have good bone structure and an oval face shape as this suits most hairstyles and is therefore creatively less limiting. The texture of the hair should be manageable, neither too thick nor too thin. But most importantly of all, the model *must* have the time for practice sessions and be willing to be adventurous with their hair colour and shape.

3 Decide on the competition to be entered; look through trade magazines then sketch out various ideas to try out.

4 Make out a time schedule for practice sessions and preparing the hair. Work back from the competition date. You will need time to practise the style, colour the hair and cut it. Hair for competition work should not be soft and silky as this is more difficult to work on, therefore, it will need time to 'settle' after the tint or bleach, but if tinted too soon there will be a regrowth!

5 Decide on the type of clothes and make-up to be worn by the model. The competition will stipulate whether the style is to be day, evening or avant garde and the make-up and the clothing should be suitable for the occasion and must also complement the colour and style of the hair. Do not choose an outfit with a collar or high neckline as this could disturb the dressing at the nape of the neck.

Designing and implementing the style

1 Wet the hair then mould it in different directions until the style evolves. Shorter hair is easier to manage unless the competition stipulates that it must be long hair. Draw the style in detail, on paper, how it was done, otherwise you may forget how you did it!

2 Set or blowdry the hair, depending on the type of competition, in the direction of the final dressing. Make a note on the drawing of any alterations you have made.

3 Once the style is decided upon, cut the hair to accentuate the shape. This may mean razor cutting or thinning out any unwanted bulk in the hair, but remember that the model must be able to wear it commercially afterwards!

4 Re-do the hair and take a note of how long it takes. The competition will have a time limit and it is therefore important to time yourself when practising.

5 Keep practising the style until you know exactly where each hair is going and that you are able to keep within the time limit. This stage will usually take weeks not days!

6 Decide on how the hair is to be coloured or bleached, as bleached hair is often easier to work on for competitions. The colours used should emphasise the movements of the style and it is worth noting that lighter, brighter colours show the hair off to its best advantage on the competition floor.

7 Have a final dress rehearsal the day before the competition to make sure that there is time to carry out any alterations to clothing or make-up. On the day, leave plenty of time to reach the venue, take lots of photos of your work and enjoy yourself!

Hair styling for photographic work

Photography for promotional purposes is a specialist skill, so unless you are a very keen amateur photographer it is much better to use an expert. Organising a photographic 'shoot' takes careful planning and many hours of preparation, therefore it is very upsetting, and indeed too late, if after the event the pictures taken do not turn out or are unsatisfactory.

Styling hair for photographic work requires imagination and often problem-solving skills too. The idea is to create an 'image' and the image can be fantasy, avant garde or for a special occasion such as a wedding in addition to commercial styles. It all depends on the type of salon image you wish to portray and what you are trying to achieve through the publicity it will generate.

Planning the photographic session

1 Decide on the 'look' that is to be created and the purpose of the photographs. Remember that any photographs can also be used as a training aid for the other staff members.
2 Sketch out your ideas. Looking at other photographs in fashion magazines often generates ideas. Note the angle and background of the shots, it will help you decide which may be the most effective for your own work.
3 Decide on the model to use. It is a good idea to use other staff members, particularly junior members if possible, as this generates a team spirit and is also a good learning experience for them. It is surprising how much they will learn through helping or just being there.
4 Practise the style(s) beforehand. Use gels, waxes, lacquers or even sugar and water to create the look you want – remember that it is an illusion you are creating and the style does not have to last. If it is only a front view then it does not matter what the back of the head looks like!
5 Make sure that the model's outfit and make-up are suitable for the hairstyle and the image being created.
6 Work out a schedule for the photographic shoot. Be organised, a photographer's time costs money, therefore have everything prepared and ready when they arrive. And finally, always allow for the session taking much longer than you thought!

Carrying out the photographic session

1 Arrive early at the venue to set everything up and get the model organised and ready.
2 Make sure that the background for the photographs is suitable. Does it contrast with the hair colour? Having a dark background with a black-haired model does not work!
3 Make sure that the lighting is adequate and that additional lighting is available should you need it.
4 Always take lots of photographs. You will find, when they are developed, that many will be unsuitable for one reason or another.
5 Keep a record of how the shoot was planned and carried out to refer to in the future. Evaluate what went well and what did not work, this will help you to improve future sessions.

Staging a hair or fashion show

This type of event is a very useful teambuilding and staff development exercise. It is also a very efficient method of promoting the salon and gaining additional clients. Even those clients satisfied with the work of their present salon will be more likely to consider your salon should they ever wish a change.

The organisation and planning of staging a hair or fashion show is covered in detail in Level 3 Unit 10, page 367.

Styling hair for special occasions

Special occasions also allow the stylist the opportunity to be creative. Very often ornamentation will also be used to allow more scope for creativity and enhance the final dressing. The 'special occasion' that most salons deal with on a regular basis is a wedding.

Bridal hairstyling

Because this is regarded as such an important day in the person's life it is essential that the ornamentation forms part of the a total 'look' together with the hairstyle and the dress. This applies to all the members of the wedding party but in particular the bride and the bridesmaids. It is also important to plan carefully beforehand to ensure that the ornamentation is suitable and to the client's liking.

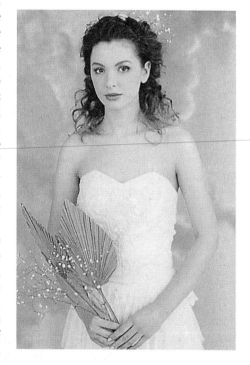

When creating a hairstyle for a bride it is useful to find out as much as possible about all the other accessories that she will be wearing, whether she will be wearing flowers, a bow or a headdress in her hair; for example, if a headdress is to be worn whether it will have a veil or not; the length and thickness of the veil will also be relevant to the choice of style. Finally, find out what type of person the client is. Is she introverted or extroverted? If she is the latter then go for an over-the-top style but if she is the former then her wedding is not the time for drastic changes in style!

The bride must portray a complete image from head to toe, therefore the hairstyle must also be in keeping with the wedding dress. Find out if it is to be classical, Victorian, modern, etc. Obviously the texture and length of the hair will influence the final choice of hairstyle but as a general rule, high necklines such as Edwardian look better with the hair off the face and neck in a roll or knot whilst a low neckline can take a style that is loose and flowing. Tailored suits look good with a sleek style such as a bob whilst a tumble of curls can look stunning with a Pre-Raphaelite style dress.

If possible encourage the client to attend the salon prior to the wedding to condition the hair so that it will look its best on the big day. Organise any cutting and perming so that it is carried out about a month beforehand with any highlighting two weeks before to allow the hair to settle and the client to get used to managing the style. A full-head tint should be carried out approximately three days before so that there will be no regrowth but still allowing the hair time to settle.

Have a 'practice run' before the day to make sure that the client is happy with the style and that it is suitable. Make sure that the bride and any bridesmaids come to the salon as early as possible on the day to help them to relax and to make sure that you have enough time to spend on their hair. If you are going to the bride's home make sure that you allow plenty of time as the bride's house on her wedding day is usually chaotic!

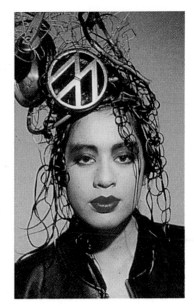

Fig. 3.50 Avant Garde hairstyling

Using added hair

Using additional hair and hairpieces can make natural hair appear longer, thicker, or almost instantly different depending on how, why and when they are used (see Fig. 3.50).

A popular type of added hair is **hair extensions** (see Fig. 3.51). These are made from synthetic fibre or real hair which is woven on to the client's natural hair either throughout the head or just where required. For example, on extremely short hair which is clipper cut at the back the client may only require the extensions at the front.

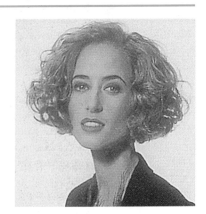

Hair extensions

Hair extensions are a specialised service which involves a very time consuming process and are usually charged for accordingly. Small meshes of hair are sectioned off and the long strands of synthetic fibre are woven into them. The extension is then sealed on to the hair with heat. This is one of the reasons why synthetic fibre is used in preference to human hair as the fibre is able to melt and fuse together thus enabling it to be more firmly anchored and secure. If real hair is used it is woven into the natural hair without sealing with heat.

The extensions should remain in the hair until they grow out. Obviously, harsh brushing or tugging on the hair will loosen the fibre so the client

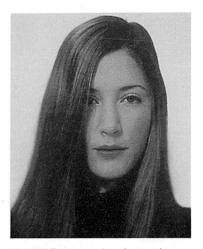

Fig. 3.51 Two examples of extensions

must be given the correct after-care advice to ensure that the extensions last as long as possible.

An extension for African Caribbean hair is shown in Fig. 3.52.

Hairpieces (postiche)

These were at their most popular during the 1960s and 70s but they are still useful today for special occasions, photographic or show work.

. They are available in various hair lengths and sizes, the choice of which depends on the finished style and how they are to be dressed. They can have either a woven base which can be hand or machine made or a knotted base which must be hand knotted. Most types of hairpiece can be obtained in both synthetic or human hair and the price will depend on the quality.

When dressing hair using hairpieces, remember to select the most suitable type of hairpiece for the effect you wish to achieve (Fig. 3.53). Postiche is like natural hair in that you can only work within the confines of what you have. Thus, if the client requires a plait then the hairpiece must have enough length to achieve this effect.

Set or blowdry the hairpiece into the required style on a malleable block. If it is made of synthetic fibre then follow the manufacturer's instructions as the fibres will usually melt if any kind of heat is used. The dressing can be carried out either on the block or on the client's head. Hairpieces can be obtained directly from the manufacturer or through the wholesaler.

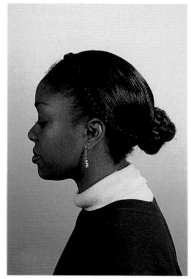
Fig. 3.52 Hair extensions used on African Caribbean hair to create a classic look

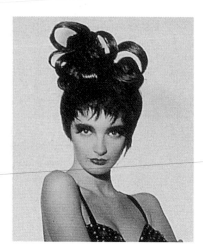
Fig. 3.53 Just one way to use a hairpiece

Attaching a hairpiece

To attach the hairpiece to the head, first brush or comb the hair in the direction of the style, decide on the position of the hairpiece on the head then section off a square mesh of hair in the centre of this position, curl it round in a pincurl and secure with two crossed hairgrips. If the base of the hairpiece has a comb this can then be pushed under the grips to hold it firm. Use hairgrips to attach the hairpiece to the scalp taking care not to harm the base. If the grips are placed correctly there should be no need to use an excessive amount, it is also useful to try to place the grips in approximately the same places each time you attach a hairpiece so that when it has to be removed you do not have to struggle to find the grips!

Backcomb/backbrush the natural hair if required (this is often done before attaching the hairpiece) then blend the hair with the hairpiece making sure that its base is camouflaged and that all hard lines and edges are also blended.

Advise the client on the care of the hairpiece and demonstrate how it is attached and removed. If the hairpiece is treated correctly it will last for many years with the minimum of upkeep.

You are asked by your salon manager to organise a photographic 'shoot'. The purpose of the event is to market your salon's new range of hair products. The manager wishes to see a layout of your plan and your ideas before it is implemented.

The following stages may help you to organise the shoot:

- Identify a suitable time and venue which will cause the minimum inconvenience and disruption to normal working practice. Decide who is to take the photographs.
- Make a list of 'objectives', that is, what you are hoping to achieve from the event.
- Write out a memo to the staff involved informing them of the event and allowing them enough time to organise their schedules, and practise the hairstyles if necessary.
- Contact all models who may be required and have a back-up in case of emergencies.
- Ensure all resources and equipment are available and in working order on the date required.
- Discuss with other staff members what incentives, if any, can be implemented to bring additional trade to the salon through the event.
- Plan how you will evaluate the effectiveness of the event.

What do you know?

Level 3 Unit 7

Explain why it is important to pre-plan any event ☐

Why is it beneficial to the salon to include junior staff members in all the events? ☐

What considerations are necessary when choosing a model for competition styling? ☐

What considerations are necessary when preparing for a photographic shoot? ☐

List the differences between commercial styling, avant garde styling and fantasy styling. ☐

Describe how you would attach a hairpiece to the client's head. ☐

AFRICAN CARIBBEAN HAIRDRESSING

Background information

The main difference between African Caribbean hair and European (Caucasian) hair is that while European hair is either fine, medium or coarse textured, the texture of African Caribbean hair varies along the actual hair shaft. This results in an uneven porosity along the length of each individual hair which creates special problems when chemicals are applied. Extra care and thought is essential before and during the treatment of African Caribbean hair to prevent damage and/or breakage to the weaker and more porous areas.

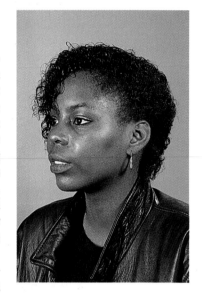

The degree of curl in this type of hair also differs from that of most European hair. African Caribbean hair has a very diffuse hair growth direction pattern which makes it difficult to manage as it does not fall in uniform waves. It is usually extremely dry and brittle which means that it can be easily broken during combing or when using heated appliances. Both the hair and the scalp should be kept well oiled and supple through the use of conditioners, oils and waxes. Because of the excess dryness, specialised products containing ingredients such as protein, lanolin, natural and mineral oils are more effective than the conditioning agents formulated for European hair.

The anagen stage of African Caribbean hair growth may last only nine to ten months and the growth rate is also often slower, therefore African Caribbean hair is considered to be long if it is 18–20 cm (7–8"). However, because of its tightly coiled nature the hair usually appears shorter than it actually is. The amount of curl present in the hair will depend on hereditary factors, e.g. African hair is very curly whilst Guyanese hair is merely curly.

When permanently changing the shape of African Caribbean hair (curling or straightening), the same structural alteration takes place as in European hair, i.e. breaking sufficient chemical bonds within the hair and rejoining them in a new shape. However, specialised African Caribbean straighteners are very strong and could easily dissolve the hair if not used correctly.

Straightening hair

This is the process of reducing curl or wave to make it straighter. Hair can be straightened either temporarily or permanently. Straightening the hair temporarily usually requires some form of heat if it is to be successful (see Fig. 3.54). The two main methods of temporarily straightening hair are:

- Wet setting; blowdrying, roller setting, etc.
- Dry setting; pulling the hair straighter using pressing combs and then curling with heated curling tongs, marcel waving irons, hot brushes or heated rollers.

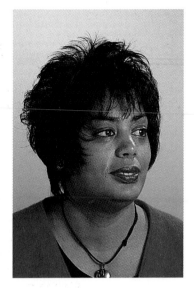

Fig. 3.54 Thermally styled hair

Temporarily straightening African Caribbean hair

African Caribbean hair can be temporarily set by either blowdrying using a wide-toothed comb attachment which is fitted to the nozzle of the hair drier or by using a pressing comb. Some of the water found naturally in the cortex is turned into steam by the heat of the drier or pressing comb. This steam breaks some of the weaker hydrogen cross-linkages. The cross-linkages re-form themselves in their new, straightened positions as the hair cools.

There are two main ways of temporarily straightening African Caribbean hair using heat:

- Soft pressing.
- Hard pressing.

Soft pressing
Sometimes referred to as single comb pressing, this is straightening the hair with the pressing comb once all over the head.

Hard pressing
This is straightening the hair twice with the pressing comb. This means that the hair has double the heat applied than when soft pressing, which makes it unsuitable for more fragile hair types. Sometimes referred to as double comb pressing.

Equipment required for pressing the hair

- Pressing combs of various sizes.
- Electric or gas heater (unless the pressing combs are electrically heated).
- Vulcanite comb.
- Protective pressing cream or oil.
- Finishing oils or waxes.
- Heated curling tongs or marcel waving irons.

Considerations before pressing the hair

Hair pressing can be damaging to the hair and scalp so it is essential to carry out a thorough hair and scalp analysis. Look closely at the hair then feel the condition, if in doubt always carry out a porosity and elasticity test. This is particularly important if the hair has had any previous chemical treatment (see Level 2 Unit 5B for how this is done). If the hair is in poor condition or very porous, recommend a course of reconditioning treatments to the client and postpone the pressing until the hair is stronger and more supple.

Examine the scalp carefully. If there are any cuts or scratches, protect with barrier cream unless they are major in which case it may be necessary to postpone the treatment. Do not carry out any hairdressing services if the client has an infectious or contagious skin condition.

Hair is hygroscopic; therefore, because the heat from the pressing comb has removed most of the hair's natural moisture from the cortex, any water or dampness in the atmosphere will make the hair revert back to its previous curly state. What is known as 'touch up' pressing of the unwanted curly parts of the hairstyle is done if this occurs.

The greater the heat used on the hair the more bonds are broken; therefore, if the pressing comb is too cool the straightening will not last but if is too hot then the hair may be burned or singed. Chemically treated hair has bonds which will break more easily, therefore additional care must be taken when dealing with this type of hair.

Contra-indications when pressing the hair

Do not straighten the hair by pressing if:

- There are any infectious or contagious conditions present.
- There are major cuts and scratches or sores on the scalp.
- The hair is in a fragile state or there is hair breakage present.
- The hair is excessively porous or highly bleached.
- The client has a headache, as the pulling action when tension is applied could be unbearable for the client.

Procedure for soft pressing African Caribbean hair

Soft pressing will remove 70 per cent of the curl.

1. Protect the client with a gown and towel.
2. Check the hair and scalp for any contra-indications.
3. Shampoo the hair with a suitable shampoo, then dry.
4. Divide the hair into four sections: forehead to nape and ear to ear, across the back of the head.
5. Starting at the nape, take a 1.25 cm ($\frac{1}{2}$″) section of hair and apply oil or conditioning cream to the section. Lift the hair away from the scalp at 90° using the index finger and the thumb.

> **SAFETY TIP**
> Excessive heat on the hair can cause scorching and loss of colour or discoloration of the hair

6 Check the heat of the pressing comb then insert the pressing comb teeth into the hair section 1.25 cm ($\frac{1}{2}$") away from the scalp.

7 Slide the comb down the hair mesh, turning it so that the back of the comb is positioned on top of the hair mesh. The angle of the comb is very important as it is the back of the comb which creates the tension and actually straightens the hair.

8 Comb each section two or three times in this manner until the hair is straight.

9 Continue towards the front of the head taking 1.25 cm ($\frac{1}{2}$") sections until the whole head has been completed.

10 Apply dressing cream or oil to the hair and brush thoroughly.

11 Style the hair with curling tongs.

12 Complete a record of work and advise the client on the care of their hairstyle including any preparations that would aid the condition of the hair and add to the longevity of the hairstyle.

Procedure for hard pressing African Caribbean hair

Hard pressing will remove almost all the curl but will also weaken the hair, so great caution is required when carrying out this service. Proceed as for soft pressing then either repeat the process or restraighten using marcel waving irons.

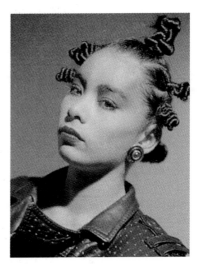

Precautions and considerations

● Check that the hair is strong enough to withstand the tension and heat needed during the process. Fine hair will require less tension and cooler temperature than coarse hair.

● Take special care with bleached or tinted hair. Remember that it is usually more fragile than untreated hair and will therefore require a cooler temperature and less tension to prevent breakage.

● Always use oil, cream or conditioner on the hair before pressing. This will lubricate the hair, make it more pliable and help prevent burning and scorching.

● During the process, ensure that the back of the comb is pulled along the top of the hair section as it is this part of the comb which smooths and straightens the hair.

● Make sure that enough tension is exerted on the hair to make it straight.

● Advise the client that pressing is a temporary means of straightening hair and will only last between seven and ten days. Any dampness in the atmosphere will cause the hair to revert back to its curly state.

● Always use a dressing cream or oil after the process to replace some of the natural oils and give the hair shine.

> SAFETY TIP
> ● Always check that the pressing comb is at the correct temperature for the type of hair. Electric pressing combs are thermostatically controlled but non-electric combs are heated by heaters and may get too hot if not properly controlled.
> ● Great care must be taken not to touch the scalp or skin with the hot comb or burning will occur.
> ● Do not attempt to straighten very short hair as there is a danger of burning the scalp and skin.

Touching up

This is carried out, between shampoos, to prolong the life of the pressing by restraightening any part of the hair which has reverted back to its curly state through water or atmospheric moisture. Sometimes it is only the roots, or a small area, which will require touching up, in which case a 'spot' touch up is all that is required. If a larger area requires restraightening, then the same procedure as for soft pressing is followed but omitting the shampoo stage.

Precautions and considerations when hard and soft pressing the hair

1 *Always* assess the hair and scalp thoroughly before pressing the hair, carry out any necessary tests before starting the treatment.
2 Coarse hair is often the most difficult to press and will require the most heat, medium textured hair responds well to pressing whilst fine hair requires less pressure and a lower heat as it could break or burn more easily.
3 Bleached, tinted or porous hair requires special attention. Use a lower heat and less pressure on this type of hair. It may be necessary to condition and moisturise the hair well beforehand.
4 Take care not to discolour grey or white hair. Use a lower heat if necessary.
5 Take all necessary precautions to avoid burning the client's skin, particularly if the hair is short. Be aware of health and safety at all times.
6 Always advise the client on the after-care of their hair. Hairsprays, oils and gloss will all help to protect the hair from the effect of atmospheric moisture, prolonging the life of the pressing.
7 Clean all tools and equipment after use. The oils used on the hair tend to burn onto the pressing comb and other electrical equipment. This causes a build up if not removed after each service and makes the equipment less efficient.

Relaxing African Caribbean hair

What happens to the hair and the method used to relax African Caribbean hair is covered in detail in Level 2 Unit 5B. But the process can be summarised as follows.

Calcium hydroxide, potassium hydroxide or sodium hydroxide are the chemicals used to relax hair although sodium hydroxide is the one most commonly used. They are extremely alkaline with a pH of between 10 and 14 and can therefore cause a great deal of damage to the hair if not used correctly and in strict accordance with the manufacturer's instructions. It is also important to use the correct neutralising shampoo for the relaxing agent otherwise there could be an adverse reaction between the chemicals used.

Unlike perming, which is a reduction then oxidation process, relaxing occurs through **hydrolysis**. This is a complicated process and is detailed in Level 2 Unit 5B.

Because of the damage that can be caused by relaxing agents, it is very important that a porosity test, elasticity test and pre-perm test are carried out before starting the treatment to make sure that the hair can withstand the chemicals. The tests will also give some idea of the development time and the strength of relaxer to use. An incompatibility test may also need to be carried out if the client has been treating their own hair with unknown chemicals. These unknown chemicals could contain metallic salts which would react with the relaxing agent. If there is any doubt, do not proceed with the relaxing treatment. A selection of possible problems, their causes and their remedies is given in Table 3.2.

Protection of the client when relaxing hair

Relaxer creams are extremely strong chemicals therefore it is extremely important to protect the client and their clothing. The client's clothing is protected with a gown and a towel tucked well down at the nape. A piece of polythene pinned to the hair at the nape, covering the neck, is also sometimes used as additional protection. The client's skin is protected with a petroleum cream which is referred to as a **base** cream. This is applied all around the hairline, ears and scalp and is known as **basing**. However, not all relaxing products need to have the whole of the scalp based, so always read the manufacturer's instructions before starting the treatment – it may only be necessary to protect the hairline and ears.

Table 3.2 Possible problems, causes and remedies

Problem	Cause and remedy
Hair reverts back to curly	• Oily barrier on the hair • Too weak relaxer used • Product is off, not correctly sealed after use *Remedy: Condition and test hair for elasticity and strength. Re-relax if the hair is strong enough*
Hair breakage	• Too much tension put on hair whilst developing • Too strong relaxer used • Development too long • Hair in poor condition *Remedy: Condition and moisturise hair thoroughly with specialised products. Hair may need cutting*
Appearance of orange bands on the hair	• Overlapping of relaxer onto previously relaxed hair – hair will break *Remedy: Condition and moisturise thoroughly with specialised products*
Skin irritation or burns	• Not enough basing cream applied to skin • Relaxer in contact with skin *Remedy: Rinse thoroughly in plenty of water. Apply neutralising shampoo to counteract alkalinity. Seek medical aid*
Hair very dry and brittle	• No pre-perm treatment used • Too strong relaxer used • Not conditioned enough after treatment *Remedy: Condition and moisturise thoroughly using specialised products*
Relaxer enters eye	• Not rinsing at backwash • Sloppy application *Remedy: Rinse thoroughly in plenty of water. Seek medical aid*
Trying to perm relaxed hair	• Do not do it, the perm will not take and the hair will be excessively damaged!

Basing method

Section the hair into four, forehead to nape then ear to ear across the back. Take small sections of hair, press the cream onto the scalp taking care not to rub or spread the cream or it could coat the hair and form a barrier. The client's body heat melts the cream enabling it to cover all the scalp.

Partial relaxing of African Caribbean hair

This is often done on shorter hair, particularly men's hair when only the longer top layers of the hair need to be straightened.

Method

1 Carry out a hair and scalp analysis and any necessary tests. Consult with the client to determine their requirements.
2 If all tests are satisfactory, proceed with the relaxing treatment.
3 Protect the client with gown and towels. Protect yourself with rubber gloves and plastic or tinting apron. Apply protective cream around the hairline and scalp if necessary (follow manufacturer's instructions).
4 Apply barrier cream or conditioner to the hair that is to be left untreated as this will protect it from the relaxer. A strip of cotton wool may also be placed over this hair as an added barrier.
5 Do not shampoo the hair unless heavily coated in oils and waxes. Apply pre-perm treatment if necessary to the hair to be relaxed. Cut the hair after the treatment when it will be more manageable.
6 Starting with the underneath hair, take sections of 1.25 cm ($\frac{1}{2}$"). Place relaxing cream on the back of the gloved hand for ease of access. Apply relaxer to the hair section, 1.25 cm ($\frac{1}{2}$") from the scalp with either a tinting brush or tail comb.
7 When application is complete, cross-check the hair to ensure an even coverage. Leave it to develop according to manufacturer's instructions. Do not be tempted to leave the relaxer in contact with the hair longer than the recommended time or it could be irreparably damaged.
8 When processed, comb through the hair gently. Then rinse thoroughly, at a back wash, in warm water using the force of the water to remove the relaxer. Handle the hair as little as possible at this point as it is in a fragile state.
9 Apply the correct acidic neutralising shampoo to neutralise the alkalinity of the relaxer. Follow manufacturer's instructions as it may be necessary to shampoo the hair two or three times. Do not rub the hair, use effleurage stroking movements to minimise any tangling or damage. Rinse thoroughly.
10 Apply conditioning or moisturising agent. This may need to be left in contact with the hair for five to ten minutes. Remove and blot the hair gently; it is important not to rub the hair at any stage of the process.
11 Cut and style into shape as required. Advise client on the after-care of their hair. Complete a record card.

Precautions and considerations when relaxing hair

1 Carry out all relevant tests before beginning the relaxing.
2 Wait at least 72 hours after tinting to relax the hair.
3 Leave braided hair unbraided for at least a week before relaxing.
4 Do not relax the hair if there are cuts and abrasions on the scalp.

5 If hair requires re-relaxing *do not* carry out the second application within one week of the first and always test the hair to make sure that it can withstand a further treatment.

6 *Do not* relax the hair if there is any breakage present. Once you agree to treat the hair, any breakage (including the previous breakage) becomes your salon's responsibility.

7 Do not shampoo the hair before relaxing; it will remove the protective layer of sebum from the scalp.

8 Always wear protective rubber gloves when carrying out the treatment.

9 Never use heat to quicken the development time.

10 Always use the weakest product possible for the hair. If development is slow, reapply with a stronger product.

11 Use the complementary neutralising shampoo for the relaxing product used.

12 Always replace the lid firmly on the relaxer cream to prevent it going off.

13 Different products do vary slightly; always follow the manufacturer's instructions very strictly together with all safety guidelines.

14 African Caribbean hair requires a higher level of moisture that Caucasian hair. Always use specialised African Caribbean products as they are specifically designed to moisturise thoroughly.

15 Keep a precise record of all work carried out for future reference and in case of any future problems.

Things to do

1 Collect pictures of African Caribbean hairstyles.

2 Mount them on plain paper then divide them under the headings: *Short hairstyles, Medium-length hairstyles, Long hairstyles.*

3 Produce an African Caribbean style book for use in your salon. You can also use this for training sessions with your junior staff members.

What do you know?

Level 3 Unit 8

State as many health and safety precautions as you can when soft and hard pressing the hair. ☐

List six contra-indications when soft and hard pressing African Caribbean hair. ☐

Which type of hair is most difficult to press? ☐

Describe what happens to the internal structure of the hair when pressing the hair. ☐

Give a brief summary of the advice you would give to a client regarding the after-care of a pressing treatment ☐

List the contra-indications when relaxing hair. ☐

What is the main active ingredient in relaxing creams? ☐

What happens to the internal structure of the hair during the relaxing process? ☐

List any possible problems that could occur when relaxing the hair. Give possible solutions to the problems you have listed. ☐

CREATIVE SETTING AND DRESSING HAIR

Creative setting

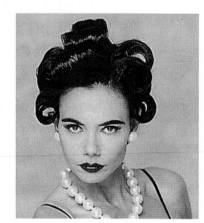

Creative setting means setting the hair imaginatively to produce an up-to-date style. This can include the use of rollers, rods, pincurls, fingers or any other suitable means to provide the desired effect, which may be flat, lifted, curly, waved, straight or a combination of any/all of these.

Setting can also be used in conjunction with blowdrying, blow waving or finger drying and can be carried out on wet, damp or dry hair. The wetter the hair, the more crisp and long-lasting the result. However, leaving the hair too wet is uncomfortable for the client and is time consuming to dry.

As with any treatment, it is important to carefully assess the hair and discuss with the client their requirements before actually starting the treatment. Consider where volume, if any, is required, hair growth patterns and the direction of any movement before deciding the most suitable method of obtaining the desired effect.

Hairstyles can be broadly divided into three main 'looks':

- Classic.
- Fashion.
- Avant garde.

Classic

This look withstands the test of time! A good example of this type of timeless style is the 'bob'. The bob of the 1960s looks just as good in the 1990s. Mature or business clients often prefer smart, classical styles which flatter their image.

Fashion

Fashion styles are the look of the moment and therefore often change quite quickly. Interestingly, classic haircuts can frequently be adapted to meet new fashion trends.

Avant garde

Unusual, different, striking and often fun are descriptions of the avant garde style. Not usually suitable for the quiet, shy type of client! However these styles are often adapted down to become the fashion styles of the future.

Setting aids

There are many products which can be used to help mould the hair and also prolong the 'life' of the set. Manufacturers all have various mousses, gels, waxes and lacquers to suit the different hair types. Choosing which to use will depend on the texture and condition of the hair and the required result (see Level 2 Unit 11).

Sectioning

The sections used will again depend on the required result and what tools are being used. Using zig-zag partings will help prevent 'tramlines' whilst square sections may be required with some winds, e.g. spiral. However, care should be taken when sectioning the hair to ensure that it is appropriate to the setting technique used and that it is an integral part of the setting process.

Creative setting techniques

Creative setting builds on the principles learnt for basic setting which are then combined and adapted to suit the needs of the finished style. Competition hairstyling is a good example of moulding the hair into the required shape and direction by adapting basic setting principles. The techniques that can be employed are therefore limitless, particularly when combining many methods on one head. Some examples of how basic techniques have been adapted are explained below.

Spiral setting

This is similar to spiral perming in that the hair is wound spirally down the length of the rod from root to point. Alternative, rectangular-shaped rods can be used to create angular shaped curls. The hair should be damp, not wet, and sections should be larger than those taken when perming, otherwise too much curl will result.

Method
1 Disentangle hair.
2 Comb in direction of final hair position with any partings or fringes, etc.
3 Apply suitable setting aid after consultation with the client to explain benefits and price.
4 Wind hair spirally on the rods, taking square sections from the nape up towards the front of the head.
5 Place client under suitable drying appliance. Spirally wound hair is very bulky and may not fit under a conventional drier; therefore a climazone, octopus or rollerball machine may have to be used.
6 When dry, dress into style usually with the fingers as combing spirally wound hair can often produce too much curl.
7 Use wax, gel, mousse or lacquer as appropriate to achieve the desired effect (see Fig. 3.55).

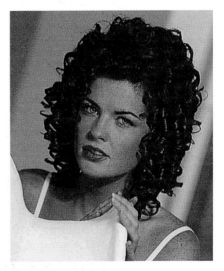

Fig. 3.55 Spiral wind – finished look

Alternating or reverse wind

This type of wind will produce volume in the hair. The rollers are placed in the direction of the finished dressing but where additional volume is required, one roller is wound up then the next down so that the curl or movement is pushed against each other creating volume in the hair. This type of wind is usually used in conjunction with other methods (see Fig. 3.56).

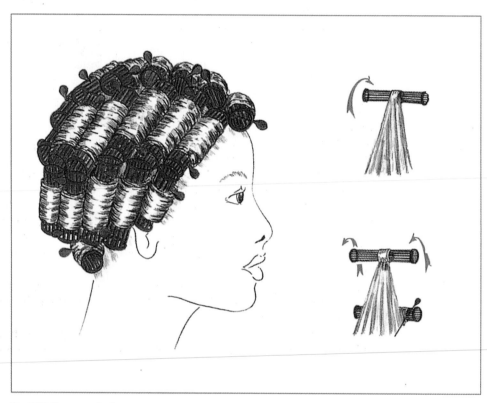

Fig. 3.56 Reverse wind

Directional setting

Comb the hair in the direction and shape of the finished dressing. Determine the amount of curl/movement, if any, required and identify where the hair needs to be lifted and where it needs to be flat. Select appropriate tools and equipment and set the hair in the direction that it has been combed. Remember that any rollers placed in the hair will give lift – controlled overdirecting or dragging of the hair at the root will give various types of lift depending on the positioning of the rollers. Experimenting with placing the rollers at different angles and base positions can create endless possibilities. It may be necessary to incorporate a variety of techniques (such as pincurling, finger waving or blow styling) into one head.

Specialised dressing of hair

Dressing hair successfully requires practice, patience and an aesthetic understanding of line and balance. The tools and products used should be carefully chosen to suit the requirements of the style and the type of hair that the stylist is working with. This may sound obvious but it is surprising how many stylists make their work more difficult by using unsuitable equipment and wrongly selected products.

Dealing with long hair

Long hair is often believed to be the most difficult to deal with and, indeed, many stylists are inhibited by this. Certainly, the styling of long hair is usually more time consuming than shorter hair, but long hair offers the stylist a whole new world of creativity and as with any other skill, the more that it is practised then the more proficient and creative the stylist will become.

Long haired blocks are ideal for practising long hair styling as they can be used whenever there is a free or quiet moment in the salon or they can be taken home to try out any new ideas.

To look its best, long hair must be shiny with no breakage or split ends; therefore, the **condition** of the hair must *always* be of the utmost importance whenever a service is being carried out.

There are significant differences between dealing with short and long hair and the following checklist (which is by no means complete) outlines the main areas to consider.

Considerations when setting and drying long hair

1 A better result can be obtained by setting the hair when it is damp as the finished result tends to be over curly if it is set from wet. Use a good, suitable setting agent such as mousse to give the hair body and protection.
2 Choose the roller size carefully. Unless a lot of curl is required, it is usual to use a large roller to achieve most effects.
3 Because of its length, long hair takes a long time to dry. Therefore, before styling, near-dry the hair first to remove the excess moisture.
4 When drying the hair it is often more efficient to use the fingers instead of a brush. Aim the air-stream down the hair shaft alternating between hot and cold air to smooth the hair.
5 Do not over-dry the hair. Leave it slightly damp before using heated rollers, tongs or hot sticks. The heat from these appliances will finish the drying process.
6 Use a diffuser attachment on the blowdrier when drying long, curly hair which requires curl in the finished style. It helps to prevent frizzing.

7 Do not set the heat of a drier too high as it can damage the hair and dry out its moisture content.

Considerations when dressing long hair

1 Always use a dressing cream, oil or wax, particularly on the ends of the hair, to replace the natural oil and give the hair shine.

2 If the dressing requires backcombing, try to keep it to the root area only (unless the style dictates otherwise) to minimise the risk of breakage or damage to the hair.

3 Make sure that smooth styles are thoroughly brushed before dressing. However, styles which are very curly are usually dressed using only the fingers or an Afro-type comb as brushing this type of style would create frizzing of the hair.

4 To prevent damage to the hair, use bands which are covered and grips which have covered ends, if they are needed, to put the hair up.

5 Trying to cope with a large amount of hair can be overwhelming for some stylists so decide on the overall effect to be achieved before starting, then break down the task into small stages.

6 Work methodically through the dressing. Don't panic!

7 Make sure that the head is kept in the correct position while dressing. For example, if it is held to one side at an angle when putting the hair up it will alter the balance of the style.

8 Because of its weight, very long hair, e.g. waist length, is often difficult to secure with hair grips and covered elastic bands. When creating chignons on this hair length it is usually easier, quicker and firmer to tie the hair *itself* into an ordinary knot then secure in position with hair grips. By sectioning the hair and knotting it in different places many different and unusual effects can be achieved.

9 When the dressing is finished, check its **shape** from all angles, particularly if the hair has been put up or drawn away from the face.

10 Aim for a 'natural' look when dressing long hair down or in a combination of up and down.

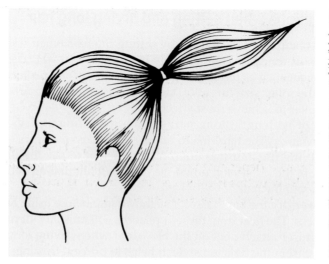

Fig. 3.57

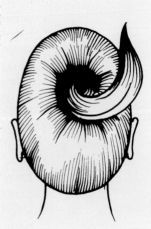

Fig. 3.58

Dressing long hair into a classic knot on the crown

1 Position the client's head at the appropriate angle. Brush the hair thoroughly away from the hairline and up towards the crown (see Fig. 3.57). Secure in a ponytail with a covered band.

2 Twist the hair in an anti-clockwise direction and secure with hair grips (see Fig. 3.58). Tuck the ends of the hair underneath the previously wound hair and make firm with hair grips (see Fig. 3.59).

Variations can be made to this method of dressing hair to produce a knot at the nape or an asymmetrical hair knot. (See Level 2 Unit 11 for other classical long hair dressings.)

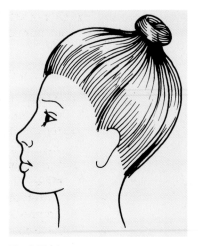

Fig. 3.59

Dressing long hair down

When dressing the hair down or partially down with some hair up, a more natural look is often required unless the client stipulates a more avant garde image, in which case added hair may also be incorporated into the dressing. The preparation of the hair before styling will determine the amount and crispness of any curl or movement. The stylist has several choices, the hair can be:

- Wet set or blowdried.
- Damp dried then set or blowdried.
- Completely dried then curled (or straightened).

Wet set or blowdried

Not recommended for very long hair as the drying time would be excessive. Moulding the hair from wet will usually make it more 'crisp' with possibly a longer lasting curl. However it can often be difficult to dress because of the amount of bounce that is produced.

Damp dried then set or blowdried

This is usually the most suitable preparation for long hair as it cuts down drying time and the hair tends to be more manageable to dress.

Completely dried then curled/straightened

This method is often used in conjunction with heated curling tongs, hot brush or straightening irons depending on the required result. It is possible to produce very effective results with this method and the hair can be made as curly or as straight as necessary, depending on the equipment used.

Setting and dressing hair creatively requires practice and skill. The following task has been devised to help you to identify and then practise certain 'looks'.

1 Collect pictures of as many hairstyles as possible.

2 Divide them into three under the headings of: *Avant garde*, *Fashion* and *Classical* hairstyles.

3 Create three style books from your pictures to use for future reference.

4 Try to emulate these styles on other staff members, friends or clients. Make sure that the style is suitable! If you are unsure of the factors to take into consideration, read through this unit again.

5 Take photographs of your work and place in your portfolio together with any other supporting evidence.

What do you know?

Level 3 Unit 9

What factors need to be considered before setting? ☐

Why is it advisable to spirally set hair which is damp not wet? ☐

Which type of setting wind produces extra volume in the hair? ☐

Which blowdrier attachment helps to prevent frizzing? ☐

List three methods of preparing long hair before dressing. ☐

Why is it necessary to keep the head in position while dressing? ☐

Give a brief description of what is meant by the following types of hairstyles:

- *Avant garde*
- *Fashion*
- *Classic* ☐

SALON PROMOTIONAL ACTIVITIES

Promotion is an important part of marketing the goods and services a salon offers. There are a variety of ways this can be carried out. These include:

- Demonstration – both for staff and in a promotional context.
- Staging displays.
- Taking part in shows.
- Use of incentives.
- Use of promotional materials.

Demonstrations, displays and shows are very similar and will all be considered under '**Demonstrating**'.

Demonstrating

The ability to demonstrate clearly a hairdressing procedure is very important in both of the following areas:

- Demonstrating practical skills to staff.
- Demonstrating to the public.

Demonstrating practical skills to staff

This type of demonstration must be carefully planned to ensure that the demonstration clearly illustrates the **key** points you wish to emphasise and the practical skills involved. It is worth remembering that an audience has a limited attention span of about 20 minutes, so the demonstration should vary in pace and allow time for the trainee to experiment or practise themselves. Learning is more efficient if the trainee is allowed to use as many of the senses as possible, including those of touch and smell as well as watching and listening.

Good preparation is the key to success when demonstrating and careful planning of specific areas, as shown in Fig. 3.60.

There are a number of ways of laying out plans for demonstrations and training. Figure 3.61 is an example of one you may wish to use.

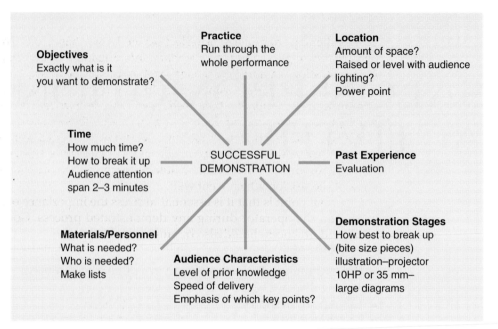

Fig. 3.60 Planning a demonstration

Title... Time allowed			
Objective	Time	Method	Materials

Fig. 3.61 Session plan

Feedback

Feedback is the information you receive from the audience during (and after) your demonstration. During the performance take care to look at the audience, to determine what signals they are sending. Are the signals negative with shifting around, talking or staring into space, or are they positive, with people giving their full attention, everyone sitting still and smiling when you make eye contact? There may be a mixture of both types of signals and it is important to assess the reasons for the differences.

At the end of the demonstration the level of questions and the length of time people linger are signs of their attitudes. Individuals may say flattering (or unflattering) things to you. However, be aware that these are probably people who feel much more strongly than the 'average' audience member. Formal feedback can be obtained using a short questionnaire on a postcard or small sheet of paper. Keep these short and clear. Try to use 'tick the box' answers for speed but allow some space for written reactions and comments.

Evaluation

This is the important stage of reflecting on 'how it has gone'. This review should be very thorough and needs to be taken into consideration when planning the next demonstration. In addition to staff and audience feedback, the model and your own evaluation of the session will help you to assess the level of success. When demonstrating to trainees, their feedback allows you to define 'success' in terms of whether you have reached the training goals with those trainees.

Always find the time to write down a summary of what went well or what did not and any lessons for the future. It may be some time before you do the same thing again and you will then be able to learn from any mistakes as well as the parts of the session which went well.

One final point is that it is essential to stress the importance of safety to both the client and the operator during any demonstrated process. Good hygiene procedures and practices should also be emphasised.

Staging and taking part in promotional shows

This is an extremely effective means of improving public relations and promoting the salon. It is also a good way to motivate the entire staff as everyone from the top stylist to the shampooist can be involved. Staging a demonstration is a stimulating experience which reinforces working together 'as a team' and encourages the stylists to give full vent to their creativity.

Hair demonstrations can be linked up with talks on different aspects of hair care or can be used as a showcase to present a specific 'look' which the salon is promoting. Demonstrations can be staged by the salon on its own or as a joint venture with another organisation. For example, boutiques or in-store fashion shows need hairdressers and make-up artists to make the most of their models and show off their fashion clothes to best effect.

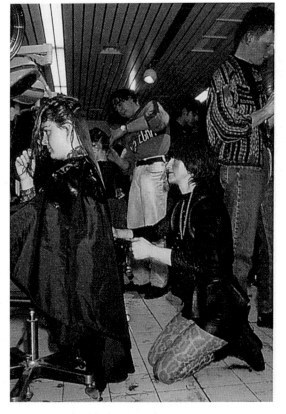

The best way to get involved with this type of work is to write to or go to see the store/boutique in question, usually in your client catchment area, taking photographs of the salon's work to give an indication of the standard and variety of work the salon can achieve. Invite relevant managers or the public relations officer (PRO) along to your salon to see the work you are doing and offer very competitive rates or, better still, do the show free of charge at first.

The type of audience you wish to attract will make a difference to the type of demonstration you present. Organising a hairdressing demonstration for younger people at a Youth Club will obviously be approached differently from staging a high-profile, expensive demonstration to a mixed audience in a top-class hotel. If the audience has paid a high price for a ticket to attend a top-class venue, then their expectations will differ from the audience that is attending a free demonstration. For this reason, it is extremely important to decide at the beginning what type of demonstration you wish to present and what the target audience will be.

POINTS TO REMEMBER

Every hair and fashion demonstration/show *must* be organised to the very last detail and timing needs to be split-second. If not, there can be embarrassing gaps in the programme, misleading information given about the hairstyles and clothes, or the wrong clothes may be worn for that part of the programme.

Organisation of tasks

Begin by delegating certain tasks and roles to a number of people. Depending on the size and type of demonstration, all or some of the following roles will have to be allocated:

- Co-ordinator.
- Compère.
- Hairstylists.
- Trainees/juniors.
- Make-up artist.
- Wardrobe mistress/dresser.
- Disc jockey (DJ).
- Models.
- Photographer.

Co-ordinator

This is the key role as the co-ordinator has overall responsibility for organising and liaising with management on the venue, music, lighting, seating, advertising, and printing and distribution of any necessary tickets. They must also make out a schedule of work and timetable both for the countdown and the actual day of the event to ensure that everyone knows exactly what they are doing and when.

Compère

This is also an important role, as the person selected will have to speak through a microphone in front of the audience. Therefore, they must have good communication skills and the self-confidence to speak in public.

They must be able to handle interruptions from the audience. Sometimes questions asked during the demonstration can be a useful means of explaining certain processes being carried out on stage, but this really depends on the type of demonstration. Too many questions may sidetrack the commentary and then become an intrusion. It may be necessary to insist that all questions be saved until the end of the session.

The compère must be sensitive at all times to the atmosphere conveyed by the audience and must be able to pitch the commentary at the correct level for the type of audience. Making the commentary too technical may bore the audience, whilst pitching it at too low a level is embarrassing and will make them feel uncomfortable.

If the audience appears restless or uninterested, then the compère must be able to regain the audience's attention by various strategies, e.g. humour; increasing the 'pace' of the demonstration; adding anecdotes; etc.

For demonstrations linked to hair care it may be possible to contact leading manufacturers to see if any of their senior sales staff would be willing to take on this role.

Hairstylists

They must be quick and efficient. If dressing the hair in public they must be confident working in front of an audience. When styling the hair for a fashion show, they often have to work in very cramped, backstage quarters. They must be able to create and convert hairstyles on long or short hair quickly, using temporary methods of curling, such as heated rollers, hot sticks, or curling tongs, as it may not be possible to wet the hair.

Trainees/juniors

They are needed to carry out any of the preliminary tasks on the hair or to help the stylists before, during and after the performance. They must make sure that everywhere is cleaned and tidied after use and check that all equipment is cleaned and returned to the salon. Often it is useful to allow the trainees to help the stylist at the demonstration, as it gives them valuable experience of working in front of an audience, boosts their confidence and makes them feel important members of the team.

Make-up artist

They must be fully briefed about the clothes and hairstyles that the models will be wearing and should be given a full list of who is wearing what, so they can make sure that the hair, clothes, colours and make-up styles all match.

If you do not know a freelance beautician, try the local press, *Yellow Pages*, or final year students on a beauty therapy course at a local college. However, always check the standard of the make-up artist's work first before engaging them, and remember that stage make-up needs to be slightly darker and heavier than normal, to counteract the strong lighting.

Wardrobe mistress/dresser

A person is needed to take charge of the clothing and accessories and to make sure that they are co-ordinated with the hair and make-up. Before a hair and fashion show, the clothing must be clean, pressed and placed in the correct order, usually on a rail in the changing room. The wardrobe mistress must then make sure that the correct outfit is worn by the correct person during the show/demonstration. All clothing should be checked and then safely returned after the event. A useful tip when having a lot of costume changes is to list (or sketch) all clothes, accessories and shoes on a piece of paper and pin this to the outside of a black plastic bag which contains all the parts of the particular outfit.

Disc jockey

The DJ must be carefully briefed on the format of the demonstration or show and should be given a list with the order of any scenes, e.g. sports, bridal, together with who will be appearing and what music is required for each particular part. Very specific instructions should also be given as to the volume of the music, and when it needs to be faded out completely – for example, whilst the compère is talking.

The music should not be an intrusion but should complement the 'looks' that are being portrayed. It must also be on cue, as any unwanted silent gaps are embarrassing to both the audience and the people involved. Always go through the music carefully with the DJ and rectify any misunderstandings or problems at the rehearsal stage.

Models

Depending on the type of demonstration or show, the models should be chosen to show off the hair and clothes to best effect. If they will be only sitting having their hair done on stage and standing at the end, then attractive clients from the salon will probably be suitable as models. However, many girls are shy and find it difficult to walk down a catwalk correctly to music; therefore, it is often better to use professional models. If this is too expensive ask at the local college, university or private modelling school to see if any of their final year modelling or fashion students would be willing to model. Often they are delighted to gain the experience and the photographs of them in action are very useful when they are creating their portfolios for use after their training.

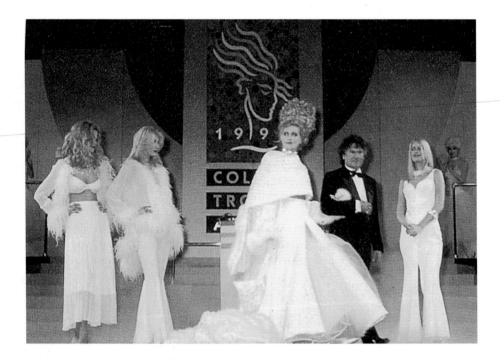

Photographer

Local newspapers can be contacted to cover the event. For added marketing impact, the event could be linked to a special offer advertisement giving discounts to those members of the public who attend the demonstration.

Always have your *own* photographer, in addition to the press, as news photographers do not always take the shots you would wish and sometimes do not even attend.

Decide on the general effect you want from the finished photographs and then, if possible, give the photographer a list of the shots you require. Remember that any good pictures can be blown up and displayed in the salon or sent to various newspapers and magazines with a short report of the event as an interest story. If it is published, this is an excellent way of promoting the salon.

A video taken of the event is a good training and evaluation aid for both present and future staff, as it can show any mistakes and where improvements can be made. If it is edited, it can be used as a marketing tool to show the standard and variety of work that can be achieved by the salon.

Planning the event

Careful planning is absolutely essential to your success; therefore, make a checklist of all the things that must be done before you start. You will need to include in your checklist:

Venue

The location will depend on the type of demonstration and the funds available. If the salon is servicing an in-store fashion show, then obviously there will be no charge. If, however, the venue is to be in a hotel or community centre, there may be a fee. So, before committing yourself, compare the prices and *facilities* of a variety of places.

Consider carefully the lighting, seating space, staging, access to water, electric sockets, changing area and fire precautions. Check what car parking facilities are available and whether the venue is easily accessible by public transport.

These issues are important as they will affect your final choice of venue. They will determine the size of your audience (fire precautions also often limit numbers) and the type of presentation it is possible to stage. For example, a big fund-raising event will require a central location, good car parking facilities, enough seating space, and adequate lighting to give good visual impact to the whole audience.

> **TECHNICAL TIP**
> Sometimes it is necessary to bring additional spot lighting. If this is the case, always make sure that the electrical systems can withstand the additional load.

Date

This may be dependent on the venue, which could have only certain dates available. If there is a free choice, then decide on the type of audience you wish to target and check local newspapers, libraries, etc., to make sure that the date you have chosen will not clash with any other events.

Consider also any holidays, such as annual or bank holidays, and the time of year. During busy summer months will your staff have *time* to put in the necessary preparation before the demonstration? In winter will the weather be too bad for people to attend?

Printing/publicity

If tickets and programmes are required, enquire into sponsorship by manufacturers or local business firms. They may be willing to print the tickets and/or programmes free of charge in return for publicity. Asking local businesses to advertise in the programme for a small fee will often offset the printing costs. Always acknowledge any sponsorship, advertising or other help received.

Publicise the event well in advance in the local press and place posters in local shops (including your own salon), local colleges, libraries and community centres. Remember that people can only attend if they know all about it well in advance.

It may also be worth while sending free tickets to local dignitaries and VIPs, as this gives added interest to the press.

After the event send photographs and a short report to your local newspaper and trade journals.

Costings

Make a list of all the 'outgoings' for the demonstration. This list could include: hire of venue; printing, publicity, flowers; materials used on the hair such as mousse, lacquer, gels, etc.; laundering of gowns and towels; refreshments; helpers' fees (e.g. make-up artist); and any other sundry expenses. Add together the outgoings and then divide this figure by the number of people you expect to attend. This will give you the *minimum* price required for each ticket. Remember that there may not be a full attendance and therefore it may be necessary to charge more, and donate any profit to charity.

Some salons prefer to stage a demonstration free of charge and offset the expenses as advertising or promotion of the salon.

Refreshments

These can be anything from coffee or cheese and wine to a full buffet, depending on the type of event, the budget allowance and when it is to be held, i.e. during the day or in the evening.

Refreshments can be served in the middle of the presentation as an interval, or at the end so that staff and models can mingle with the audience to answer any questions and talk about the hair salon. This part of the event can be especially good for the salon's public relations!

Schedule of work

Make out a list of the people needed to help with the demonstration and then make out a detailed timetable for practice sessions and rehearsals, ensuring that everyone attends.

Work out a 'countdown' timesheet and then a timetable for the actual day of the demonstration. Everyone involved in the demonstration *must* know not only their own role but also where they fit into the programme as a whole. So, to keep the event under control, write down each production number in order, together with the following information:

- Music for the scene.
- Names of models.
- What clothes they will be wearing.
- What accessories, e.g. shoes, hair ornaments.
- What hairstyle for each model.
- Prices, if necessary.

Give a copy of this information to the compère, DJ, hairstylists, make-up artist, wardrobe mistress and models. Pin another copy next to the door in the changing room for communal reference so that everyone knows the schedule and exactly what is going on.

Preventing RSI
If the event has been carefully prepared beforehand, there will be less chance of excessive stress on the day.

Evaluation and feedback

This can be both during and after the event. During the demonstration the audience will express either positive or negative reactions. Positive reactions can be determined by the way in which the audience listens attentively, asks relevant questions when appropriate, and can also be felt in the general atmosphere. Negative reactions can be very noticeable – if the audience fidgets in their seats, lacks concentration and attention, talks together or walks out either during the demonstration or at the interval.

Walking amongst the audience after the demonstration will also give a good indication as to whether the event has been successful or not. If the audience is enthusiastic and wanting to know more about the hairstyles, the clothes and the salon, then this is usually an indication of a successful event. If, however, the audience is non-committal, unwilling to give an opinion or avoids eye contact, this could be an indication that they have not enjoyed themselves.

It is *very* important to have a debriefing session with the entire staff as soon after the event as possible to find out what worked well and what problems there were.

Write down all the important points to use for future reference and give an indication of how to improve future performance. Keep a record of all transactions and costings to evaluate whether your predictions were accurate. Make notes on any improvements or savings that could be made.

Feedback from clients may take a period of time. Regular clients are usually delighted that 'their' salon has a high profile. However, other members of the audience may be perfectly happy with their current salon, but may become a new client much later. Staff should be encouraged to ask any new clients whether they attended the event, in order to determine its impact on the local community.

Sample timesheet for a hair and fashion show

Night before
Collect clothes, accessories and any props. Check that all equipment, tools and materials needed for the hair are clean and ready.

8.00 a.m.
Arrive at venue. Divide clothes into production numbers or 'looks' and place in order on the rail. Pin up the schedule on the wall.

8.30 a.m.
Models, hairstylists and make-up artist arrive.

9.00–10.45 a.m.
Rehearsals. Make sure that everything is in the correct order and that the compère and DJ have been fully briefed.

Anything that goes wrong or missing can be rectified at this stage.

Dress models. Do hair and make-up. Check that programmes are laid out on the audience's seats.

Make sure that the photographer and local press are positioned where they can see. Also check that the compère's script has the details about any VIPs or sponsorship, and all credits for make-up artists, boutique or fashion house, and hair salon.

12.00–12.45 p.m.

The Presentation.

12.45 p.m. onwards

Refreshments. Models and stylists mingle with the audience, answering any questions on the hair and salon. Make a note of all comments made by the audience for the future debriefing session.

3.00 p.m.

Collect all clothes and equipment and check that nothing is missing.

Using incentives

Incentives are designed to get people to try something. These can be anything – limited only by imagination, appropriateness and finance! Staff can also be offered incentives through 'commission'.

Many salons offer incentives to clients through:

- Reduced prices.
- Reduced rates to particular groups.
- Providing 'extras' in a set price such as 'free' conditioner after a perm, etc.

The basic idea is to tempt clients into the salon and so impress them that they will not only return but publicise the salon's goods and services to their friends!

Promotional materials

As with incentives the same marketing limitations apply. Again, there are lots of types to choose from, from inserts in local papers to leaflets through doors/under car windscreen wipers, etc. These often include a 'money off' or 'free' voucher but to be effective any form of promotion or advertising must be carefully planned and professionally carried out otherwise it will lose prospective clients instead of attracting them.

There are many methods of advertising, some of which are more suitable for the salon than others. Factors which will influence which type of advertising to use are:

- Cost.
- Target population.
- Product.

Cost

Any type of advertising must be cost effective and the overall price of the advertising campaign must be measured against the potential profit from selling the goods. A large organisation may have more funds at their disposal than a smaller salon. They may also have a certain amount set aside for advertising which has been built into their yearly budget.

Target population

This is the category of client that is most likely to be attracted to the product. They may be within a local area or available nationally. The type of potential client and where they live will greatly influence where and how the goods are advertised.

Product

The **type** of product will also influence the type of advertising necessary. For example, demonstrating toupees at an all-women WI meeting would not be particularly effective as the target population for toupees is usually men.

Methods of advertising

Once the factors of cost, target population and product have been decided then it is possible to consider the most appropriate method of advertising to give the best results. The following options are available:

- Newspapers and magazines.
- Direct mail and leaflets.
- Posters.
- Business directories.
- Local radio and cinema.
- Transport advertising.
- Demonstrations.
- Window display.
- Personal selling.

Newspapers and magazines

There are four types of newspapers available: nationals, regional dailies, local weeklies and free newspapers. The cost of advertising in these papers will vary but usually the national press is the most expensive. Any newspaper advertisement should be noticeable but easy to read and understand. The price of the advertisement will depend on the number of words; therefore keep it brief, snappy and to the point! The following points should be considered when selecting which newspaper to use.

1 A local paper would be the most suitable for a local target population as a national newspaper would not be selective enough.
2 Local weekly papers have a reading life of one week or more therefore the advertisement will have more chance of being seen.
3 Advertisers have to pay to advertise in the free papers but research indicates that they are read by a high percentage of the population in each delivery area.

National magazine advertising is usually well out of the price range of most salons, but other magazines such as parish magazines, carnival programmes and cinema, theatre or bingo programmes are worth considering if the target population is local. An advertisement placed in any of these magazines should have visual appeal as this type of literature is usually hastily read.

Direct mail and leaflets

This can be a good way of informing local people of the services that the salon offers. The literature must be well produced and visually interesting so that it is noticeable and creates a good impression. Care should be taken with the wording to ensure that all the information is clearly stated and precise without being too long winded. If too much information is crammed onto the sheet no one will bother to read it.

There are sometimes offers available for salons using direct mailing for the first time (e.g. free postage on first mail shot). A specialist mailing house will provide a mailing list and will also produce and mail the publicity material for the salon. However, some salons prefer to produce their own material, particularly those with access to word processing or desk-top publishing facilities, in which case the electoral register may be used for the mailing list.

Leaflets can be delivered locally by hand and there are various organisations who are willing to carry out this task for a donation. Sometimes, for a fee, a local newsagent (or local newspaper itself) will slip a leaflet inside each newspaper before it is delivered.

Posters

These are used to attract local trade and can be displayed at local halls, bus stops, and businesses including the salon. They must look professional and be designed to attract attention. It is often worth enlisting the help of a graphic artist or art student from a local college. Desk-top publishing can also produce professional posters which can be enlarged on a photocopier.

Business directories

These list businesses together under their specialist areas to enable consumers to easily find the service they require (e.g. *Yellow Pages*). These are good for long-term publicity as they are delivered to all homes within the locality that have a telephone. However, the salon will be listed with other competing salons therefore the entry has to be carefully worded.

Local radio and cinema

Advertising on the local radio has the advantage that their audiences vary throughout the day therefore it is possible to target potential customers. However, it is cost effective only in areas of high population such as cities or large towns. Advertisements in local cinemas last approximately 15 seconds and the commercial itself is usually a generalised, pre-recorded one on hairdressing which is then personalised with the salon's name, address and services offered. The salon has to enter into a contract with the cinema so this is more of a long-term commitment and, unless the cinema is situated near the salon, could have little effect.

Transport advertising

Advertisements can be displayed on either the inside or outside of buses, trains, taxis, tubes or cars. Commuters do tend to read what is displayed about them while they are sitting immobile during transit. Advertisements appearing on the outside of transport must be visually exciting with a simple message so that they are easy to see and read. However, to be effective, the transport must travel through the salon's area so that it can be easily identified by potential clients.

Demonstrations

This is an extremely effective way to promote the salon's services and image. It gives potential clients a very clear indication, at first hand, of what the salon can achieve. It also allows the consumer the opportunity to see what is on offer without any obligation or commitment to buy the goods. However, to be successful and to attain the desired result, the demonstration must be carefully planned and professionally executed irrespective of the size of audience or venue.

Window display

This is also known as point of sale advertising and can be carried through to the reception area with displays and special offers. Local events, national incidents and seasonal displays (e.g. Christmas) can all be used as a vehicle for the display or promotion. All displays should be changed regularly otherwise they lose their impact and prospective clients fail to notice them. Large stores are extremely conscious of the power of an effective window display and use various devices to entice the consumer into the shop. Next time you walk down the high street, notice how many people are looking in the shop windows and try to see what has attracted them. See Level 2 Unit 11 for a more detailed explanation.

Personal selling

Personal selling is one of the most important forms of advertising but is very reliant on the expertise of the stylist, receptionist and other staff members as sales people. The whole process is far more personal and allows the client to find out more about the product/service by being able to ask questions. However, to be effective the staff must be aware of the importance of their role and must also have adequate product/service knowledge to give informed advice to the client. The staff should be encouraged to wear different forms of false hair themselves if this is the salon's specialism, for example hair extensions, which will enable the client to see a finished product and also enable the staff to discuss and advise the client from first-hand experience. If this is not possible, for example with toupees or specialised wigs which may be only suitable for certain people, then the staff must be given adequate training so that they have the necessary knowledge to carry out the service and advise the client.

POINTS TO REMEMBER

Marketing is a highly professional and expensive area. It is very easy to produce materials or use incentives which are not particularly good or effective. We are all constantly bombarded with marketing ploys of all kinds. Many of these have involved very large expenditure which a salon could not hope to match. Remember: the most effective 'marketing' is word of mouth – personal recommendation. Making sure *each* client is satisfied with the service and treatment they have received repays *all* the effort put into ensuring a highly professional and top quality experience for the client.

You are asked by your salon manager to organise a day or evening of staff development, to take place within the salon, in conjunction with a manufacturing firm's technical services team. The purpose of the event is to acquaint all staff with a new range of products. The manager wishes to see a layout of your plan and your ideas before it is implemented.

The following stages may help you to organise your session:

- Identify a suitable time and date which will cause the minimum of inconvenience and disruption to the normal working week.
- Make a list of 'objectives', i.e. what you hope to achieve through the session.
- Contact the manufacturer to determine availability of a technician on the chosen date and time.
- Write out a memo to all staff informing them of the event and allowing enough time to organise their schedules.
- Contact any models who may be required and have a back-up in case of emergencies.
- Ensure all resources and equipment are available and in working order on the date required.
- Plan how you will evaluate the effectiveness of the session.
- Plan how you can motivate the staff to provide ideas for incentives to market the new products to their clients.

What do you know?

Level 3 Unit 10

What is meant by 'marketing' a salon's services? ☐

What can be used as incentives in marketing? ☐

Why is personal recommendation so important in publicising a salon? ☐

What is 'evaluation'? ☐

What is 'feedback'? ☐

*List **four** ways of obtaining feedback from a training programme.* ☐

What is the best way to get involved in outside hair demonstrations? ☐

What could happen if a hair demonstration was not organised down to the very last detail? ☐

List the tasks and roles that should be delegated to people when organising an outside demonstration. ☐

*List **seven** areas that need to be carefully considered when planning a demonstration of the salon's hairdressing skills to an outside audience.* ☐

INSTRUCTING AND DEMONSTRATING

There has been a great deal of research which has produced a large amount of material on the development of individuals and teams. The reason for this is that improving 'performance' improves business, profitability and staff morale. Learning and improving skills are important to the development of both teams and individuals.

The important thing is to be as CLEAR as possible as to what 'improved performance' actually means. The better you can define this the easier it will be to plan activities and processes to bring this about. The basic steps in this can be framed in three questions.

1 **Where are we now?** (present situation)
2 **Where do we want to get to?** (improved performance)
3 **How do we get there?** (planning the development of team, individuals and self)

One definition of *management* is 'utilising and facilitating the use of resources to maximum effect'. In other words, the manager's role is to seek to achieve the *objectives* of an organisation by controlling and organising its resources, including human resources, in the most efficient way possible.

The word **objective** is important here. What are the objectives of a hairdressing salon? One definition is *to provide a quality service which is profitable and professional*. There would be little argument with this, but it is a very broad statement. Unless this is broken down into more *specific objectives* it is hard to plan for an improvement in performance.

It is often helpful to think of specific objectives at different 'levels' in the organisation of the salon. These can be:

Organisational objectives
↓
    Team objectives
    ↓
        Individual objectives

The more exactly these objectives can be identified and written down the easier the planning towards achieving these objectives will be.

How to develop specific objectives

If these are not already established in the salon it is well worth carrying out a 'SWOT' analysis. This is a thorough and honest review of the salon's:

- **Strengths** – what are we good at? For what do we enjoy a good reputation? What are the particular strengths of our team operations, individuals or the staff? In which areas do we compete successfully with other salons?
- **Weaknesses** – what are these? Are there other salons we are not competing successfully with? Why not? What aspects of team/individual operation are we not so good at?
- **Opportunities** – what areas can we develop? Services to clients, potential in the salon staff, skills gaps?
- **Threats** – what are these? Are there events which would threaten the salon's profitability?

The outcome of this analysis will be a number of areas where action is needed. It will provide a framework derived from the salon's general objectives which may be a combination of:

- Long-term or short-term objectives.
- Individual or team objectives.
- General salon operation.
- Qualifications.

These can be used to develop a training and development plan to:

- Capitalise on 'strengths'.
- Reduce/eliminate 'weaknesses'.
- Make best use of 'opportunities'.
- Reduce potential or actual 'threats'.

Training and development plans

Training and development plans are really 'action plans' based on outcomes of a 'SWOT' analysis or other types of review activities. They often come down to the same three questions:

1 'Where are we now?' What skills/expertise/knowledge do we have? What is our **current competence**?
2 'Where do we want to get to?' What do we need to develop? What is our **potential competence**?
3 'How do we get there?' The writing of a **training** or **development** plan.

The specific objectives of this plan, however they are arrived at, need to be clearly stated. There is a natural tendency to rush into planning 'actions' often before it is entirely clear what the plan is supposed to do. It is well worth spending significant time on *carefully* stating *exactly* what the objectives of the plan are and this will be a tremendous help in deciding how best to get there. Make sure that the plan is:

S   Specific

M   Measurable in its outcomes (how will you judge if the objectives have been met?)

A   Achievable } with the potential of the individuals involved and the
R   Realistic   } resources available

T   Time limited (carried out within a particular length of time)

The starting point of 'Where are we now?' is a key part of managerial/supervisory activity. Assessment of potential performance and learning ability is very important in making sure that the plan is 'achievable' and 'realistic'. The best method is to encourage staff through listening, support and review meetings, in order to identify training and development needs. This will ensure a commitment to the process and encourage staff motivation. In addition, any planned outcomes need to be worked out by the individual or team concerned so that they feel an 'ownership' of the process, The NVQ training base can be very useful in helping people identify what they can or cannot do. Competency statements mean staff can 'tick off' those areas where they consider themselves to be competent and thus identify areas for development.

There will be times when there are tensions, or even conflicts, between some of the specific objectives used to develop training and development plans. Long-term objectives may not fit well with short-term ones, individual needs may not rest within those identified for the team, etc. There will also be constraints on **resources** such as time, materials, money which will need to be considered. The strategy here is to **prioritise** – decide which are the most important and put these top of the list. This should be a team-based task and discussed openly and fairly. Staff morale can be severely damaged if decisions are perceived as being made 'behind closed doors'. In addition, teams are a good way of sorting out such complex issues.

Updating and improving development plans

It is good practice to review planned activities at regular intervals. The more clearly the specific objectives, activities and outcomes have been planned the easier this review will be. The review process is a chance to evaluate effectiveness, sort out problem areas and move on. It fits into the **management cycle** as shown in Fig. 3.62.

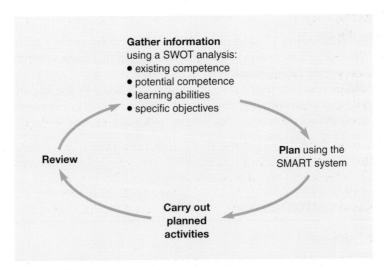

Fig. 3.62 The management cycle

Training and development activities

These are the particular actions designed to fulfil the objectives identified by individuals and/or teams to improve their performance. The choice of activity will depend on the experience and expertise of staff, their personal preference, suitability and cost to the organisation or individual. These may include a combination of one or more of:

- **Particular work activities** – such as arranging for certain individuals to work together in order to share experience and skills between them. Other work activities can be individual meetings and/or team meetings.

- **Training courses/seminars** – these can be in-house within the salon or outside at a local college or other training provider. They can provide specific update in both practical skills, product development and legislation/guidelines on subjects such as health and safety.

- **Open learning activities** – these are available on a flexible basis, often with the individual carrying out the activities without the direct supervision of the training provider. Advantages of open learning are that they:
  - are student centred
  - are flexible to fit in with other commitments
  - allow students to work at their own pace

- **Assignments/projects** – these can be used where individuals (or teams) investigate a particular area and present some type of report.

- **Coaching/mentoring** – these are 'one-to-one' techniques where one individual takes responsibility for developing the competence of another. *Coaching* means encouraging an individual to develop their potential in a series of steps organised by the 'coach'. *Mentoring* is 'looking after' someone, in that the mentor is present as a resource which the other individual can draw upon as and when they wish.

- **Job rotation** – as the title implies, involves moving people around the various tasks/operations in the salon. This will depend on the individuals involved and may very often involve a period of tuition by the more skilled staff before a person begins.

- **Job shadowing** – is an interesting method of observing a more skilled and experienced person in action and provides a rich learning environment for trainees. The person being 'shadowed' must obviously agree and support the procedure and provide the right sort of example! A useful outcome of job shadowing is that the person being observed benefits from the experience as it reinforces good practice and facilitates reflection and thought about the 'why' as well as the 'how' of hairdressing operations.

Organising the training

There are four key areas in successful training:

- Planning and preparing for the training session/programme.
- Carrying out the training: coaching the trainee.
- Assessing and recording trainee performance.
- Evaluating the training.

Training is a skill and like all skills a good performance is smooth, polished and 'looks easy'. Think of occasions when you would say 'that was really good'.

Reflect on *why* this was in terms of the technique and delivery. You will probably find that it involved all of the items listed above. Experienced trainers often do much of their preparation, responding to trainees during the session, and assessment and review of their own performance automatically (almost unconsciously), but to begin with it is necessary to plan these stages.

Planning and preparing for the training session/programme

Planning and preparation are extremely important to the success of a training programme. Care and attention to detail at this stage is very worthwhile.

The place to start planning is at the **specific objectives** level, as discussed earlier. In other words, what is it exactly that the trainee should be able to do at the end of the session that they could not do, or could not do to a sufficient level of competence, at the start?

The more precise you are about this, the easier the planning of the stages to achieve objectives will be. A useful aid in planning to reach a training objective is to bear in mind 'BEEP', a system which can be used for whole programmes, individual sessions or parts of sessions.

B *Before the training*
What is the level of existing competence? Are the trainees starting from nothing or do they have previous experience?

E *Experience*
Practice and experimentation must be built into the training programme to enable the trainee to achieve the desired level of competence.

E *Environment*
Where is the training to take place? What equipment and other resources will be needed from both within the salon and/or from outside?

P *Performance*
What are they to be able to do and to what standard, using which procedure and in what length of time?

The following notes should help you in planning and preparing better training sessions:

1 Specific descriptions of competency levels and how to measure these are given in the Hairdressing Training Board's publication on the National Vocational Qualifications (NVQ) in Hairdressing. The NVQ is based on 'competence statements', and includes very useful analyses of what is needed to be 'competent' in the major hairdressing operations.
2 Having identified what you want to achieve, this clarifies and informs you on what to do. Your planning should identify the key stages in the learning and concentrate on these. Exactly what these are will depend on the level of previous experience of the trainee.
3 Having planned what you want to achieve and the steps needed to get there, you need to decide 'how' you are going to achieve it. What facilities will you need? While the essential facilities and equipment will be those always available in a salon, basic visual aids could be included such as videos, colour slides, wall charts, training manuals, articles cut from magazines and trade journals.
   Help can also be obtained from outside the salon from manufacturers' training schools, short courses in your local Further Education college, textbooks, video

games, demonstrations by manufacturers' technicians, day seminars, and workshops held by leading stylists and private hairdressing schools.

4 Does the trainee receive training from another organisation, such as off-the-job training at college? If so, make sure you are fully aware of the content of the programme. There may be flexibility in these programmes to meet your trainee's needs and it will be worthwhile finding out if their analysis of the training needs of the trainee agree with yours.

In general, it is very useful to make contact and co-operate with others who provide hairdressing training for your trainees.

5 Will the material you have selected for your training be suitable for a wide range of trainees: male as well as female; older people; people from various ethnic groups? It is very easy to see hairdressers as 'stereotypes' – being young, white and female. Always bear this in mind, not just because of the desirability (even legal requirement) of 'equal opportunities' but so that your time and effort in planning and preparing the session materials can be used as widely as possible.

Carrying out the training: coaching the trainee

Having set clear objectives, carefully planned your delivery in terms of content, pace and resources/facilities needed, and organised these resources and facilities, you are ready to run the session. The best training sessions involve:

- Learning by doing (activity learning).
- Tolerance of mistakes/errors.
- Responding positively to individuals.

Plan your session to involve as little 'showing' and as much 'doing' as possible. Use as much time as possible on one-to-one discussions if working with a group. Be active and vigilant and respond positively to any request for help or further information. Provide positive feedback. Encourage progress by praise and general positive reinforcement ('that's good!, 'well done', 'you're doing well'). Avoid the negative. If a trainee is not getting much out of the session, try to analyse where the problem is or who is at fault.

Assessing and recording trainee performance

If you have clear definitions of your competency goals (such as those used by the National Vocational Qualification) then you have a structure with which to work, both in terms of checking competence (can they do it to the right standard in the required time?) as well as a system of recording achievement.

There are a variety of systems for keeping records. The City and Guilds/ Hairdressing Training Board uses a 'tick the box' type based on observation of practical skills and on oral and written assessment. This is a good starting point although you may wish to adapt it to the salon's requirement. The important point is that the system of recording progress is quick, clear and can be modified if required in the future. When a recording system is established it provides a structure for reviewing the training requirements with a trainee.

A **review session** should be carried out on a one-to-one basis and in a situation where disturbance and interruptions are minimal. Both the trainee and the supervisor should prepare for the review session. If you have a clear set of criteria for competence in an area, the trainee can independently assess their own level of competence and then compare this with the supervisor. This encourages the trainee to feel they have some role in the process and to take it seriously. In addition, it concentrates time on the areas of 'mismatch' where the supervisor's and trainee's opinions vary. If both assessments agree then the review can move straight on to producing a plan to achieve the missing or underdeveloped skills.

Evaluating the training

Evaluation is judging the worth of something (its value) and any evaluation of training hinges on whether it has been 'worthwhile' and has achieved its objectives. Even if it has, could it be improved? Perhaps it could be more efficient (using less time and resources) or more effective (with better learning opportunities)?

As much time needs to be spent on a detailed evaluation as on the planning stage. There is a tendency to 'finish and run', that is, to finish the programme and let that be the end of the supervisor's involvement. This is particularly so if the training has been successful. Post mortems should not be reserved for the bad ones!

A careful, step-by-step review of all parts of the programme using **feedback** from the trainees, management and the supervisor's own feelings and perceptions can save time in the future and improve even the most successful programmes.

This feedback will arise:

- During the sessions – verbal and non-verbal communication of the level of involvement, enjoyment and learning.
- During the review – with trainees before and after the programme.
- During discussion with salon management on the content and outcomes of the training.

You can also use questionnaires to obtain anonymous feedback from participants, session by session if required. However, if questionnaires are used they should be short and 'tick the box' type responses, with some space allowed for a written comment.

Following the evaluation, ensure that notes on improvement, etc., are kept for reference in the future. It is surprising how even the best memories lose details of the evaluation after six busy months. Writing short notes will ensure that lessons learnt are taken into consideration and do not have to be relearnt at a later date.

Influences on training and development activities

The influences are factors which produce a need for training and may well form part of the content of the activity.

There are a large number of such influences, as shown in Fig. 3.63.

Key areas for training

There are three other important areas which will involve training in addition to the training of practical skills:

- Inducting new staff.
- Developing up-to-date product knowledge.
- Client care.

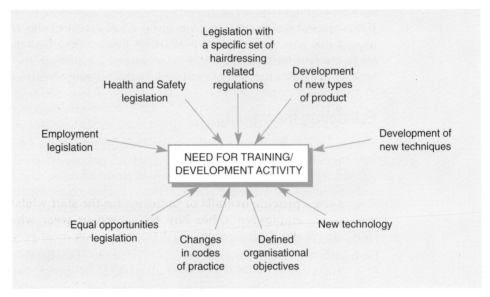

Fig. 3.63 Influences on training and development

Inducting new staff

This means giving a new employee all the information they will need and settling them into their new environment as quickly and painlessly as possible. Starting somewhere new can be a bewildering process and a lack of induction can leave the employee feeling confused, anxious and frustrated.

Very often, a large amount of information needs to be taken in at once so an induction programme spread over a period of time is a useful way to ease the learning process. Some salons have a 'probationary' period of about three months during which time the salon and the new staff member can decide whether they are compatible with one another. Any induction programme should be well planned with sessions built in to assess how the new employee is coping with their new environment and whether there are any problems. Solving any initial difficulties quickly prevents problems becoming insurmountable and also helps to create a bond between the employee and the organisation.

The induction programme should include the following:

- General salon rules and procedures.
- Contract of employment.
- Protective clothing and use of equipment.
- Roles and responsibilities of the staff.
- Training, monitoring and appraisal systems.
- Reception duties (if applicable).

General salon rules and procedures

Each salon will have its own rules and procedures and these should be clearly stated at the beginning to prevent misunderstanding at a later date. Issues such as laundry, cleaning rotas, safety precautions, use of hazardous substances and security procedures for handling cash and stock should all be carefully explained to all new members of staff. It is also a good idea to display notices on important procedures (such as what to do in case of fire or accident) in a prominent position in the staff-room as a constant reminder that can be easily referred to at any time.

Contract of employment

This is a signed contract between the employer and the employee which is required by law and is legally binding by both parties. It states the conditions of employment and responsibilities of the employee in terms of hours of work, holiday entitlement, grievance procedures, health and safety, codes of conduct, notice of intention to leave employment, equal opportunities, discipline and dismissal procedures, and it usually includes a restraint on working in another salon via a 'radius clause'. Thus, it is in the interests of both the employer and employee to ensure that the contract and its contents are fully understood and agreed upon before it is signed.

Protective clothing and use of equipment

Some salons provide overalls or uniforms for the staff whilst others do not, in which case employees either buy their own or wear whatever they wish. However, it should be remembered that the salon must project a professional image and to do so the staff should be dressed accordingly. A salon uniform helps to maintain this professional image and also protect clothing from the effect of strong chemicals such as bleaching and tinting agents.

All new staff should be shown how to safely use and maintain each piece of salon equipment to minimise the risk of any accidents. All staff should be encouraged to report any faulty equipment so that it can be rectified immediately.

Roles and responsibilities of the staff

All new staff members must be encouraged to acquire a thorough knowledge of the work of the team, the policies of the organisation and how they themselves fit into the organisation's structure. They must also know what responsibilities they have towards their peers, seniors, clients and the salon. A job description is useful to enable the employee to know their duties exactly and to establish who is responsible for what. If staff do not know what they are supposed to do then it is difficult for them to do it well.

Take time introducing new staff to the other team members and use everyone's names as often as possible. It can be embarrassing at first to try to remember names, particularly in large organisations. Asking a more experienced member of staff to act as a 'mentor' to the new member can sometimes help them to settle in more easily and quickly. This system helps a new person to become part of the team more quickly and to ask questions which they may be reluctant to ask an employer or senior member of staff. Remember that a new team member can be a little disturbing to established relationships so it is important to give existing staff time to adjust.

Training, monitoring and appraisal systems

Training has been described as the transfer of knowledge/skills from one person to another. It plays an important role in any organisation as it is the mechanism which enables each individual to be effective and produce work of a high standard. A new member of staff must be made aware of the salon's training programme and how it is to be implemented. New senior staff will need to be aware of work to meet changing demands.

Staff must also be aware of the salon's system of monitoring and assessing their progress and performance to enable them to measure their success and increase their motivation.

Appraisal systems are a useful way of monitoring staff performance. Their aim is to identify strengths and weaknesses and provide a means of setting goals and improving performance standards.

Reception duties (if applicable)

Larger organisations employ a receptionist who takes over these duties in their entirety. However, in smaller salons the reception duties may be carried out by all members of staff, so guidance must be given on the salon's policies and procedures regarding the use of the telephone, booking and cancelling appointments, behaviour towards clients, taking messages and handling cash. Most salons have strict rules regarding these areas and each system should be carefully explained to avoid future mistakes.

Product knowledge

There is a constant flow of new products onto the market. Updating on these can be obtained from:

- Trade journals.
- Manufacturers' marketing materials and representatives.
- Seminars.

Product knowledge is essential in order to:

- Meet client requirements.
- Sell the product.
- Protect the client against possible hazards.

The key areas of product knowledge required are

- Applicability.
- Cost effectiveness.
- Health and safety implications (if applicable).

These are best discussed with the supplier or the company directly. All of these factors are important in providing the best standard of client care.

Demonstrating

Demonstrating is a technique which combines oral explanation with the handling or operation of equipment to teach or show a skill. It can be carried out on a one-to-one basis or to a group. When using demonstration as an instructional technique to trainees, there are essentially **three** different types:

- Demonstration to help familiarisation – an example of this would be showing a trainee how to carry out a conditioning treatment.
- Demonstration to aid understanding of concepts and principles – showing a trainee, on a hair cutting, what happens to the hair if it is over-processed would be an example of this.
- Skills demonstration – can be used as instruction to trainees or for promotional purposes, as when putting on a hair show.

There are three stages to providing a demonstration for trainees, and indeed when any form of more formal instruction takes place. These three stages consist of:

- Preparing for the demonstration.
- Delivering the demonstration.
- Evaluating the end of the demonstration.

Preparing for the demonstration

Any instructional technique is always more effective if it is well planned in advance with clear objectives or outcomes. These should be written down in simple terms, stating exactly what you want the trainee to know, or be able to do, at the end of the demonstration. The following guidelines may be useful when planning a demonstration for trainees.

1 Decide on the **specific** outcomes (objectives) for the trainee.
2 Explain the **purpose** of the demonstration to the trainee. They need to fully understand exactly what is expected of them and why.
3 Plan the most effective and efficient time to carry out the demonstration.
4 Carefully plan the content of the demonstration to have a clear introduction with each stage of the process logically sequenced. List the **key** points you wish to make to prevent them being missed out during the demonstration by mistake.
5 Estimate the time needed for the demonstration. Remember that additional time should be included to allow the trainee practice-time for the skill afterwards.
6 Consider the room/surroundings where the demonstration will take place.
7 Familiarise yourself with the equipment you will use, making sure that it complies with health and safety and is in good working order.
8 Make sure that any additional visual aids, such as posters, videos, shade charts, etc., are up to date and available.
9 Have completed examples of the finished result, or product, to enable the trainee to see exactly what they are aiming for. This need not be too complex, a magazine picture or completed practice head would be sufficient.

Delivering the demonstration

Demonstrating is more complex than it seems. Experienced stylists often assume that their trainees know more than they actually do. Think back to learning a new skill yourself, driving a car is a particularly good example, not enough hands and too much to remember is usually the first reaction!! It becomes obvious, therefore, that to learn effectively, the trainee needs to be taken through the process of the skill they are learning stage by stage, in small steps. To help their understanding, it is important to be very clear and precise about **what** you are doing and **why**. Encourage lots of questions and stress any key points, including health and safety, continually throughout the demonstration. Other points to consider are:

1 Make sure that everyone can see and hear.
2 Talk to the trainees **not** the equipment!
3 Explain fully any new or unfamiliar terms or processes.
4 Clarify in simple terms any difficult or complicated areas.
5 Relate facts to the trainee's own experiences wherever possible.
6 Move at the correct pace for the skill demonstrated.
7 Ask trainees to predict outcomes and give solutions to hypothetical questions.
8 Watch out for signs of confusion or inattention.
9 Summarise key points and health and safety at the end.
10 Provide opportunity for practice.

Evaluation at the end of the demonstration

Check whether the outcomes and objectives set for the trainees have been met. To improve future demonstrations, it is also necessary to evaluate your own performance and ask yourself whether your delivery has helped the trainee learn in the way you had hoped. At the end of the demonstration it is helpful to:

1 Encourage the trainees to practise the skills immediately afterwards (and during the demonstration too if possible).
2 Ask questions.
3 Allow trainees to demonstrate procedure.
4 Test understanding and knowledge, particularly of key points, health and safety and any legislative requirements.

Things to do

1 You have been asked to help organise the training of a trainee in fashion colouring techniques. What method (or methods) of training would you use? Explain your choice.

How would feedback on the person's performance be provided?

2 List:

- Those areas of the salon's activities which are fully under your control.
- Those areas decided jointly by yourself and salon management.
- Those areas decided by management.

What do you know?

Level 3 Unit 11

What is meant by the **induction** of new staff? ☐

List **six** areas that an Induction Programme may cover. ☐

List the most important rules/guidelines which exist in your salon. ☐

What is a training plan? ☐

What is usually included in a training plan? ☐

Give your ideas of how staff within your organisation could be made more aware of Health and Safety within the salon. ☐

State the staff members of your organisation and list their specific responsibilities. ☐

What is the main aim of any review system? ☐

What are the key areas of product knowledge? ☐

ASSESSING

Assessing candidate performance

Part of the role of the manager or supervisor within an organisation is to monitor the progress, efficiency and effectiveness of their working team. This is carried out by **assessing** performance, which is something that we do all the time – not only in the work situation. For example, when someone is seen for the first time, judgements are made about that person through the clothes that they wear, the way that they talk and their manner, etc. These judgements are usually very **subjective** – in other words, they are only a **personal** opinion, and may be totally incorrect. The old saying 'never judge a book by its cover' shows that snap judgements are not very desirable and in some cases can be damaging. Indeed, subjective judgements of staff *could* have far reaching implications in terms of their future training and career prospects.

Assessments involve making judgements about someone's ability to carry out specific tasks or work roles to a specified standard. The **criteria** for making judgements as to whether a person is competent as a hairdresser have been devised by the Hairdressing Training Board, which is the **industry lead body** for hairdressing, and the strategies used for testing these criteria have been designed by the **awarding body** (City and Guilds of London Institute) who are also responsible for the application and verification of all the assessments. The standards required by industry are built into the criteria and these are referred to as **National Standards**.

Assessment, if carried out correctly, is a means of ensuring **quality control** within the organisation and will also help to determine future **training needs** of the staff. However, to be effective the assessment process has to be fair, valid, efficient and reliable.

Fair assessment

The assessment can only be fair if it is carried out by a person qualified to National Standards. In other words, the assessor should have adequate experience in the industry and should have had training in assessment procedures and methods to be able to make convincing judgements. In addition, the person being assessed should have access to the **criteria** by which they are being judged so that they know in advance what is expected of them. It is unrealistic and unfair to expect anyone to succeed if they do not know what it is they are supposed to be doing and what exactly the assessor is looking for.

Valid assessment

This means that the assessment is sound and that it tests what it is supposed to test. For example, if a trainee was questioned on how to brew tea this would not be valid as it does not test their practical hairdressing skills! For certification purposes, staff should be assessed to the criteria specified in the National Standards, and *only* to these criteria, to make sure that the assessment is carried out **objectively**. Assessing to the National Standards makes the assessments valid because it tests what the hairdressing industry has decided are the skills necessary for their trained workforce. In addition, having a National Standard means that everyone's competence/skill is measured to the same standard. Thus, it is the same throughout the country and should not matter whether the assessment is carried out in salons, colleges or training centres as the outcome should be identical.

Reliable assessment

To be reliable, the assessment should have the same outcome (result) no matter who assesses, where the assessment is carried out or when. Again, by using *only* the criteria stated in the National Standards and by having **trained assessors** the assessment becomes as reliable as possible.

Efficient assessment

Assessment that is cost effective and tests what it is supposed to test in a productive manner can be claimed as efficient. Carrying out the assessment with as little disruption as possible to normal routines and incorporating the assessment into the normal working week both at the salon and/or at the college or training centre will encourage the assessment to become an integral part of the training process and ongoing staff development.

Before anyone can begin to assess, however, it is necessary to have some underpinning knowledge of the systems and structure of the standards to be achieved. Without an overall understanding of the system it is very difficult to carry out the assessments in the correct manner. Thus, it is perhaps useful at this point to take an overview of the National Vocational Qualification system and its historical perspective.

Overview of National Vocational Qualifications

In 1985 the government proposed a review of all vocational education and training. This led to the setting up of the **National Council for Vocational Qualifications (NCVQ)** which in turn led to the reform and rationalisation of existing vocational qualifications. A new framework of qualifications was introduced called **National Vocational Qualifications (NVQs)**. These qualifications are based on **standards of competency**, which indicate whether someone is skilled in their work role. These standards are defined by industry through their Industry Lead Body (ILB), and in the case of hairdressing this is the Hairdressing Training Board.

The framework has **five** levels which create a system allowing for progression upwards, or across to other work areas, e.g. from hairdressing to beauty therapy or retailing, etc. It also provides a national and clear indication of the level of attainment achieved by those completing their award.

Definitions of each of the five levels are defined by the NCVQ as follows:

Level 1

Competence in the performance of a range of varied work activities, most of which are routine and predictable.

This first level is particularly useful for staff who carry out an **assisting** role and are not expected to make decisions, e.g. Saturday staff.

Level 2

Competence in a significant range of varied work activities performed in a variety of contexts – some of which are complex and non-routine, involving some individual responsibility.

In other words, this level is concerned with the knowledge of how to carry out basic hairdressing skills **without supervision**.

Level 3

Competence in a broad range of varied work activities performed in a wide variety of contexts, most of which are complex and non-routine. There is considerable responsibility, and control and guidance of others is often required.

Level 3 begins to look at the **managerial** role, the **training and assessing** of others, and the more intricate and **specialised practical hairdressing** skills.

Level 4

Competence in a broad range of technical or professional work activities performed in a wide variety of contexts and with a substantial degree of personal autonomy and responsibility. Responsibility for the work of others and the allocation of resources is also important.

This level is **management**-orientated and is therefore particularly relevant to those who are aspiring to be, or already are, salon owners.

Level 5

Competence which involves the application of a significant range of fundamental principles and complex techniques across a wide variety of contexts, substantial personal autonomy, responsibility and accountability.

This is the highest standard attainable and is equated with the academic standard of postgraduate studies.

Requirements of a National Vocational Qualification

The NCVQ do not write the content of the qualification – this is done by the industry in partnership with the examining body. However, the NCVQ provides the quality seal of approval if the qualification satisfies their criteria. Their criteria states that an NVQ should:

- Be based on national standards required for performance in employment – standards written by industry for industry.
- Be based on an assessment of the **outcome** of learning – what the trainee can **do** regardless of when and how it was learnt.
- Be awarded on the basis of sufficient, valid and reliable assessment of current competence.
- Be of no set duration of study – candidates work at their own pace.
- Allow open access – no age barriers, no specific entry requirements, no specific ways of studying.

- Enable a system of credit accumulation. Candidates can be accredited for the units they wish to achieve then build on these as and when they wish.
- Be assessed when the candidate is ready, in the workplace or in a suitable, realistic, simulated environment.

This new framework has many implications for the hairdressing industry. Firstly, trainees can learn their skills wherever they wish and the length of time it takes them to become competent becomes their own responsibility. Therefore, how quickly they attain the desired level of competence depends on their commitment and level of skill.

It is also the responsibility of the trainee to decide when **they** think they are competent enough to be assessed and this assessment can take place in the workplace, often referred to as 'on-the-job', or in a simulated environment such as a college or training centre which is known as 'off-the-job'. Because of this often 'split' method of assessing, trainees will be assessed by different people in different locations – hence the need for trained assessors both on and off the job who understand the underlying principles of assessment and who know what, when, and how they are to assess.

The structure of National Vocational Qualifications

There is a formal structure for all NVQ (competence-based) schemes outlining what stages a candidate has to go through to gain their award.

Each NVQ is given a **title** which will identify the job role it relates to and the **level** within the NVQ framework, e.g. 'NVQ Level 3 in Hairdressing'.

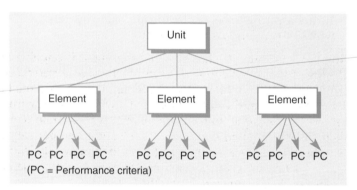

Fig. 3.64 NVQ structure

The NVQ is then subdivided into **units** (Fig. 3.64). A unit is like a mini qualification because each unit can have separate accreditation; therefore it is possible for an individual to build up separate units in their own time at their own pace until they have been accredited enough units to make up a qualification. Thus, the unit structure of NVQs allows individual choice and enables the candidate to select relevant units to suit their individual requirements. The final certificate will show each successful unit obtained, e.g. Level 3 Unit 12, Assessment.

Each unit is broken down into what is referred to as **National Standards**. These standards are used to describe what performance is expected of the candidate in the working environment. In other words, what a competent person would be expected to be able to do in the salon and what is considered to be an acceptable level of performance by the hairdressing industry. Each standard has three components:

- **Element titles** – for example, Level 3 Unit 12.4 'Giving feedback and keeping records'.
- **Set of performance criteria** – each of the performance criteria (PC) describe one characteristic of satisfactory performance of the element. All the performance criteria of the element have to be met in order to claim competence and all of the elements have to be completed to pass the unit. Each performance is judged on a 'can do/cannot do yet' basis, and there are no grades or marks.
- **Range statement** – each element is accompanied by a range statement which describes the various circumstances in which the competence must be applied. It may refer to differences in physical location, employment contexts, equipment used, etc.

Assessing the competence of a candidate

Competence is concerned with what people can do and if the assessment is carried out correctly it becomes not only a means of judging that person's skill, but also a very valuable 'learning tool'. Most of the time, in everyday life, we learn through our mistakes – a small child learns by this method constantly – therefore, if the assessment is carried out in a supportive and non-threatening manner with mistakes treated as a means of improving future performance then the assessment process becomes a valuable experience instead of a fearful one.

Types of assessment

There are two main forms of assessment:

- **Formative assessment** – this type of assessment is ongoing and means that the candidate has not yet fulfilled all the performance criteria over the full range. Anyone in training will need to prove that they can do the task/skill in a variety of situations and can transfer the knowledge learnt from one situation to another. For example, to be a competent 'permer', one would expect a candidate to be able to perm hair of different lengths and porosity in a variety of curl strengths. Formative assessment allows the candidate to learn from their experience and when used in conjunction with summative assessment can provide evidence of their competence over the full range.
- **Summative assessment** – this is the **final** assessment (summing up) when a candidate has met all the performance criteria over the full range and has produced all the relevant evidence. They are therefore ready to be accredited in that particular unit. Thus, if a candidate **has not yet** satisfied all the performance criteria it is a formative assessment, whilst if they **have** satisfied all the performance criteria it is a summative assessment.

What makes an effective assessor?

To be effective, an assessor **must** be fully aware of the performance criteria, range statements, and what evidence is required from the candidate to prove their competence. The candidate will also need to be asked either oral and/or written questions to test their 'underpinning knowledge' which in general terms means, do they know and understand what they are doing – this is not always the case!

The candidate must also have a clear understanding of why they are being assessed, by what criteria, when and by whom. This means that they should have an opportunity to discuss these issues and be given the relevant guidance and documentation to help them to understand how the assessment will operate. As mentioned previously, it is far easier to arrive if you know where you are supposed to be going and are given a route to go by!

Letting people know where they have gone wrong and how they can remedy any faults is not easy but it is an essential, and perhaps **the** most important, aspect of the assessment process. Always comment on the task, **not the person**, and use only the performance criteria, not your own personal preferences (again, this tends to be difficult when first assessing). Limit any comments to praise of where the candidate has been successful and constructive suggestions of how they can improve where they have not. Make specific references to the performance criteria, as it reinforces that this is the standard that the candidate should be working towards and it also takes some of the 'blame' away from you personally if they have been unsuccessful.

The feedback given on any performance should be a two-way process to allow the candidate the opportunity to question any assessment decisions. Encouraging them to identify how they think they have performed in relation to the criteria and allowing them to suggest ways in which they could improve will help them to make their own decisions and be more responsible for their own actions in the future.

Interpersonal skills are extremely important when assessing. A good assessor is firm and fair but also supportive and approachable. Remember, that effective assessment should also be used as an aid to learning and, as such, it should leave the candidate feeling that they are able to move forward in a positive way.

Assessment procedure

It is important to bear in mind that assessment is not a competition and is certainly not a method of catching people out. It should be a well-planned operation that enables people to be accredited for their achievements and encouraged to improve. There are four broad areas of activity involved (see Fig. 3.65) to ensure that the assessment is carried out fairly and effectively:

1 Preparing for the assessment.
2 Observing the evidence.
3 Testing knowledge and understanding (underpinning knowledge).
4 Giving feedback and keeping records.

Preparing for the assessment
(Unit 12.1 and TDLB Element D32.1)

This is planning the actual assessment with the candidate. It is very important that the candidate is fully involved in this stage of the procedure as it is **their** responsibility to decide when they are competent. To make sure that everyone knows what they are expected to do it is necessary to draw up an **ASSESSMENT PLAN** which is negotiated between both the assessor and the candidate.

When the plan has been finalised it should be agreed by both parties and anyone else who may be affected to make sure that it causes the minimum disruption to normal working duties and makes the best use of situations which occur naturally such as assessing shampooing competence when a candidate is carrying out a shampoo on a regular client, etc. Make sure that the assessment is carried out in a suitable place and at a suitable time.

If the assessor is unsure when a candidate offers alternative forms of evidence ('Is a roller set on a practice block a suitable form of evidence?' for example) then expert advice should be sought. The awarding body scheme notes, the internal verifier, the external verifier and the awarding body are all sources of expert advice if there are any difficulties.

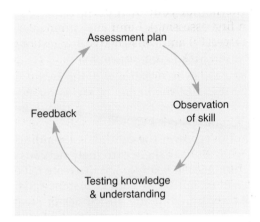

Fig. 3.65 Assessment process

Drawing up the assessment plan

The following information should be included in the plan: **When** the assessment is to take place; **Where** (either workplace or college/training centre); **Who** will be carrying out the assessment; **What** evidence the candidate can provide to support their claim of competence. In addition, to make sure that the assessment procedure is fully understood and documented, it is necessary to make a note of the following:

- **Who** is the candidate being assessed?
- **What national standard** is the candidate being assessed against? (e.g. Hairdressing Level 2)
- **What elements** of competence are being assessed?
- **What** are the **assessment requirements** of the elements?
- **What opportunities** will be used for the assessment? (e.g. simulation, practical activity, case study, work experience)
- **What assessment methods** will be used to assess the candidate? (e.g. observation, review of video events, discussion of written work, review of answers to questions, review of records, examination of product/final result, etc.)

Observing the evidence
(Unit 12.2 and TDLB Element D32.2)

Watching people work, judging their capabilities and asking them questions about what they are doing is an activity that we carry out all the time, particularly if we are watching someone carrying out a skill. For example, anyone baking a cake in the home could be asked questions such as 'What type of cake is it?', 'What's in it?', 'Will it have cream on top?', etc. These questions check what the cake will be like and whether the person knows what they are doing – they also provide a yardstick which enable you to judge the final result and see whether it has turned out as predicted. Exactly the same process is used when assessing a candidate's performance but because it is about their work role, it is done in a more specialised way.

Judging the performance

At the start of the observation, encourage the candidate to explain what they are going to do and how they are going to do it. If you are not actually able to see them carry out the task then it is important to make sure that the work or evidence they are submitting is actually theirs. This can be done by obtaining signed statements from people involved, e.g. employers or clients, to verify the truth of the claim.

The evidence or performance must **only** be judged against the performance criteria within the national standards, making sure that the judgements are accurate and any tests or simulations are in accordance with the awarding body guidelines (all information regarding the implementation of the assessment can be found in the Scheme Notes which are issued by the awarding body). In other words, you are not allowed to make up your own rules!

The assessor should not overpower the candidate. Standing next to them and watching their every move will make them extremely nervous and prevent them from giving a natural performance. It is important therefore to be as unobtrusive as possible although there will obviously be certain instances when a close look at what they are doing will be required. If any difficulties or misunderstandings do occur then it is always better to ask an appropriate authority – ultimately, a final decision will always rest with the awarding body after weighing up all the evidence.

Testing knowledge and understanding
(Unit 12.3 and TDLB Element D32.3)

Anyone can be taught to demonstrate a skill – animals are frequently used to carry out specific roles or tasks either to entertain or to help the human race. However, this does not automatically mean that they also understand what they are doing or why. By watching someone 'do' something we often presume or infer that they are competent, but how do we know whether they truly are? A hairdressing candidate could prove a positive danger to the client if they were not aware of the effects of the chemicals they use or do not have a full understanding of what they were doing in addition to their practical skills. Therefore, to prove that a candidate really is competent they also have to demonstrate their knowledge. This can be done in two ways:

- Written evidence.
- Oral evidence.

Written evidence

Written evidence of underpinning knowledge can be supplied in many different forms, through projects, assignments, case studies, reports, testimonials, diaries/appointment books, job appraisals/specifications, letters, minutes/agendas, action plans, assessor-devised written questions, etc. In some instances the awarding body supply their own written questions which must be completed before competence can be claimed by the candidate.

Written questions are usually carried out after the observation of the candidate's practical skill but within a certain time limit so that the theory of the task is easily related to what they are doing – it should never be thought of as a separate entity. Specific guidelines on how to administer these written tests are *always* stipulated by the awarding body and must be *strictly* adhered to at all times. Traditional examinations were always administered and marked by the awarding body but this is inappropriate for candidates on a competence-based scheme where they work at their own pace. Consequently, the responsibility now rests with the assessor, together with the incumbent ethical and moral issues.

The candidate must sit the written test in a quiet place, away from any distractions, and they must be invigilated/supervised by the assessor to ensure that the work is theirs. Books or other aids are not allowed and the assessor should not help with the questions. The test should be completed within the stipulated time scale, then the answers collected and marked as soon as possible. Marked papers must be kept in a locked, secure place and filed as evidence that the external verifier may wish to see on their verification visit.

Oral evidence

This takes place either during or just after the observational assessment. Questions should be phrased so that the candidate understands exactly what is being asked, but if there is any misunderstanding of the question it should be worded differently. It would be very unfair for the candidate if they were penalised because of this. Alternatively, the questions should not 'lead' the candidate; in other words, they should not tell them the answer in a roundabout way otherwise there would be no point to the questioning.

Do not harass the candidate whilst they are trying to demonstrate their competence. If the questioning seems to be affecting their performance either by making them nervous or distracting them, then the questions should be asked when they have finished – again, in a quiet, private area without distractions – the assessor is not supposed to be an inquisitor!

As is the case with written questions, oral questions should also be relevant to the task/skill and should not be personal opinions but based on the performance criteria of the national standards.

It is possible for the assessor to devise their own written and oral questions which can be used as forms of evidence, but if this is the case then they must make sure that the questions are unambiguously worded and are testing what they are supposed to test according to the specifications contained within the performance criteria. It is not permissible to test people on your personal preferences! When devising the questions it is always useful to look at the 'range' that has to be covered by the candidate and to use questions that test their understanding in these areas.

Giving feedback and keeping records
(Unit 12.4 and TDLB Element D32.4)

Giving feedback

This is a very, very important part of the assessment process for it is at this stage that the candidate will gain the most learning from their experience. Think of your own past experiences – how did you feel when you were praised? How did you feel when you were criticised? How did you feel when no one would tell you if you had done something wrong? You need to bear these feelings in mind when you are giving feedback. It is important to all of us to know what we do well and what we need to improve on because if we never know these things then we will never be able to give a better performance.

Feedback should always be given as soon as possible following an assessment otherwise both the assessor and the candidate will have forgotten a good proportion of what happened and also the momentum will be lost. Again, the session should not be an ordeal for the candidate and the aim should be to give encouragement and advice where needed.

POINTS TO REMEMBER

- Encourage the candidate to carry out a self-evaluation of their performance at the beginning of the session.
- Always begin the feedback with a positive statement of the candidate's performance.
- Comment only on the **task not the person**.
- Go through the performance criteria identifying weak and strong areas. This process should also lead to discussion regarding further training, practice and progression.
- Encourage the candidate to ask questions and identify ways in which they can improve.
- Keep a record of the discussion for future reference and review sessions.

Keeping records

Record keeping is extremely important because the awarding body will require evidence that the assessor is carrying out duties correctly and in accordance with awarding body specifications. Records also enable the assessor to keep track of how the candidate is progressing and where they need additional training, as well as providing a basis for future discussions.

Records are private documents and as such must not be used for general viewing. The candidate should have the right of access to them whenever they wish excepting the awarding body written answer sheets which should be stored in accordance with their specifications. However, if the assessments have been carried out correctly there should be no secrecy regarding what the candidate has attained.

All records MUST be clear, legible and accurate, particularly dates. They must be completed in accordance with verification requirements otherwise they could be considered invalid by the awarding body and the candidate will fail to gain their certificate. When completed, records are usually passed on to the person in overall charge of the assessments – usually the Internal Verifier – and to ensure that their records are up to date it is necessary to pass on the results of a successful assessment as soon as possible.

Things to do and **What do you know?** – see Level 3 Unit 13, page 405.

ASSESSING: SPECIAL CONSIDERATIONS

Assessing candidates using differing sources of evidence (TDLB D33)

There are many ways of assessing a trainee, three of which have been covered previously; that is, by observation of a natural performance and by oral and written questioning. However, there are other sources of evidence that can be shown to the assessor to prove that a trainee can carry out the requirements of their work role competently, to the required standard. Other evidence includes:

- Simulations.
- Projects and assignments.
- Case studies.
- Trainee reports and written statements.
- Witness testimonies (peer and client reports).
- Videos.
- Trainee prior achievement and learning (APL).

Simulations

To gain an NVQ qualification, a trainee must show that they are able to competently meet all of the performance criteria over the stated range. However, in certain circumstances it may not be possible to have access to the necessary specialised equipment or situation to enable the trainee to do this, for example, using an electronic till or fax machine. If this is the case then it will be necessary to devise a suitable 'simulation' of the real situation.

Any simulation **must** be carefully planned to enable the trainee to practise the required skills beforehand to be ready to be actually assessed when the simulation is carried out.

Projects and assignments

These are a means of encouraging trainees to actively find out relevant information and gain the underpinning knowledge needed to understand more fully what they are doing and why. However, trainees will not automatically know where and how to gather the information they require and it is the responsibility of the person delivering the training to give adequate support and guidance on the necessary study skills. Study skills could include how to:

- Use a library.
- Extract information from textbooks, magazines or journals.

- Use a computer (CD ROM, internet).
- Summarise information.
- Write for information from manufacturers and other sources.
- Present their findings.
- Work fairly and effectively as a team member if a group project is devised.

Themes for projects and assignments may be either negotiated with the trainees or devised by the tutor/trainer/supervisor or they may be supplied by the Awarding Body. However the project theme is arrived at, it is very important that sufficient information is given to the trainee to ensure that they fully understand **exactly** what the expected outcomes are and how they should go about this. The project/assignment criteria should be very specific to aid objectivity when assessing, and should also be in writing to enable the trainee to refer to them as and when necessary.

Case studies

These are a useful means of enabling the trainee to look at and solve difficult situations and potential problems. They also allow practice in 'working things out for themselves', encouraging autonomy and less reliance on senior staff members. Case studies enable trainees to practise dealing with problems in a safe environment without the additional stress and responsibility of a 'real' situation. In this way, should an accident or problem *actually* occur, it is less traumatic for the trainee and they will be more confident and competent to deal with it.

Providing evidence via case studies helps to illustrate the depth of understanding and knowledge of the trainee, particularly if used in conjunction with oral questioning.

Trainee reports and written statements

These are explanations of the process or processes that have been carried out and why certain techniques were used. They are often submitted as evidence with photographic proof of competence. A photograph by itself may not prove either that the trainee actually carried out the work or that it was what the client wanted. Thus, a written statement or report is a means of helping to ensure **sufficiency** of evidence to enable the assessor to make an informed judgement through the additional evidence.

Witness testimonies (peer and client reports)

These can be used by the employer to state that they believe the trainee is competent if the employer/manager/supervisor is not a qualified assessor. They can also be used by clients to show that they are satisfied with the service they have received and they can also be done by the trainee's colleagues. Allowing trainees and other working colleagues to assess each other's performance is a good learning tool, in that it again increases autonomy, and also responsibility, on behalf of all the staff members. It is worth remembering that trainees need to be able to make objective judgements about themselves and others if they are to develop and improve.

Any witness testimony must be relevant to the NVQ criteria and should include the name of the trainee, the date of the assessment, what was carried out, the name and status of the witness and any other relevant information. There are often special proformas that can be easily filled in which are supplied by the Awarding Body for greater coherence and ease.

Videos

If a trainee cannot be directly observed, a video of them carrying out the skill or process can be a very effective form of evidence. Very often a lot of evidence can be generated if the salon carries out a promotional hair show which is videoed. However, to be valid, the video needs to show the trainee actually carrying out the task and this may require close-ups. It is therefore useful to bear this in mind when organising what type of photographic shots are needed prior to the event.

Trainee prior achievement and learning (APL)

This is a means of accrediting people for what they have already achieved or what they can do. Sometimes this is quite easily done by matching any previous certification to the current performance criteria of the qualification they wish to gain. However, it can be very time consuming as it is usually carried out on a one-to-one basis and the trainee usually requires a great deal of help and guidance in deciding what past experience is relevant and what is not. It is also important that all of the evidence is current as well as relevant.

After an initial consultation, the trainee usually tries to match any evidence they may have against the performance criteria and range statements. An individual training plan is then negotiated to provide training and/or assessment of any 'shortfall' or areas where the performance criteria and range cannot be met by past experience. The main points to consider are whether the evidence is:

- Current enough.
- Sufficient.
- Authentic.
- Valid.

Assessing a trainee who is lacking in confidence

A trainee who is nervous will not perform to the best of their ability particularly if the assessor increases their nervousness through an unsympathetic, abrupt manner. The trainee should never feel intimidated by the assessor either before or during the assessment process and the feedback given should emphasise strengths and provide guidance on ways of eliminating any weaknesses. Nothing succeeds like success and it is possible to increase trainee confidence by providing a supportive and positive environment for them.

Trainees with special assessment requirements

All trainees are special and therefore all require individual support and guidance. However, some trainees have obvious disadvantages and an example of this would be deafness or dyslexia. These trainees should never be penalised or patronised because of their disability and ways must be sought to enable them to succeed in spite of their difficulties. Any queries regarding problems with any trainees should always be referred in the first instance to the Internal Verifier, and if not resolved then the External Verifier.

Summary

The process for assessing trainees using different sources of evidence (TDLB D33) is slightly different to assessing the trainee by merely observation and questioning (TDLB D32). The process can be summarised as shown in Fig. 3.66.

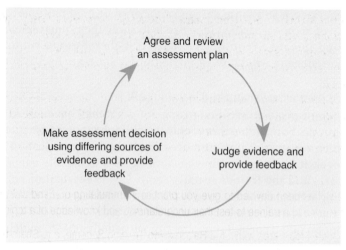

Fig. 3.66 Agreeing and reviewing an assessment plan

The main points to remember when dealing with different sources of evidence are:

- Does the evidence belong to the trainee?
- Is there enough evidence to be able to make a truthful decision?
- Is it valid evidence, or in other words, does it show what it is supposed to show?
- Is it reliable in that other assessors, including the Internal and External Verifiers, would agree with your decision?

If in doubt always seek advice from other assessors to ask to see additional evidence as proof of competence until you are satisfied. BUT remember that the trainee must always be assessed to the national standards for their qualification and not yours!

Compiling a portfolio of evidence

The amount of evidence produced for any portfolio depends on the individual. However, the evidence should be:

- **Valid** – relate only to the elements and performance criteria used.
- **Sufficient** – enough to cover the scope and conditions outlined in the range statements for each element.
- **Reliable** – must belong to the person presenting it.

Before starting the portfolio, read through the performance criteria and range statements of each element thoroughly to be familiar with what is required. It is then useful to prepare a file to collate the evidence. Divide the file into the required elements *before* beginning to collect the evidence which will enable it to be systematically filed in the correct place as it is collected. Each piece of evidence should be labelled to correspond with the relevant element and performance criteria and filed accordingly. In the final portfolio there should be a contents list and an indexing system to enable all the evidence to be easily found.

When all evidence has been collected, it is usually necessary to describe how the evidence matches the performance criteria. This provides written evidence of understanding the performance criteria and is often referred to as an **achievement record**. Below is an example of what an achievement record may look like:

Level 3 Unit 12.1 Agree and review a plan for assessing performance

The evidence I am submitting for 12.1 can be found in Appendix 1 of the attached file.

Sample 1 shows the assessment plans drawn up by me and vocational candidate Karen Barrell on [date]. These are submitted as evidence for performance criteria a, b, c and d.

Sample 2 shows observation notes made by my assessor on [date] when she observed me drawing up an assessment plan with vocational candidate Karen Barrell. It shows how discussion between myself and the candidate was used to identify assessment opportunities and is submitted as evidence for performance criteria a, b, d, e and f.

Things to do

Level 3 Units 12 and 13

This task has been devised to give you practice in formulating oral and written questions which can then be given to a trainee to test their understanding and knowledge of a topic area.

1 Choose a topic area within the Hairdressing Training Scheme, e.g. Shampooing. Read the performance criteria for the topic area thoroughly and carefully devise:

- 10 questions that you could ask the trainee *orally*
- 10 questions that would require a written response by the *trainee*

2 Write out, type or word process the questions then try them out on a trainee in the workplace.

3 Evaluate whether the questions were suitable by discussing the outcome of the test with the trainee. Were the questions **valid** and **reliable**?

Useful guidelines

- Make sure that the questions relate to the performance criteria, i.e. they test what they are supposed to test.
- Make the questions *clear*.
- Do not use language that the trainee finds difficult to understand – do they understand the terminology used?
- Do not make the questions too long or complicated.

What do you know?

Level 3 Units 12 and 13

Explain the difference between a **subjective** and **objective** judgement. ☐

What **four** things are necessary to ensure that the assessment process is effective? ☐

What is the meaning of a **valid** assessment? ☐

Give the definition of Level 3 as defined by the NCVQ. ☐

What is the Industry Lead Body for Hairdressing known as? ☐

What is a **range statement**? ☐

Explain the difference between a formative and summative assessment. ☐

What makes an effective assessor? ☐

List the **four** areas of activity for the assessment procedure. ☐

List **six** points to consider when giving feedback. ☐

Glossary

Acid Any substance which when dissolved in water gives off hydrogen ions. It produces a solution with a pH value below 7.

Acid conditioners Conditioners which help to restore the hair to an acid state.

Acid mantle Idea that natural oil (sebum) and sweat produce a slightly acid condition on the skin.

Acid perms Perms which operate at an acid pH. Cause less damage to hair than traditional alkaline perms.

Action plan A detailed plan of what is to be done, how it is to be carried out, by whom and by what date.

Activators *see* boosters.

Added hair Extra pieces of hair wound or plaited into the client's style.

Aesculap scissors Scissors which have one (or both) blades serrated.

Afro comb A comb with thick, large prongs usually made from vulcanite that can be used to create volume without frizz on African Caribbean or extremely curly hair.

Afro hair African Caribbean hair which is usually extremely curly and brittle.

AIDS Stands for Acquired Immune Deficiency Syndrome. This very dangerous disease could possibly be transmitted from one person to another in the salon by blood contamination. For example, when someone is cut by a razor and the razor is not cleaned, and then it is used again and cuts another person. There is some risk but there have been no recorded cases of transmission in this way in the hairdressing salon.

Alkali *see* base.

Alkaline bleach A type of simple bleach using an alkali to speed up the bleaching action.

Allergic dermatitis *see* dermatitis.

Allergy test *see* skin test.

Alopecia The general name for hair loss or balding. There are a number of different types including:

> **alopecia areata** hair loss in patches, cause not known.
> **Circatrical alopecia** on scars and scar tissue.
> **alopecia diffusa** general thinning of hair, can be due to a number of causes, e.g. some drugs.
> **traction alopecia** hair is pulled out by tension applied to the hair, e.g. some hairstyles.

Alternative tools, equipment and techniques The improvised use of tools, equipment and techniques to enable an effect to be achieved which cannot be achieved using conventional means.

Amino acids Building blocks of protein. They make up polypeptide chains.

Ammonium sulphite Used in some hair straighteners (relaxers).

Ammonium thioglycollate Active ingredient in traditional alkaline (pH 9.5) perm lotions. Acid perms contain glycerol thioglycollate.

Anagen Actively growing phase of the hair growth cycle.

Appraisal An assessment of staff performance, potential and action planning to encourage development.

Arrector pili muscle A small muscle in the skin which is connected to the hair follicle. When it contracts it pulls the follicle upright and produces 'goose pimples' (goose flesh) and causes the hair to rise.

Assessment (of client) Judging a client's requirements in terms of their face, shape, lifestyle, hair types and condition before a treatment.

Assessment (of staff) Often called **appraisal.** This should be done against specific criteria and is a positive process of finding out what staff can or cannot do well.

Back brushing Pushing the hair back on itself using a brush to create volume to the hair-style when dressing hair.

Back combing Pushing the hair back on itself at the roots to produce a padded effect which gives volume to the hairstyle. Backcombing on top of the hair mesh to blend the hair is termed 'teasing'.

Bacteria Type of micro-organism which can be neutral or useful or harmful (pathogenic) and cause disease.

Balance Term used in hairdressing to refer to the shape of the final hairstyle in relation to the client's face, head, neck and body. The silhouette of a hairstyle helps to show up any defects in its balance.

Balding/baldness *see* alopecia.

Barber's itch (sycosis barbae) Caused by staphylococci bacteria which cause inflammation of the beard hair follicles.

Barrier cream A cream used to protect the client's skin when carrying out processes which could cause skin irritation or staining, e.g. when perming, tinting or bleaching.

Base Any substance which can react with an acid to form a substance called a salt and water. Soluble bases are called alkalis and have pH values above 7.

Bevel cutting Club cutting the hair on a curve. The hair is held between the fingers and then bent up and in towards the scalp; when this hair is then cut straight across, graduation is created on the ends of the hair.

Bleach Chemicals used to lighten or decolorise the colouring pigment of the hair. Types include simple, oil, powder (or paste) and emulsion bleaches.

Blepharitis *see* styes.

Block colouring A fashion colouring technique usually used to emphasise the shape of a short hairstyle by graduating various colours in 'blocks' through the hair from the nape through to the front of the head.

Blowdrying A method of drying the hair with the aid of brushes, combs and/or hands to create a natural, soft effect which can be either curly or smooth depending upon the desired result.

Blow waving A method of waving the hair with the aid of a comb or brush and the heated air from a hand drier.

Boil (furuncle) Caused by staphylococci bacteria. Symptoms are red, round area which is very sensitive with a central core containing pus.

Boosters (activators) Oxidising agents which add to the action of the main oxidiser (often hydrogen peroxide).

Brighteners (brightening shampoos) Mild bleaches which lift the hair base colour shade slightly.

Canities Technical name for hair growing without pigment. Produces 'white' hair.

Catagen A stage in the hair growth cycle where old hair is replaced.

Chipping in Haircutting technique used to remove bulk or weight from the ends of the hair and for softening the outline shape of the haircut.

Chopsticks A perming rod which produces a considerable volume with uniform angular curl.

Circuit breakers (earth leakage devices) Automatic switches which switch the electrical supply off in the event of overloading or a fault.

Citric acid Technical term for lemon juice.

Client care All the aspects of making a client feel valued, satisfied with the service received and protecting them from hazards in the salon.

Client image That which is projected through personality, appearance and lifestyle.

Club cutting Cutting the hair straight across to remove length but not bulk.

Cohesive set (wet setting) Hair that is wet then moulded and dried in the moulded position, e.g. setting, blowdrying.

Cold sores (herpes) Caused by a virus. The symptoms are cracking and oozing of skin around the mouth.

Colleagues People who form the staff in the salon.

Colour flashes Fashion tinting technique of lightening a band of hair around the front hairline.

Colour reducer Used to remove unwanted artificial colour pigments from the hair.

Communication The key process of passing information from one person to another. Sounds easy but is not.

Compound henna An inorganic dye which is a mixture of vegetable henna and a metallic dye. It reacts with hydrogen peroxide and is therefore not used in salons any more as the chemical processes available to the client are severely restricted if the hair has been treated with metallic salts.

Concave cutting *see* inversion

Condition An overall summary of the client's hair type, damage (if any) to the hair and amount of oil present, etc.

Conditioner A product designed to leave the hair in good condition. Types include: oil-based (emollients), substantive and mild acid rehabilitating rinses .

Conjunctivitis Eye infection which causes a general inflammation and weeping of the front of the eye.

Consultation A detailed discussion and assessment of the client and the client's requirements.

Contact dermatitis *see* dermatitis.

Contagious Spread by direct or indirect contact, e.g. touch.

Contingency plans Plans ready for likely but unpredictable events. Staff off ill is a good example.

Contra-indications Things to look for which would prevent hairdressing operations .

Conventional tools, equipment and techniques Those which are commonly used in a traditional way by the hairdressing profession.

Cornified layer Dead, protective outermost layer of the skin.

Cortex *see* hair cortex.

Covering dyes Dyes which tint hair darker or a similar shade (tone) to the natural, base colour shade of the hair.

Cow's lick Hair tending to stick up around the crown. Caused by hair growth pattern.

Creativity The individual's ability to express their own and the client's wishes artificially through their work.

Critical influencing factors Anything that could affect a given service.

Croquignole A term used for winding the hair from the hair points down towards the roots.

Cross-checking A procedure to check that a hairdressing treatment, e.g. cutting, tinting, bleaching, has been thoroughly and correctly carried out.

Cross-linkages (cross-links) Hold the polypeptide chains in place in the hair cortex.

Curl test Used to monitor reagent action during perming or relaxing/straightening hair.

Cuticle *see* hair cuticle.

Cutting comb A pliable comb that is smaller and thinner than most other combs to enable the hair to be cut nearer to the scalp when using the 'scissor over comb' method of cutting hair.

Damaged cuticle Caused by chemicals or physical damage. Causes hair tangle.

Dandruff *see* pityriasis.

Decolorising Removal of colour from a pigment by either oxidation, e.g. bleaching or reduction.

Delivery note A document that is usually received with an order. The contents of each should be checked not only against one another but also against the original order to ensure that the correct stock has been delivered in good condition.

Depilatory A product used to remove hair. Generally works by breaking down the hair structure so that the hair disintegrates.

Demonstrations Are very effective if properly planned. They can be used to show staff techniques and to promote/publicise the salon.

Density *see* abundance.

Dermal papilla A bundle of blood vessels and fat cells in the centre of the hair bulb. It provides the chemicals for hair growth.

Dermatitis Inflammation, swelling and cracking of the skin: contact dermatitis is a response to a substance (called the primary irritant) which may need previous exposure until body 'over-reacts' to it, i.e. a period of sensitisation .

Dermis Inner layer of the skin which gives it its elasticity.

Development (developing) Producing the final colour of hair tints and bleaches or the transition from straight to curled hair during the softening and moulding stages of perming.

Development plans *see* training plans.

Diagnostics Means looking at the client's hair and scalp. Recognising skin and scalp condition and knowing what to do about them. Particularly important is knowing which conditions prevent hairdressing operations and which do not.

Disciplinary procedures A statement of the steps involved in taking such action against someone.

Double crown Two crowns, caused by hair growth patterns.

Dressing comb A comb (usually made of vulcanite) with a fine end and a rake end that is used for disentangling and dressing the hair.

Dressing hair The final stage of the hairdressing process when the hair is arranged into the finished style using a variety of techniques (brushing, combing, teasing, etc.), tools (brushes, combs, fingers), and dressing aids (dressing creams, sprays, etc.).

Earthing A part on an electrical system that provides an 'easy' route for electricity into the ground. It helps to prevent electric shock.

Eczema Similar to dermatitis, words are often used interchangeably. The general distinction is weeping of the skin and eczema is caused by internal factors .

Effleurage Hand massage involving slow, stroking movements. Used at the beginning and end of every massage treatment.

Elasticity test Test of hair conditioning by stretching it and allowing the hair to return to its unstretched length.

Electrode Used in conjunction with the high-frequency machine. The electrodes used on the scalp are usually the rake, used for general thinning, the bulb for spot baldness or the saturator for general thinning or as a 'tonic' to aid hair condition.

Emollients *see* conditioners.

Emulsions Droplets of one liquid suspended in another. **Emulsifying agents** help this process.

Epidermis The upper layer of the skin which has an outer horny layer of dead, flattened cells that are constantly flaking off to be replaced by cells that have been produced in the basal, the lowest layer of the epidermis.

Evaluation A judgement (or series of judgements) about somebody or something based on specific criteria.

Exothermic perm A perming technique which uses heat.

Feedback Obtaining information about performance. How well something has gone.

Finger waving Setting the hair using 'S' shaped movements formed with the fingers and a comb.

First Aid Measures designed to help an injured person until help arrives.

Fish-hook ends Hair points which are bent back on themselves. Creates a 'frizzed' look on the ends of the hair which can be removed by wetting when caused during setting but can only be removed by cutting if the hair has been permed in this position.

Flea (pulex irritans) A blood sucking parasite on the body, in clothing, bedding etc. Moves by jumping.

Flying colours *see* painted lights.

Foam perm A perming technique where the perm lotion is applied as a mousse.

Follicle *see* hair follicle.

Folliculitis Swelling and reddening of the hair follicle often with pus formation .

Formative assessment Judgements made about a process while it is happening.

Fragilitis crinum (split ends) Where the points of the hair fray and split. No 'cure': they must be cut off.

Freehand The cutting of hair without holding it in place not to be confused with texturising).

Fresh air Air which is usually cool, dry and free from contamination.

Fungi (tinea) Are plants made up of tiny threads called hyphae, some of which are parasites on humans, e.g. ringworm.

Furuncle *see* boil.

Gel A thickened liquid (technically, a liquid with high viscosity).

Germinative layer Growing layer of the skin epidermis.

Glimmering (polishing) Adding colour to the hair using tin foil painted with tint in a polishing motion.

Graduation A hair cutting term used to describe the effect created when the top layers of the hair lie above the underneath layers. A steeply graduated haircut is referred to as high layering, while very little graduation in a haircut is referred to as low layering.

Grievance procedure A statement of the steps to be taken if someone has a grievance against something or somebody.

Hair bulb Bulge on lower part of the hair root. The area from which hair grows.

Hair colour restorer Metallic dye containing lead acetate and sodium thiosulphate.

Hair cortex Inner bulk of hair made up of fibres.

Hair cuticle The outer layer of the hair, made of overlapping scales.

Hair cuttings Cuttings of hair taken from various parts of the head to enable certain tests to be carried out, e.g. incompatibility, porosity, elasticity, etc.

Hair extensions/hair pieces Additional pieces of hair woven in the client's hair as part of the hairstyle design.

Hair fixing sprays Developed from plastic polymers dissolved in alcohol which coat the hair with a plastic film.

Hair fly When hair tends to lift away from the scalp due to static electricity.

Hair follicle Tiny pit in the skin from which hair grows.

Hair growth cycle Consists of three phases (stages): anagen – active growth; telogen – resting; catagen – hair replaced by new one.

Hair growth pattern The growth direction of the hair due to the angle of the follicle in the scalp.

Hair medulla Possible third, central area of hair.

Hair mesh A section of hair gathered together in some way for a hairdressing operation.

Hair root The part of the hair which is buried in the skin.

Hair root sheath Lining of hair follicle which holds the hair in the skin.

Hair shaft The part of the hair which is visible beyond the skin surface.

Hard pressing A hair straightening technique where more heat is used, which consequently removes more of the hair curl.

Hazards Potential or actual risks to people's health and safety. They may be biological, chemical, or physical.

Head louse *see* lice.

Hepatitis A very dangerous disease which can be transmitted in the salon.

Herpes simplex *see* cold sores.

High-frequency treatment Uses a high voltage machine (apparatus) which produces a warming of the skin and encourages blood flow.

Highlighting Technique of lightening fine strands of hair using bleach and/or tint.

Hirsutism Literally means 'very hairy'. What happens in practice is that the areas which usually have the fine vellus hair grow darker, thicker secondary hair.

Hone To sharpen, e.g. a razor, before shaving.

Horny layer *see* cornified layer.

Hydrogen peroxide An effective oxidising agent which decomposes to produce water and oxygen. Used for oxidising permanent waves, para dyes and bleaches.

Hydrometer Used for measuring the density of liquids. One type, a peroxometer can be used for direct measurement of the strength (concentration) of hydrogen peroxide solutions.

Hygiene Practices likely to reduce the chances of infection or infestation.

Hygrometer Device for measuring the amount of water vapour (humidity) in the air.

Hygroscopic Ability of some materials (including hair) to absorb water vapour (moisture) from the air.

Hyperaemia Increased flow of blood to the skin. Can cause the skin to redden. The most common form of this phenomenon is a 'blush'.

Hypertrichosis The growing in specific place of thick pigmented hair in areas where usually only fine vellus hair grow.

Images *Fantasy* – that which is extreme, imaginative and often theme-based. *Avant garde* – that which is a fore-runner of fashion. *Commercial* – that which is popular with the mass market.

Impetigo Caused by staphylococci bacteria. Characteristics include blisters and weeping, formation of yellow crusts. Common as a secondary infection.

Incompatibility test A test to determine whether the hair has been previously treated with an incompatible chemical (e.g. metallic dye); if positive, hairdressing treatments should be avoided.

Induction The process where a person new to a salon is informed on the policies, procedures, work patterns, etc.

Infection Invasion of the body by pathogens (germs).

Infectious Of a disease spread by air or water.

Infestation Animal parasites living on the body. Sometimes used to refer to premises, e.g. a house 'infested' with mice.

Inversion (concave) Refers to a rounded inwards shape that is cut into the hair.

Invoice A document which lists and gives the price of the various products contained in an order. It should be checked against the delivery note to ensure that the order is correct before paying for the goods.

Itchmite (sarcoptes scabiei) Causes scabies (or the itch). Very small parasites which are almost invisible to the unaided eye. The females burrow into the skin and lay eggs which causes intense itching (usually at night). Scratching often leads to secondary infections, e.g. impetigo.

Job role/job description A detailed description of a person's role and responsibilities in the salon.

Karaya gum An Indian gum used in some setting agents. Requires a preservative to prevent it going mouldy.

Keratin Hard, fibrous protein found in hair, skin and nails.

Keratinisation Process by which skin, hair, and nail cells become filled with keratin.

Lanolin A wax which is obtained from sheep's wool, and is often used in traditional conditioning agents, shampoos and hand creams.

Lanugo hair The first hair produced by babies, often while in the womb.

Layering A form of graduation. **High layering** has steep graduation. **Low layering** has very little graduation.

Legislation Laws affecting the conduct of business, the premises or working environment, persons employed and systems of work.

Leuco-compounds Breakdown products produced by decolorising (removing colour) from a developed para tint.

Liaison Communicating with someone, working with them.

Lice Parasitic insects (all have six legs, none can fly). Headlouse (pediculus capitis) produces an infestation called pediculosis. The adults are small and lay pearl-coloured eggs (nits) which are cemented to the hair shafts particularly in the nape and behind the ears. Other types of lice include the body louse (pediculus corporis) and pubic louse (phthirus pubis).

Lightening dyes Para dyes which tint the hair lighter than the hair's natural colour.

Limits of own authority Individual's extent of responsibility as determined by own job description and organisational policy.

Line and balance The relationship between the finished hairstyle and the shape of the client's face, facial features and body size.

Local by-laws Special rules, issued normally by a local authority, affecting certain parts of the business and often relating to health and safety.

Looks *Classic* – that which is recognised by clients and the profession as having timeless appeal. *Fashion* – that which is recognised by clients and the profession as being currently in vogue. *Avant garde* – that which is a fore-runner of fashion.

Lowlights Adding small strands of colour to the hair either throughout the head or where necessary to emphasise and enhance the finished hairstyle .

Male pattern baldness An inherited condition that affects approximately 40% of males by the age of 40.

Management All the processes and methods used to ensure a salon operates effectively, efficiently and economically.

Massage The general name for rubbing and kneading actions. It generally increases blood flow to the massaged area.

Medulla A third central layer sometimes present in hair.

Melanin Black/brown natural pigment in the hair and skin.

Melanocytes Cells which produce and lay down natural pigments in the hair and skin.

Mesh (or section) *see* hair mesh.

Monilethrix A rare condition where there are bead-like swellings along the hair shaft.

Mousses Foams produced by a propellent gas blowing through a liquid.

Nape whorls Patterns of hair growth.

Nascent oxygen Single atoms of oxygen (unlike oxygen gas which has two atoms, O_2). Highly reactive and responsible for developing tints, bleaches and oxidising ('neutralising') perms.

National Vocational Qualifications A national system of vocational qualifications.

Neutralisation The oxidation stage of perming/straightening where the hair is fixed in the new style.

Nits Eggs of the parasitic louse (*see* lice).

Non-verbal communication The very powerful transfer of information by body movements, eye contact, facial expression and tone of voice.

Normalisation A term sometimes used in perming to mean 'neutraliser'.

NVQ *see* National Vocational Qualifications.

Oil bleach A bleach contained in an oil emulsion.

Operational requirements A statement of what is needed and/or what needs to be done for a particular salon operation.

Oral communication Spoken words, often less important than **non-verbal communication**.

Organisational requirements Procedures and arrangements issued by a given salon management, affecting the conduct of its business.

Oxidation The addition of oxygen or the removal of hydrogen from a substance. Chemicals that can do this are called oxidising agents or oxidisers.

Painted lights (flying colours) The technique of tinting fine strands of hair using a 'vent' brush, wide-toothed comb or fine artist's brush to emphasise the shape of a hairstyle.

Para dye (aniline dye) Permanent, semi-permanent, synthetic, organic dye. Must be mixed with hydrogen peroxide to be effective.

Parasite A living thing that lives on or in another living thing (called the parasite's host).

Patch test *see* skin test.

Pathogenic Disease causing. Pathogenic micro-organisms (pathogens) are germs .

Pediculus capitis Infestation of the scalp by head lice (*see* lice).

Percentage strength (%) A way of expressing strength (concentration) of hydrogen peroxide solutions (see volume strength). Based on parts per hundred (%) of 'pure' peroxide in a solution.

Performance criteria The specific method and standard to which something is to be done.

Perimeter lines Important in cutting in the outside profile or shape of the haircut.

Peroxometer *see* hydrometer.

Petrissage Massage movements involving kneading actions.

pH balance A product designed to leave the hair/skin slightly acid.

pH scale A scale of acidity or alkalinity. Has 14 points; 7 is neutral (neither acid nor alkaline), below 7 is acid and above 7 is alkaline.

Pheomelanin Red/yellow natural pigment in the hair and skin.

Pin curls Type of setting where the hair is wound flat. Types are: clockspring, barrel spring, stem and sculptured curls.

Pityriasis (full name pityriasis simplex) The technical name for dandruff (scurf) due to the flaking of the scalp skin.

Plaiting Various techniques where the hair is weaved together.

Pointing *see* chipping in.

Policy A statement (written or oral) issued by a given salon management, setting out its considered approach to the conduct of its business. It may be required by legislation, e.g. a Health and Safety policy.

Polypeptide chains The smallest chains in the hair cortex made up of amino acids .

Porosity test A test to assess the state of the hair cuticle. The more open or damaged it is the more porous is the hair.

Portfolio A set of evidence of competence in a particular area. Can be used as a basis for assessment.

Post-damping Applying perm reagent to the curlers after they have been wound.

Postiche Collective name for wigs and hair pieces.

Posture The way in which someone stands.

Powder bleach Where the liquid bleach is made into a paste with a powder.

Predisposition test *see* skin test.

Pre-perm test A test cutting perm carried out before perming the whole head.

Prepigmentation Tinting bleached hair to its original colour.

Pre-saturation Applying perm reagent to the hair mesh as it is wound.

Pressing combs Used for straightening hair.

Primary colours The three colours, yellow, red and blue, from which all others can be made.

Primary irritant *see* allergy and dermatitis.

Professional image of the salon That which the salon wishes to portray to achieve a targeted position within the commercial market.

Promotion A variety of techniques designed to market the salon and its services.

Psoriasis A non-infectious skin condition. Often seen as silvery scales with red skin underneath; the silvery scales flake off when rubbed.

Pulex irritans Human flea. It has long back legs which allow it to jump from one person to another.

Pull-burn A burn on the skin caused by winding the hair too tightly when perming.

Reduction The opposite of oxidation. It involves removal of oxygen from or addition of hydrogen to a substance. Chemicals that do this are reducing agents .

Reduction dye A metallic dye which uses pyrogallol as a reducing agent.

Regrowth The hair nearest the scalp which has grown since the last hairdressing treatment, therefore has natural colour and wave.

Rehabilitating rinse *see* conditioners.

Relaxer cream Reagent for straightening hair.

Relaxing hair *see* straightening.

Repetitive Strain Injury Painful reaction to using the same muscles and joints with a high frequency over a long period.

Restructurant Type of conditioner which is substantive, 'adds to' the hair shaft. Makes hair less porous.

Re-style A change of look which is significantly different from that which existed before cutting commenced.

Retouch Applying a chemical treatment to a regrowth.

Reverse graduation A haircutting term used to describe the effect created when the top layers of the hair lie below the underneath layers.

Ringworm (tinea) Caused by a parasitic fungus. When present on the scalp it produces reddened, round patches with a stubble of hair. Tinea capitis – fungal infection of the scalp.

Risk assessment The process of looking at the hazards and chances of accidents in the salon.

Roller setting A wide variety of setting techniques using rollers (rods).

Root *see* hair root.

Root sheath *see* hair root sheath.

Rota A list of the duties of salon staff at different times.

Salon requirements Procedures and arrangements issued by a given salon management, which must include the minimum health, safety and hygiene requirements of the service being provided.

Saponification Technical name for soap making process.

Saprophyte Bacterium which feeds on and causes the decay of dead, organic material.

Sarcoptes scabiei *see* itchmite.

Scabies An infection of the skin caused by the itchmite. Causes intense itching.

Schedule *see* rota.

Scrunching When used in relation to fashion colouring it is a method of lightening the ends of the hair using either tint, bleach or a combination of both.

Scurf *see* pityriasis.

Sebaceous cyst (wen) A raised lump on the skin caused by a blockage of the sebaceous gland.

Sebaceous gland Produces natural oil sebum which coats the hair and the skin. A blocked gland can lead to a build up of sebum in a wen (sebaceous cyst).

Seborrhoea Is an overproduction of sebum. Causes oily hair and skin, it can be triggered by hormone changes at puberty. It may also cause swelling, itching and reddening on the scalp, called seborrhoeic dermatitis.

Sebum Natural oil made by sebaceous gland in hair follicles. It waterproofs and conditions the hair and skin.

Secondary hair Sometimes called terminal hair. It is the thick, usually darker hair on the scalp and body.

Secondary infection It occurs where an earlier infection produces conditions which encourage a second type of pathogen to invade the body, e.g. impetigo is a common secondary infection of scabies caused when the skin is broken through scratching.

Self-development The process of increasing knowledge, understanding and skill level.

Selenium sulphide A substance used in shampoo to combat dandruff. It reduces the activities of the germinative layer of the skin thus reducing flaking .

Sensitisation *see* allergy and dermatitis.

Sensitivity test *see* skin test.

Setting Various methods both wet and dry, used to give hair a temporary style. Setting aids help to produce and prolong the set.

Shampoo A solution for cleaning hair. Usually a soapless base containing a mixture of ingredients to remove dirt and oil from the hair.

Shimmer lights A tinting technique that produces a similar effect to painted lights. The hair is combed into position with a gel, then the raised part of the ridges has tint applied to it with a fine brush.

Shingle A graduated hair cut where the nape hair is cut extremely short, usually with the clippers or scissors over comb.

Simple bleach A bleach made with hydrogen peroxide as a liquid.

Skin epidermis The outer part of the skin, made up of layers. The bottom layer (germinative) grows and moves towards the surface, eventually producing the dead outer layer of the skin (cornified).

Skin test A test taken to see if a person has an allergy to a substance. The material to be tested is placed on the skin and checked to see if a 'rash' develops. If such a reaction takes place the person is probably allergic to that substance.

Slicing (tramming) A method of tinting whereby slices of colour are placed in the hair where required.

Slither cutting *see* tapering.

Soft pressing A relaxing technique where heat is used to produce some hair straightening.

Specified procedures Those requirements which relate to the conducting of tests carried out on hair, skin and scalp and are in accordance with manufacturer's instructions.

Spot tinting/bleaching Tinting or bleaching the hair where required to correct uneven colour faults.

Sterilisation A process which kills all micro-organisms.

Stock control Procedures designed to ensure that stock is available when needed and is rotated to ensure it is used before deterioration.

Straightening (relaxing) hair Methods used to remove curl/wave from the hair.

Strand test A test used to monitor the development of the hair colour during tinting.

Streptococci Bacteria which cause infections, e.g. sore throat. Divide to form chains.

Strop A leather strap used to sharpen open, cut-throat razors.

Styes (blepharitis) Caused by bacteria invading the hair follicle of eye lashes (commonly of the lower eyelid) causing reddening and swelling.

Substantive Something which joins with or enters the hair shaft. *See* conditioners .

Sulphide dye An inorganic metallic dye.

Sulphur bonds Cross linkages that hold the polypeptide chains, sometimes referred to as 'S' bonds', di-sulphide bonds, cystine linkages or sulphur bridges.

Summative assessment The final stage in an assessment of performance. Based on the whole process and overall performance.

Supervisor A person with a degree of responsibility. Generally concerned with carrying out policies rather than determining them.

Sycosis barbae *see* barber's itch.

Tail comb A comb used for sectioning, lifting or weaving the hair. It has a fine end and a tail end. A variation of the tail comb is the pin-tail comb which has a thin, metal, stiletto tail end.

Tapering (slither cutting) A method of cutting hair using a 'slithering' movement which removes bulk and length.

Technical services The group name for the large range of services a salon may offer.

Telogen The stage in the hair growth cycle where hair growth stops; a resting stage.

Terminal hair *see* secondary hair.

Test cutting Taken before a hairdressing process to ensure the best choice, and to determine the effects of the products to be used on the hair.

Texture The texture of the hair refers to its diameter. Fine hair is narrow in diameter while thick hair has a much larger diameter.

Texturising Cutting into the hair to increase movement, volume and create a non-uniform effect.

Thinning A haircutting method that removes weight and bulk from the hair .

Tinea *see* ringworm *and* fungi.

Tints Dyes used to colour the hair. They can be lightening or covering, temporary, semi-permanent or permanent.

Toners Tints used to 'mask' unwanted colour tones.

Tortoiseshell highlights Woven strands of hair which are then tinted with three or four different colours throughout the head or where required.

Traction alopecia *see* alopecia.

Tragacanth gum White powder obtained from the bark of a shrub grown in Turkey, which can be used in setting agents.

Training plan A statement showing the steps to meeting a person or staff team's identified training needs.

Tramming *see* slicing.

Translucent Allows light to pass through, and scatters (diffuses) it.

Trichorrhexis nodosa Condition where hair splits and frays at swellings along the length.

Ultra violet radiation Part of electromagnetic spectrum not visible to the eye, which is used in UV sterilisers and triggers melanocytes in the skin, producing a sun-tan.

Uni perm A perming technique using heated rollers.

Vegetable dye A dye obtained from plants, e.g. camomile.

Vellus hair The fine, often unpigmented (or slightly pigmented) downy hair, e.g. present on the female face.

Verrucae *see* warts.

Vibro machine A mechanical form of massage. The machine has various attachments, the most common of which are the spiked applicator, the sponge applicator and the bell-shaped applicator. It is used in conjunction with hair/scalp treatments to stimulate blood flow, and promote healthy hair.

Virus The smallest type of micro-organism; it cannot survive long outside the body. It causes colds, 'flu, 'cold sores' (herpes) and some types of wart.

Volume strength (vol. strength; 'vols') A way of expressing strength (concentration) of hydrogen peroxide solutions. It means the number of volumes of oxygen gas given off by one volume of peroxide. For example, when completely broken down 1 cm^3 20 vol. hydrogen peroxide would give off 20 cm^3 of oxygen gas.

Warts (verrucae) Some warts are caused by a virus (papova virus) which makes the skin produce raised lumps. On the feet, the pressure of the body weight can cause the wart to grow inwards creating a verruca (plantar wart).

Wen *see* sebaceous cyst.

Wet setting *see* cohesive set.

Widow's peak A natural wave in the fringe area caused by hair growth direction.

Winding Term for insertion and rolling up of rollers, curlers, etc., in the hair.

Zinc pyrithione Substance found in medicated or anti-dandruff shampoos.

Index